Rapid and Practical Interpretation of Urodynamics

Eric S. Rovner • Michelle E. Koski
Editors

Rapid and Practical Interpretation of Urodynamics

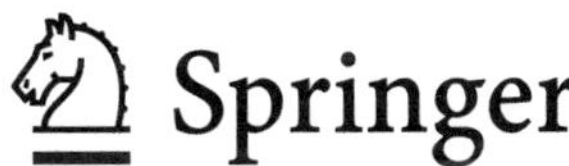 Springer

Editors
Eric S. Rovner
Department of Urology
Medical University of South Carolina
Charleston, SC, USA

Michelle E. Koski
Department of Urology
Medical University of South Carolina
Charleston, SC, USA

Department of Urology
Kaiser Permanente Southern California
San Marcos, CA, USA

ISBN 978-1-4939-4673-0   ISBN 978-1-4939-1764-8 (eBook)
DOI 10.1007/978-1-4939-1764-8
Springer New York Heidelberg Dordrecht London

I would like to dedicate this book to my loving family. It is my beautiful, brilliant wife Michelle, and my two wonderful children, Alex and Brooke, who constantly challenge, motivate, and inspire me at home and at work. Without their steadfast support and understanding this work would never have been completed. I can only hope that the final result is worth the nights and weekends that I spent working on it, instead of spending precious time with them.

Eric S. Rovner

It is with great honor that I dedicate my work on this book to my teachers and mentors. Dr. Joseph Smith, Dr. Roger R. Dmochowski, Dr. Chris Winters, and Dr. Melissa R. Kaufman—thank you for your education through lesson and example in medicine, life, and humanity. Thank you to Dr. Eric S. Rovner for the opportunity to work on this project, your adroit contributions to other works, and your excellent advice on all topics. A very special thank you to my husband Josh and to my son Alden for their love and unwavering support.

Michelle E. Koski

Foreword

The foreword is a strange literary custom. It doesn't contribute any additional information about the book's subject matter, but serves essentially to introduce the author and content. In the case of Dr. Rovner and his new book, it is a pleasure and honor for me to do both.

I have had a long and close relationship with Dr. Rovner since he completed our Fellowship program in Pelvic Medicine and Reconstruction at UCLA. I have rarely encountered a person with the academic vision, personal integrity, commitment to education, dedication to his patients, and surgical skills that Dr. Rovner possesses.

His book, accordingly, is outstanding. Until now there was no comprehensive resource to learn in a systematic and practical way the quick evaluation and analysis of urodynamics. Dr. Rovner has brought together the best specialists in the field to write *Urodynamics: rapid and practical interpretation*. This book sheds a very timely and needed light on the occasionally shadowy field of urodynamic studies.

The book is cleverly organized to help the reader learn procedures and interpretation in stages. The first part of the book is a guide to the performance of urodynamic studies, with sections for equipment, technique, indications, artifacts, and even coding for the studies. The second part is about interpretation, with sections for bladder capacity, sensations, involuntary contractions, changes in compliance, obstruction, and stress incontinence. The third and most innovative section is dedicated to the examination of sample cases by which the reader can test his or her knowledge.

The organization of the book provides the reader with a methodology for reading and interpreting the UDS tracing in a structured, reproducible, and accurate way. Unlike virtually all previously published UDS books, which are organized around disease states and applicable urodynamic findings, this book breaks down the urodynamic tracings into their component parts and salient features and then applies these findings to various disease states. For the first time, we are offered an objective diagnostic approach that accurately represents how EKG tracings are actually interpreted.

While the book is not primarily meant to teach urodynamic techniques, there are chapters on a number of related areas including: purchasing a urodynamics machine, billing for the studies, recognizing artifacts, and optimizing the diagnostic value of the UDS study. The selected urodynamic cases are challenging and interesting, most of them are straightforward examples of specific pathology. These cases were carefully selected to illustrate most clearly the salient points under consideration in each section.

In this book, Dr. Rovner has continued in his quest to explore new theories and ideas with clear and practical answers that everyone can comprehend. While it is directed to general urologists, gynecologists, and residents, it will be of great value to trainees in Pelvic Medicine and Reconstructive Surgery and specialists in the field as well. The casual reader will be impressed by the book's readability and comprehensiveness, while practitioners will be astonished by its depth of detail. This remarkable book is a must in the library of any physician performing urodynamic studies.

Los Angeles, CA, USA   Shlomo Raz, MD

Preface

Urodynamic studies have been widely utilized in both Urology and Gynecology for decades. Such tests provide critical information about the function, physiology, and, in some instances, the anatomy of the lower urinary tract including the urinary bladder, urethra, and surrounding soft tissues including pelvic floor muscle, nerves, and connective tissue. Although urodynamics have been performed for decades, there is not a well-established or standard method of interpretation of these studies. Several seminal documents from the ICS, IUGA, SUFU, and AUA over the past two decades have guided performance of the study and standardized terminology, but none provide specific organization or direction in the reading and interpretation of these complex studies [1–4].

Urodynamic studies are expensive and invasive and yet few practitioners may consider themselves truly expert in their performance or especially their interpretation. Beyond the basic interpretation of studies, subtle nuances in the tracings can impart important meaning in the reading of the test. A well done and properly read urodynamic study yields meaningful clinical information which has significant impact on the individual's healthcare. However, a poorly performed study, or a misinterpreted or incompletely read study, is not only uncomfortable and morbid for the patient, but can also result in misdiagnosis and inappropriate interventions.

Rapid and Practical Interpretation of Urodynamics brings a simple, quick, and very practical approach to the understanding and analysis of urodynamic studies. There have been several urodynamics texts published over the past few decades. Without exception, these encyclopedic textbooks are written and categorized by disease or condition. This structure is not consistent with the paradigm in which urodynamics are most often performed and interpreted in practice. The urodynamics study is commonly done in patients who have symptoms but do not yet carry a diagnosis, or who have not appropriately responded to initial therapy. The study is therefore used as a means to define their condition, prognosis, or direct management. Furthermore, in patients with lower urinary tract symptoms presumably due to a defined clinical condition, such as Parkinson's disease, the urodynamic studies are performed to confirm the expected findings as well as exclude confounding conditions.

However, ultimately the management is directed by the urodynamics and thus the complete and accurate interpretation of the study is critical.

Instead of the disease specific approach to the interpretation of urodynamics, *Rapid and Practical Interpretation of Urodynamics* is structured around specific types of patterns seen on urodynamic tracings. The majority of the textbook consists of actual urodynamic tracings annotated and fully interpreted by the authors. Multiple examples of each type of finding are provided with attached expert commentary. The expert commentary expands on the potential clinical significance of the tracing and, where appropriate, discusses its importance diagnostically, prognostically and the implications for clinical management. The emphasis in this book is on the interpretation of actual patterns seen on such tracings and their meaning, as well as the identification of potentially misleading artifacts or "look-alikes." This is a distinctly innovative method to learning urodynamics. The tracings will be interpreted and then associated with the disease/condition ("ground-up approach") as opposed to the disease/condition being associated with the tracing ("top-down approach").

The approach utilized in this book is novel to learning urodynamics but is not unique in medical education. As compared to the pressure-flow urodynamic tracing, an analogous graph/tracing type of diagnostic study is the electrocardiogram (ECG). The classical textbook on ECG from which many medical students first learn interpretation of these studies is Dale Dubin's "Rapid Interpretation of EKGs," now in its sixth edition from Cover Inc [5]. This textbook teaches the interpretation of EKGs from the perspective of the tracing and then relates such findings to potential disease states. This format is readily adaptable to urodynamics.

Rapid and Practical Interpretation of Urodynamics consists of three parts. Part I, Urodynamic Basics, is an overview of urodynamic studies along with practical information on the performance and selection of these tests. Part II, Interpretation of Tracings, forms the majority of the textbook. This portion of the book is organized into sections: (1) the normal study, (2) abnormalities of bladder filling and urinary storage, and (3) abnormalities of bladder emptying. Overall the emphasis in this section is on the interpretation of multi-channel pressure-flow urodynamics tracings. Fluoroscopic images are also included. This section consists of actual urodynamics tracings, annotated, highlighted, and interpreted by the chapter author. Using a combination of the functional classification of voiding dysfunction as popularized by Wein [6], and a simple to remember acronym, "the 9 C's of Urodynamics" (see Chap. 2), all the aspects of a proper and complete interpretation of the pressure-flow urodynamic study are well organized within an easy to understand framework. Part III, Final Examination, consists of a series of "unknowns." Part III will allow the reader to test their newly acquired skills in interpreting urodynamic studies.

It is hoped that this book will assist practitioners in helping a broad population of patients who are currently being underserved or suboptimally treated. This book is applicable to any reader who is interested in this standardized approach, but will be especially useful to the practitioner who desires more practical knowledge in the performance of urodynamics. *Rapid and Practical Interpretation of Urodynamics* provides practitioners with a practical, easy-to-read, and well-organized approach to the performance and analysis of pressure-flow urodynamics.

Charleston, SC, USA   Eric S. Rovner, MD
San Marcos, CA, USA   Michelle E. Koski, MD

References

1. Haylen B, de Ridder D, Freeman RM, Swift SE, Berghmans B, Lee J, Monga A, Petri E, Rizk DE, Sand PK, Schaer GN. An International Urogynecological Association (IUGA)/International Continence Society (ICS) joint report on the terminology for female pelvic floor dysfunction. Int Urogynecol J. 2010;21:5–26
2. Abrams P, Cardozo L, Fall M, Griffiths D, Rosier P, Ulmsten U, van Kerrebroeck P, Victor A, Wein A. The standardization of lower urinary tract function: report from the Standardisation Subcommittee of the International Continence Society. Neurourol Urodyn. 2002;21:167–78
3. Schafer W, Abrams P, Liao L, et al. Good urodynamic practices: uroflowetry, filling cystometry, and pressure-flow studies. Neurourol Urodyn. 2002;21:261–74
4. Winters JC, Dmochowski RR, Goldman HB, Herndon CD, Kobashi KC, Kraus SR, Lemack GE, Nitti VW, Rovner ES, Wein AJ. Urodynamic studies in adults: AUA/SUFU guideline. J Urol. 2012;188(6 Suppl):2464–72
5. Dubin, D. Rapid interpretation of EKG's. 6th ed. Tampa: COVER Publishing, Inc.; 2000
6. Wein A. Classification of neurogenic voiding dysfunction. J Urol. 1981;125:605–9

Acknowledgments

The editors, Eric Rovner and Michelle E. Koski, first acknowledge the chapter authors with great thanks. We owe them a substantial debt of gratitude for the time and effort put forth into their outstanding contributions. The book is structured in such a way that it would not have been possible to produce without the authors' expertise, excellence in the field, and intellectual skills. Additionally, we would like to thank the Springer publication staff, including Richard Hruska and Andy Kwan, for making this book happen, and especially Mariah Gumpert, whose editorial assistance and organizational skills greatly enhanced the production of this work.

Contents

Contributors

Michael E. Albo, MD Department of Urology, UC San Diego Health Systems, San Diego, CA, USA

Chasta Bacsu, MD, BSc Department of Urology, UT Southwestern Medical Center, Dallas, TX, USA

Elizabeth Timbrook Brown, MD, MPH Department of Urology, Louisiana State University School of Medicine, New Orleans, LA, USA

Benjamin M. Brucker, MD Department of Urology, New York University Langone Medical Center, New York, NY, USA

Chong Choe, MD Division of Urology and Renal Transplantation, Department of Urology, Virginia Mason Medical Center, Seattle, WA, USA

J. Quentin Clemens, MD, FACS, MSCI Division of Neurourology and Pelvic Reconstructive Surgery, Department of Urology, University of Michigan, A. Alfred Taubman Health Care Center, Ann Arbor, MI, USA

Teresa L. Danforth, MD Department of Urology, SUNY Buffalo School of Medicine and Biomedical Sciences, Buffalo General Hospital, Buffalo, NY, USA

Department of Urology, Keck School of Medicine of USC, University of Southern California, Los Angeles, CA, USA

Roger R. Dmochowski, MD MPH Department of Urology, Vanderbilt University Medical Center, Nashville, TN, USA

Ahmed El-Zawahry, MBBCh Department of Surgery, Incontinence Center, Southern Illinois University, Springfield, IL, USA

Lynette E. Franklin, MSN, APRN-BC, CWOCN-AP, CFCN Wound Ostomy & Continence Nursing Education, Emory University, Atlanta, GA, USA

Denise Lynn Gartin, AAS, CPC Department of Urology, Vanderbilt University Medical Center, Nashville, TN, USA

Physician Billing Services, Vanderbilt University Medical Center, Nashville, TN, USA

David Ginsberg, MD, DSc Department of Urology, Keck School of Medicine of USC, University of Southern California, Los Angeles, CA, USA

Howard B. Goldman, MD Cleveland Clinic, Lerner College of Medicine, Glickman Urologic and Kidney Institute, Cleveland, OH, USA

Alexander Gomelsky, MD Department of Urology, Louisiana State University Health – Shreveport, Shreveport, LA, USA

Angelo E. Gousse, MD Herbert Wertheim College of Medicine, Florida International University, Memorial Hospital Miramar, South Broward Hospital District, Miramar, FL, USA

Cory Harris, MD Department of Urology, Memorial Hospital Miramar, South Broward Hospital District, Miramar, FL, USA

Kristi L. Hebert, MD Department of Urology, Louisiana State University School of Medicine, New Orleans, LA, USA

Jack C. Hou, MD Department of Urology, UT Southwestern Medical Center, Dallas, TX, USA

Kelly C. Johnson, MD Department of Urology, Medical University of South Carolina, Charleston, SC, USA

Ying H. Jura, MD Department of Urology, Stanford University School of Medicine, Stanford University, Stanford, CA, USA

Melissa R. Kaufman, MD, PhD Department of Urologic Surgery, Vanderbilt University Medical Center, Nashville, TN, USA

Kathleen C. Kobashi, MD Division of Urology and Renal Transplantation, Department of Urology, Virginia Mason Medical Center, Seattle, WA, USA

Michelle E. Koski, MD Department of Urology, Medical University of South Carolina, Charleston, SC, USA

Department of Urology, Kaiser Permanente Southern California, San Marcos, CA, USA

Gary E. Lemack, MD Department of Urology, UT Southwestern Medical Center, Dallas, TX, USA

Lara S. MacLachlan, MD Department of Urology, Medical University of South Carolina, Charleston, SC, USA

Alana M. Murphy, MD Department of Urology, Thomas Jefferson University, Philadelphia, PA, USA

Victor W. Nitti, MD Department of Urology, New York University Langone Medical Center, New York, NY, USA

David J. Osborn, MD Department of Urology, Vanderbilt University Medical Center, Nashville, TN, USA

Christopher K. Payne, MD Department of Urology, Stanford University School of Medicine, Stanford University, Stanford, CA, USA

J. Todd Purves, MD, PhD Department of Urology, The Medical University of South Carolina, Charleston, SC, USA

Ross Rames, MD Department of Urology, Medical University of South Carolina, Charleston, SC, USA

Shlomo Raz, MD Division of Pelvic Medicine and Reconstructive Surgery, Department of Urology, David Geffen School of Medicine at UCLA, Los Angeles, CA, USA

W. Stuart Reynolds, MD, MPH Department of Urology, Vanderbilt University Medical Center, Nashville, TN, USA

Eric S. Rovner, MD Department of Urology, Medical University of South Carolina, Charleston, SC, USA

Ariana L. Smith, MD Penn Medicine Division of Urology, University of Pennsylvania Health System, Perelman Center for Advanced Medicine, West Pavilion, Philadelphia, PA, USA

Philip P. Smith, MD Department of Surgery, University of Connecticut Health Center, Farmington, CT, USA

Department of Urology, Connecticut Children's Medical Center, Hartford, CT, USA

Center on Aging, University of Connecticut Health Center, Farmington, CT, USA

Andrew A. Stec, MD Department of Urology, The Medical University of South Carolina, Charleston, SC, USA

Anne M. Suskind, MD, MS Division of Neurourology and Pelvic Reconstructive Surgery, Department of Urology, University of Michigan A. Alfred Taubman Health Care Center, Ann Arbor, MI, USA

Mary Y. Wang, MSN, CRNP Penn Medicine Division of Urology, University of Pennsylvania Health System, Perelman Center for Advanced Medicine, West Pavilion, Philadelphia, PA, USA

Alan J. Wein, MD, PhD(hon), FACS Penn Medicine Division of Urology, University of Pennsylvania Health System, Perelman Center for Advanced Medicine, West Pavilion, Philadelphia, PA, USA

J. Christian Winters, MD Department of Urology, Louisiana State University School of Medicine, New Orleans, LA, USA

Part I
UDS Studies

Chapter 1
Urodynamic Studies: Types and Indications

Benjamin M. Brucker and Victor W. Nitti

Introduction

The origin of the word "urodynamics" dates back to 1954, when David Davis used this term while presenting work on upper tract pressure and renal injury [1]. Since that time our understanding of the urinary tract, the equipment used to test, and even the definition of urodynamics (UDS) has expanded significantly. Now "urodynamics" refers to a collection of tests that aim to provide the clinician information about the lower urinary tract during bladder filling/storage and emptying [2].

There are numerous conditions and diseases that affect the lower urinary tract and disrupt the storage and/or evacuation of urine. This can lead to bothersome symptoms (e.g., urinary incontinence or pain from failure to empty) or, in some cases, potentially harmful sequela. Depending on the complexity of the symptoms, condition, or patient, varying degrees of precision may be required to assess urine storage and emptying to optimally treat patients. UDS is the dynamic study of the transport, storage, and evacuation of urine. It is comprised of a number of tests that individually or collectively can be used to gain information about urine storage and evacuation. UDS involves the assessment of the function and dysfunction of the urinary tract and includes the actual tests that are performed (UDS studies) and the observations during the testing (UDS observations) [3, 4]. The actual UDS studies chosen will depend on the amount of information and degree of precision required to comfortably treat a patient.

B.M. Brucker, MD (✉) • V.W. Nitti, MD
Department of Urology, New York University Langone Medical Center,
150 East 32nd Street, Second floor, New York, NY 10016, USA
e-mail: Benjamin.brucker@nyumc.org

© Springer Science+Business Media New York 2015
E.S. Rovner, M.E. Koski (eds.), *Rapid and Practical Interpretation of Urodynamics*, DOI 10.1007/978-1-4939-1764-8_1

UDS are considered an interactive diagnostic study of the lower urinary tract [5]. The clinician should be using these "tests" to answer a specific question (or questions) about normal function and/or dysfunction. The clinician needs to first understand the tools that make up UDS, so that the appropriate evaluation can take place. We follow three important rules before starting the UDS evaluation [6]:

1. Decide on questions to be answered before starting a study.
2. Design the study to answer these questions.
3. Customize the study as necessary.

Before the clinician can know what test to perform, a clear history and focused physical examination are needed. The more salient information the clinician has prior to testing, the more effective they can be at tailoring tests toward an individual patient. Frequency–volume charts or bladder diaries are very useful tools that help ensure that other urodynamic tests provide meaningful information. A bladder diary provides useful real life information of how often a patient voids, what his/her functional bladder capacity is, and on the volume of fluid intake and urine output. Correlation of UDS findings with a bladder diary can help to avoid errors of interpretation. This is especially important when one considers that UDS is preformed in an "artificial" environment where we try to obtain "real life" information.

There are three critical "good urodynamic practice elements" [7]:

1. Have a clear indication for, and appropriate selection of, relevant test measurements and procedures.
2. Ensure precise measurement with data quality control and complete documentation.
3. Accurately analyze and critically report results. *This includes interpreting UDS in the context of a patient's history and symptoms.*

It is important that the staff involved with patient preparation for UDS (especially invasive testing) is well trained, attentive, and supportive. The person performing the actual study, if different from the clinician ordering the study, should have a clear understanding of why the tests are being performed and what critical information is necessary. Finally, patients should be properly prepared and told why the test is being done, how the results may affect treatment, and what to expect during the actual UDS test.

Components of UDS

Post Void Residual

Post void residual (PVR) refers to the volume of urine left in the bladder immediately after voiding. It is one of the most basic and widely used urodynamic tests [8]. The PVR value can be obtained by ultrasound (bladder scan) and/or catheterization. The advantage of ultrasound is that it is less invasive and can usually be done promptly to avoid additional input from the upper urinary tract that occurs if there is a delay prior to obtaining a catheterized specimen [9]. The bladder scan has been shown to correlate well with urine volume obtained from catheterization in many, but not all patients [10]. A PVR should ideally be obtained immediately after a "normal" void. Forced voids (i.e., when a patient does not have a desire to void) can lead to falsely elevated PVR. There are some situations where obtaining or interpreting bladder scans can be difficult (i.e., significant abdominal ascites, obesity, large fibroids) and a catheterized PVR is favored.

Elevated PVR is suggestive of detrusor underactivity, bladder outlet obstruction, or a combination of both [5]. PVR alone cannot differentiate between the two. However, knowing that a patient does not empty completely may prompt further testing (see below), when it is important to determine the cause of the incomplete emptying. It is often difficult to determine what a "significant" PVR is and even the recently published AUA/SUFU UDS Guideline states that a definition of exactly what constitutes an elevated PVR has not been agreed upon [5]. However, urologists generally agree that in some patients, an elevated PVR may be harmful. Therefore, when considering what an elevated PVR is and whether or not it is significant, it must be considered in the context of a particular patient and his/her clinical presentation. Unfortunately, there is not a lot of high-level evidence that correlates PVR with treatment outcomes. PVR can be falsely elevated in some patients who may not empty completely in the clinic setting or who were asked to void without a normal desire. PVR may vary in the same patient and an elevated PVR should be confirmed with a second measurement, especially if treatment is being considered based on the elevation.

Uroflowmetry

Uroflowmetry, or uroflow is an objective way of "observing" the act of micturition [11]. Uroflow assesses the rate of urine flow over time. When possible this test should be done free of any catheters, in a private room at a time when the patient feels the "normal" desire to void [8]. This allows for the clinician to assess a "normal" void. Patients should also be asked if the void was representative of their usual toileting [12].

There are multiple data points that can be reported from non-invasive uroflowmetry. These include:

Voided volume (VV—mL)
Flow rate (Q—mL/s)
Maximum flow rate (Q_{Max}—mL/s)
Average flow rate (Q_{ave}—mL/s)
Voiding time (total time during micturition—s)
Flow Time (the time during which flow occurred—s)
Time to maximum flow (onset of flow to Q_{max}—s)

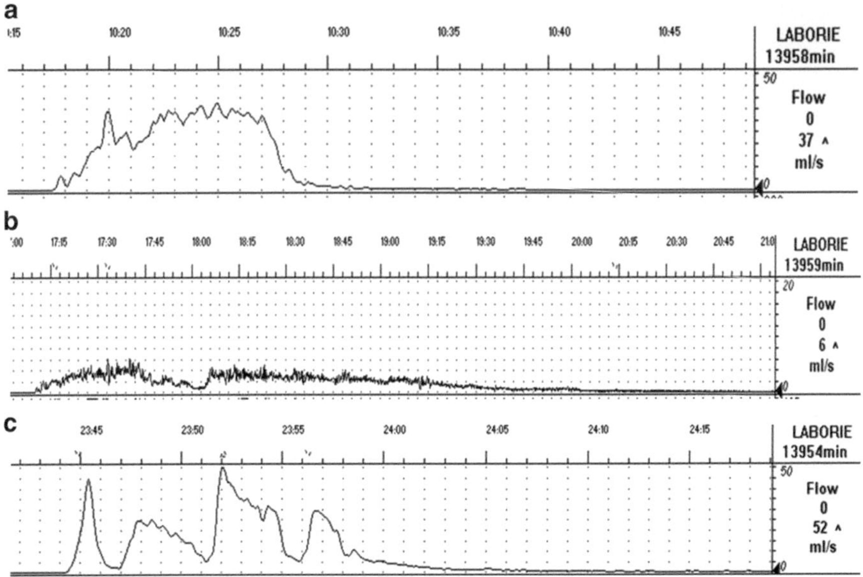

Fig. 1.1 Three examples of uroflow patterns: (**a**) Normal bell-shaped. (**b**) Obstructive pattern. (**c**) Straining pattern

In addition to these objective measurements, it is also important to observe the pattern or shape of the uroflow curve. A normal uroflow curve is bell-shaped (Fig. 1.1). Uroflow curve interpretation is somewhat subjective because of difficulty in qualitatively judging a pattern [11]. While certain patterns are suggestive of certain voiding dynamics (e.g., an interrupted or straining pattern with detrusor underactivity and a flattened pattern with a fixed obstruction) one cannot definitively identify specific underlying abnormalities without detrusor pressure data (see invasive pressure-flow UDS below).

It is helpful to obtain a PVR after completion of uroflowmetry in order to fully understand bladder emptying. In addition, bladder-emptying efficiency can be calculated using the formula: VV/(VV + PVR). Voided volume will have a large impact on flow rate and can lead to variability in an individual patient. It has been suggested that maximum flow rates are not meaningful at voided volumes of less than 150 mL because of the hyperbolic relationship that exists in men between the two variables (maximum flow rate and voided volume) [12]. However for patients who cannot hold 150 mL, obtaining an "accurate" uroflow can be impossible. In some patients uroflow with voided volumes of <150 mL may not have to be discounted, but interpreted with caution.

Today, most uroflowmetry equipment utilizes one of two transducer types. The first is based on weight. After setting the density of urine, the voided weight is measured and as this changes with time a flow rate is determined. The urine is voided into a container that sits on top of the weight transducer. The other method relies on a rotating disk. Here the voided urine is directed toward a spinning disk and alterations of the disk's speed (and the electrical energy needed to keep the disc spinning at a constant rate) are converted into electrical signals that represent flow rate [13]. Other methods of uroflow data collection are also available, but may have more limited practical application [14].

Abnormalities in non-invasive uroflow indicate that voiding phase dysfunction may exist. Figure 1.1 shows examples of an abnormal elongated flow curve and an interrupted/straining that suggest voiding phase dysfunction. However, uroflowmetry, like PVR, does not allow the clinician to determine the cause of an abnormality (e.g., if slow flow is secondary to outlet obstruction, detrusor underactivity, or a combination of both).

Electromyography

Pelvic floor muscles and the striated urethral sphincter both have a critical role in bladder storage and emptying. Electromyography (EMG) is the test that best evaluates these muscles. EMG is the study of electrical potentials generated by the depolarization of muscles [15]. In the setting of UDS, EMG is recording the motor unit action potential; this is the depolarization of the striated muscle fiber that occurs when the muscle is activated by the anterior horn nerve cell. Needle electrodes or surface electrodes can record the action potential. The quality of EMG has often been cited as variable or problematic because of a poor signal source. Needle electrodes are thought to be superior, however are often avoided because of patient discomfort and logistical difficulty [16]. The more commonly used surface EMG was described in 1980 to determine relaxation of the pelvic floor as an indirect measure of the simultaneous relaxation for the external sphincter [17].

EMG testing can be performed in isolation, however this test is usually combined with other UDS tests. As an isolated test, EMG can allow the clinician to assess the voluntary contraction of pelvic floor muscles, confirming that the corticospinal tract is intact and the cortical function required to initiate the contraction of the external sphincter is working.

Passive continence does not require external sphincter activity in most cases. However, there does exist a somatic passive guarding reflex that causes sphincter activity to increase as the bladder fills. Accurate measure with needle electrodes will often show a gradual increase in EMG activity with filling until a voluntary void is initiated. When using surface electrodes, one may not always see this pattern and may rather see a consistent signal. The EMG signal, assuming appropriate recording, should transiently increase if the patient performs a stress maneuver, i.e., straining or coughing (Fig. 1.2). When a voluntary void is initiated the first UDS evidence of this is relaxation of the external sphincter and a decrease in EMG activity (Fig. 1.2). This is then followed by an increase in detrusor pressure and initiation of flow. In a neurologically normal person, failure of the external sphincter to relax will result in inhibition of a detrusor contraction.

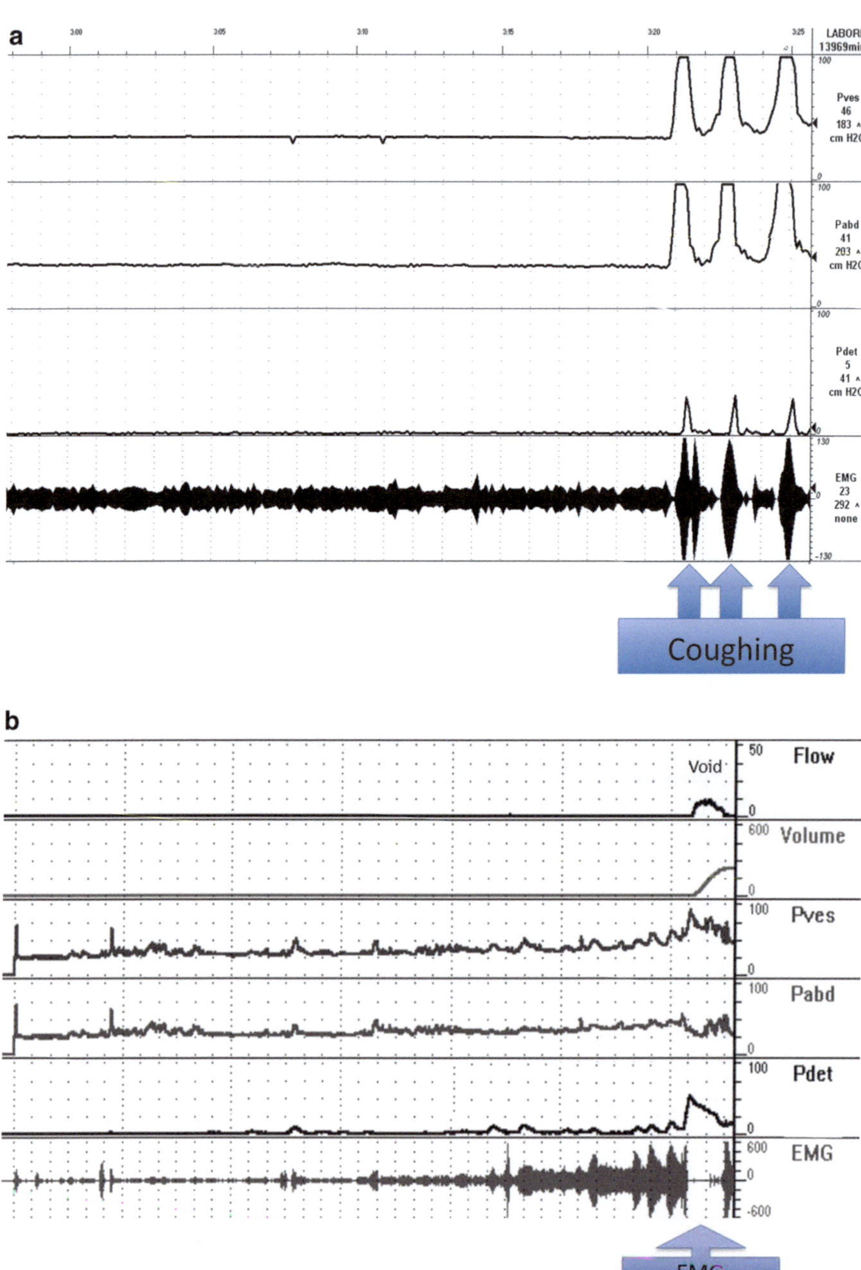

Fig. 1.2 Three examples of EMG activity: (**a**) Normal activity with increase due to coughing. (**b**) Appropriate relaxation of the EMG signal with voluntary voiding. (**c**) Increase of the external sphincter activity with voiding

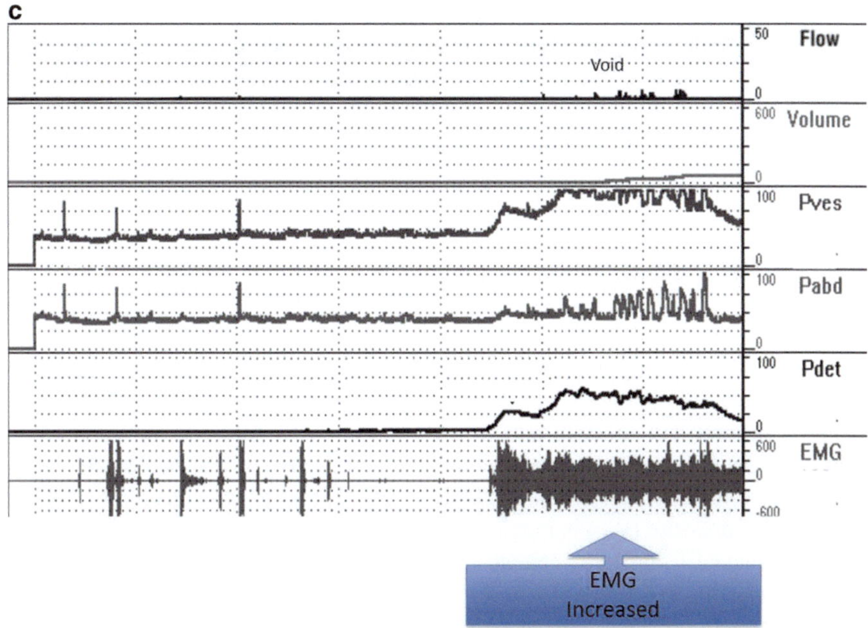

Fig. 1.2 (continued)

Normal EMG studies can lead to the exclusion of some diagnoses. However, the diagnostic utility is seen best in cases where it confirms neurological or functional causes of voiding phase dysfunction [5]. When not attributed to artifact, inappropriately increased EMG activity during the voiding phase is known as detrusor-external sphincter dyssynergia (DESD), when a neurologic lesion that can explain the dyssynergia exists (typically a suprasacral spinal cord lesion) (Fig. 1.2). When there is no underlying relevant neurologic lesion, the failure of external sphincter relaxation (or increasing EMG) leads to a diagnosis of dysfunctional voiding (a learned behavior of failed external sphincter relaxation during voiding). It is difficult to accurately predict when EMG information is going to be needed to explain voiding abnormalities. Thus, because of the relatively easy methodology and low morbidity of obtaining a surface EMG, EMG is often included as a channel in multichannel pressure-flow UDS studies [18].

EMG activity can also be increased during micturition because of external factors or artifact, sometimes called "pseudo-dyssynergia." This includes abdominal straining, movement, guarding reflex, painful urination due to the presence of a urethral catheter, and wet or dislodged electrodes [19]. The interpretation of the study therefore should include all other available information. For example, if fluoroscopy (discussed below) is obtained during voiding on studies where EMG contains artifacts, it may be used to discriminate between voiding patterns that would otherwise be differentiated by their EMG signals, i.e., dysfunctional voiding

(EMG activity is expected to be increased during voiding) and primary bladder neck obstruction (PBNO) (where EMG signal is expected to be quiescent) [7, 16]. Also, a completely normal uroflow (Q_{max}, Q_{ave}, and pattern) usually will exclude significant sphincter activity during voiding. EMG and/or uroflow abnormalities seen on invasive UDS should be confirmed with non-invasive uroflow.

Cystometry

The cystometrogram (CMG) assesses the bladder's response to filling. The CMG can measure filling pressure, sensation, involuntary contractions, compliance, and capacity. Sensation is the part of cystometry that is truly subjective and therefore requires an alert and attentive patient and clinician. The filling phase starts when filling commences and ends when the patient and urodynamicist decide that "permission to void" has been given. The CMG is ideally started with an empty bladder. The bladder pressure (P_{ves}) is monitored and fluid is infused into the bladder. This can be achieved using two separate catheters, or more commonly, a dual lumen catheter (usually 6–8 French) usually placed transurethrally (or much less commonly via a suprapubic stab incision). Guidelines exist regarding the technical specification of these catheters [7]. It is important to note that changes in bladder pressure can represent a change in detrusor pressure (P_{det}), for example from a bladder contraction voluntary or involuntary, or a change in abdominal pressure (P_{abd}), for example from movement, Valsalva, etc. Though single channel studies that monitor only P_{ves} can provide information about bladder function, the recommended method to measure bladder pressure includes simultaneously measuring P_{abd}, usually by placing a balloon catheter in the rectum or vagina. When both P_{ves} and P_{abd} are measured, the P_{det} can be calculated by using the equation: $P_{det} = P_{ves} - P_{abd}$.

In addition to recording pressures during filling, the CMG study also should record the volume infused into the bladder during filling. Filling rates [1], fluid temperature [7], and fluid type [8] all need to be considered. Today most cystometry is done with liquid (most commonly saline or radiographic contrast in cases where fluoroscopy will be used). The practice of gas CMG was historically described [20–22], and is rarely performed any longer as it does not allow for studying the voiding phase.

Normally detrusor pressure should remain near zero during the entire filling cycle until voluntary voiding is initiated. That means baseline pressure stays constant (and low) and there are no involuntary detrusor contractions (Fig. 1.3a). Involuntary bladder contractions can occur with filling and are seen as a rise in P_{ves} in the absence of a rise in P_{abd}. Urodynamically, this phenomenon is known as detrusor overactivity (DO). DO may be accompanied by a feeling of urgency or even loss of urine (Fig. 1.3b). Another important parameter that the CMG measures is bladder compliance, the relationship between change in bladder volume and detrusor pressure. Normally the bladder is highly compliant and stores increasing volumes of urine at low pressure. However certain conditions may cause the bladder

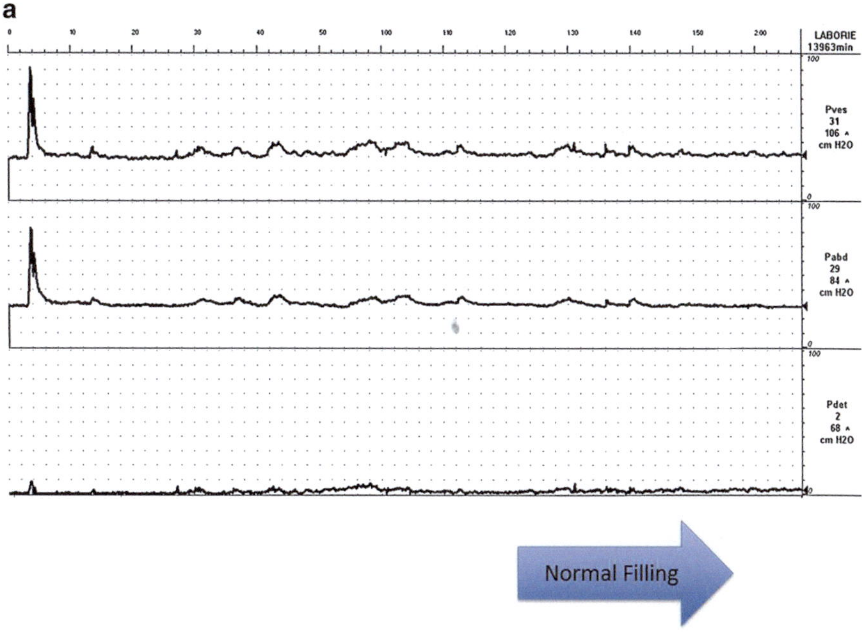

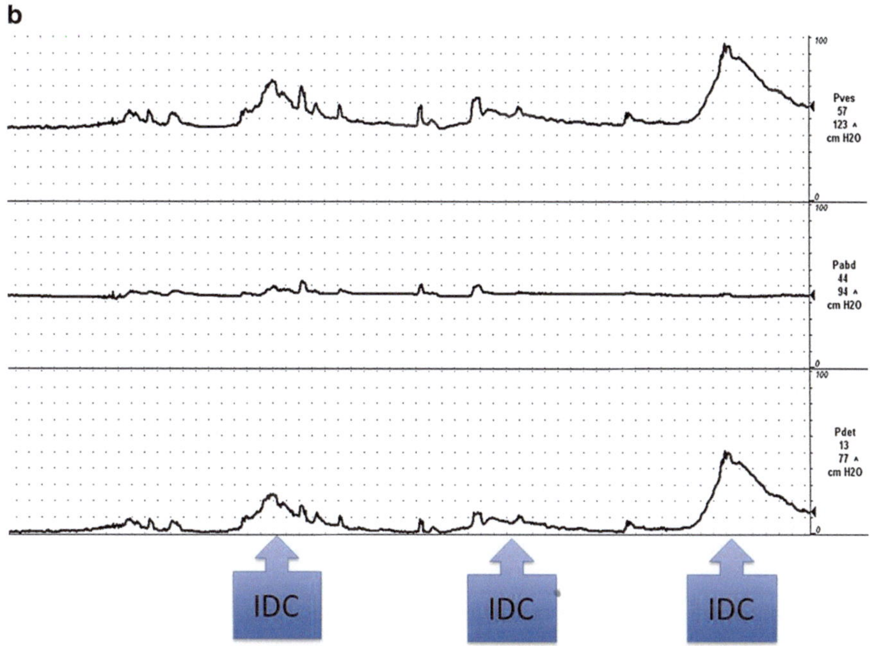

Fig. 1.3 Cystometrogram. (**a**) Normal low pressure filling. (**b**) Involuntary detrusor contraction (detrusor overactivity), there is a rise in P_{ves}, but not P_{abd}. (**c**) Impaired or low bladder compliance, with end filling pressure of over 40 cm H_2O

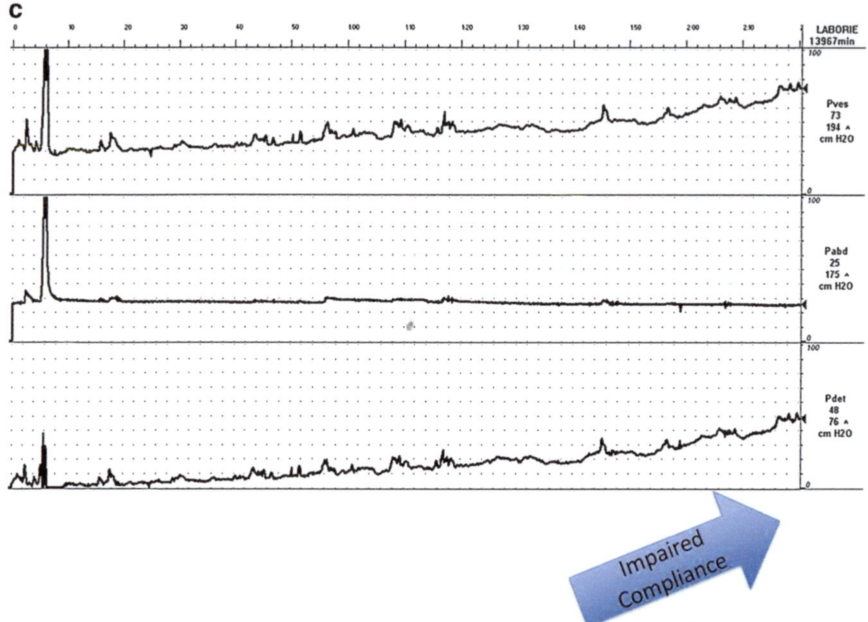

Fig. 1.3 (continued)

pressure to rise in the absence of a distinct detrusor contraction. This is known as impaired compliance (Fig. 1.3c) and can pose danger to the kidneys when this pressure is transferred to the upper urinary tracts. It is difficult to define what "normal compliance" is in terms of mL/cm H_2O. In the literature mean values for normal compliance in healthy subjects range from 46 to 124 mL/cm H_2O [23–25]. Various definitions of impaired compliance have been used (i.e., between 10 and 20 mL/cm H_2O), however there is not a consistent definition based on mL/cm H_2O. Stohrer et al. have suggested that a value of less than 20 mL/cm H_2O is consistent with impaired compliance and implies a poorly accommodating bladder [26]. However, examples can be cited (i.e., small cystometric capacity) where this may not be the case. Therefore, in practical terms, absolute pressure is probably more useful than a "compliance number" or value. For example, it has been shown that storage >40 cm H_2O are associated with harmful effects on the upper tracts [27].

For patients who have incontinence, provocative maneuvers can be performed during CMG to assess urethral competence and diagnose stress urinary incontinence (SUI). Patients can be asked to Valsalva or cough during filling. The abdominal leak point pressure (ALPP) is a measure of sphincteric strength or the ability of the sphincter to resist changes in abdominal pressure [28]. ALPP is defined as the intravesical pressure at which urine leakage occurs due to increased abdominal pressure in the absence of a detrusor contraction [1]. This measure of intrinsic urethral function is applicable to patients with stress incontinence. An ALPP can only be demonstrated in a patient with SUI. Conceptually the lower the ALPP, the weaker the sphincter.

In addition to providing information of filling pressures, the CMG can assess coarse bladder sensation and capacity. The International Continence Society (ICS) defines the following measures of sensation during bladder filling [1]:

First sensation of bladder filling is the feeling the patient has, during filling cystometry, when he/she first becomes aware of the bladder filling.

First desire to void is the feeling, during filling cystometry, that would lead the patient to pass urine at the next convenient moment, but voiding can be delayed if necessary.

Strong desire to void is defined, during filling cystometry, as a persistent desire to void without the fear of leakage.

Urgency is a sudden compelling desire to void.

Maximum cystometric capacity, in patients with normal sensation, is the volume at which the patient feels he/she can no longer delay micturition (has a strong desire to void).

Various methods exist, but ensuring quality control and adhering to standardized practices and interpretation guidelines can achieve good inter-rater reliability [29].

Voiding Pressure-Flow Study

Once the bladder is filled to cystometric capacity, the voiding portion of the pressure-flow study can begin. This examines the emptying phase of micturition. The same bladder and rectal (or vaginal catheter in women) catheters are used while simultaneously collecting pressure data along with uroflowmetry (Fig. 1.4). Ideally, such a study should assess a voluntary void. When there is flow of urine during an involuntary detrusor contraction patients may contract the pelvic floor to prevent leakage. Such an event should be annotated on study. In addition, some subjects may have a difficult time voiding on demand in a public setting and with invasive monitoring in place. These stressors and the artificial environment of the testing need to be accounted for when interpreting the test. For example, some patients cannot voluntarily void during an urodynamic study due to discomfort or psychogenic inhibition. Therefore the lack of a voluntary voiding bladder contraction during UDS does not always indicate that a patient has a truly a contractile bladder. Such a finding needs to be placed in the context of other parameters (i.e., non-invasive flows, history, PVR, etc.) to determine if it is, in fact, testing artifact. Remember that in order to answer a clinical question, the symptom(s) should be reproduced during the study. For example if a man has a complaint of a slow urinary stream, and his pressure-flow study reproduced the slow stream which occurs with a high pressure detrusor contraction, this is assumed to be an accurate depiction of an obstructive process.

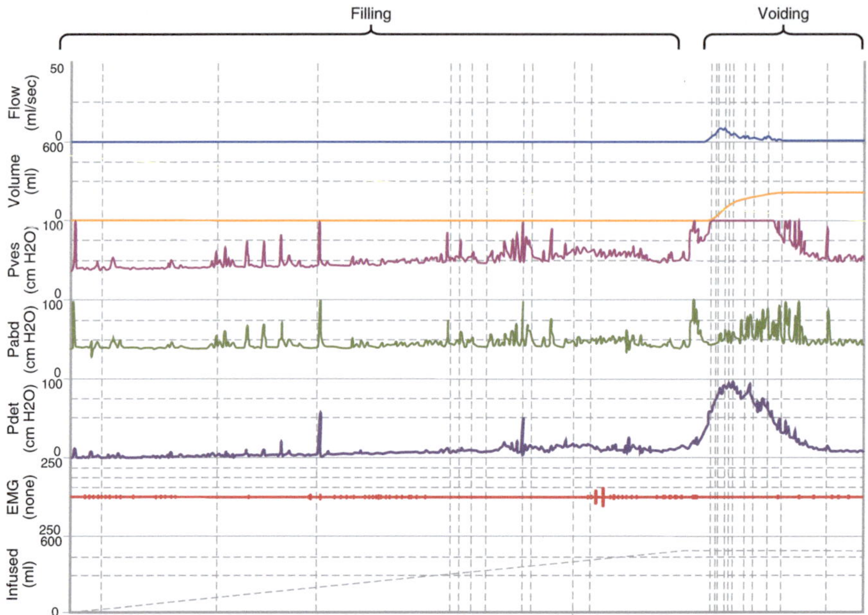

Fig. 1.4 This image shows a printout of a multichannel urodynamic study. The channels are labels and the filling and voiding phases are labeled

However, if a woman, who complains of urinary incontinence and has no reported difficulty with voiding and a low PVR, is unable to generate a voluntary detrusor contraction, it is less likely to have clinical significance. In these cases a poor flow rate can be confirmed or refuted with a non-invasive uroflow done in a private setting.

The voiding phase of a pressure-flow study helps assess two critical parameters related to the bladder and bladder outlet: detrusor contractility (normal vs. impaired) and outlet resistance (obstructed vs. unobstructed) [30]. Combinations of these two features will be discussed in Chap. 2 as contractility, coordination, complete emptying and clinical obstruction. In general the pressure-flow study can identify three fundamental conditions [30]:

1. Low (or normal) detrusor pressure and high (or normal) flow rate (normal, unobstructed voiding).
2. High detrusor pressure and low (or normal) flow rate (obstruction).
3. Low detrusor pressure with low flow rate (impaired contractility).

The most widespread application of pressure-flow studies has been to determine the presence of bladder outlet obstruction, most commonly in men. Starting in the early 1960s [24] nomograms were developed to standardize the definitions of obstruction and bladder contractility [31–33]. These nomograms are well established and broadly accepted in men (because of a single highly prevalent condition, benign prostatic obstruction—BPO). However pressure-flow nomograms are less widely agreed upon for use in women (due to the lack of a single highly prevalent condition causing obstruction) and as such have not gained widespread utilization in clinical practice [34–38].

Not all pressure-flow studies fall neatly into the three fundamental conditions. An example is a man with a poorly contractile bladder from long-term outlet obstruction. His bladder may not be able to generate a sufficient pressure to have his condition classified as obstruction, even though it is a progression of a process that occurred as a result of BPO. In such cases, it is once again important to consider all aspects of the patient's evaluation and come to a consistent clinical conclusion.

Urethral Pressure Profilometry

Urethral pressure profilometry (UPP) was popularized by Brown and Wickman [39] as a method to determine resistance provided by the urethra. Using a small catheter with lateral apertures through which fluid is continuously infused, simultaneous bladder and urethral pressure is measured as the catheter is slowly withdrawn along the course of the urethra. The urethral pressure transducer measures the fluid pressure required to lift the urethral wall off the catheter side holes and thus evaluates the circumferential and radial stresses induced by the presence of the catheter in the urethra and the slow urethral perfusion. Thus, urethral pressure is defined as the fluid pressure needed to just open a closed urethra [1].

Several parameters can be obtained from the UPP:

The urethral closure pressure profile (UCP) is given by the subtraction of intravesical pressure from urethral pressure.

Maximum urethral pressure (MUP) is the highest pressure measured along the UPP.

Maximum urethral closure pressure (MUCP) is the maximum difference between the urethral pressure and the intravesical pressure.

Functional profile length is the length of the urethra along which the urethral pressure exceeds intravesical pressure in women.

UPP has been mostly used as a measure of urethral resistance in women with SUI. Despite an abundant literature on urethral profilometry, its clinical relevance is controversial. Many urologists do not routinely perform urethral profilometry. In 2002, the ICS standardization sub-committee concluded that the clinical utility of urethral pressure measurement is unclear [40]. Furthermore, there are no urethral pressure measurements that (1) discriminate urethral incompetence from other disorders; (2) provide a measure of the severity of the condition; (3) provide a reliable indicator to surgical success, and return to normal after surgical intervention [40].

Videourodynamics

Videourodynamics (VUDS) consists of the simultaneous measurement of UDS parameters and imaging of the lower urinary tract. It provides the most precise evaluation of voiding function and dysfunction. VUDS are particularly useful when anatomic structure in relation to lower urinary tract function is important, for example in localizing bladder outlet obstruction (particular in women) or in assessing vesico-ureteral reflux in relation to storage and/or voiding pressures. VUDS can be performed using a variety of different methods. Most commonly fluoroscopy is employed using a C-arm that gives the most flexibility for patient positioning. However a fixed unit with fluoroscopy table that can move from 90° to 180° may also be used. It is important that the patient be able to be positioned properly to evaluate the desired function and anatomy.

The technique of obtaining fluoroscopic imaging during multichannel UDS was popularized in the United States by Tanagho et al. [41] and in Europe by Turner-Warwick [42]. Over the years, the value of adding this functional and anatomical picture to multichannel UDS studies has been described in various situations [35, 43–45].

In isolation, pressure-flow UDS can identify if obstruction is present, but cannot determine where in the lower urinary tract the obstruction is located. Simultaneous fluoroscopy can provide that information. Another benefit of fluoroscopy is the identification of vesico-ureteral reflux (Fig. 1.5). The detection of VUR can be critical in patients with high storage pressures such as certain types of neurogenic bladder as well as other conditions that can lead to impaired bladder compliance. During bladder filling, storage pressures may appear low (a safe situation), but poor compliance and high bladder filling pressures may be masked by a "pop-off" valve due to reflux into a dilated upper urinary tract. This is a situation that is accurately diagnosed with VUDS. Compared to a voiding cystourethrogram alone, the simultaneous pressure and volume readings during VUDS provide information about the pressure and volume at which reflux occurs, which can direct management.

Fluoroscopic imaging can also have a role in the diagnosis of urinary incontinence. Images can help identify small amounts of urinary leakage [46]. The level of continence is also assessed during bladder filling (e.g., open or closed bladder neck at rest or straining). Furthermore, the function of the bladder neck and external urethral sphincter can also be assessed during the voiding phase. This can be especially important in cases where EMG readings are difficult to interpret. Finally, in some cases of voiding dysfunction in women, the fluoroscopic images can be used to define as well as localize obstruction [35].

Other Urodynamic Tests

This chapter is not meant to be an exhaustive list of all technology used or investigated in the evaluation and management of disorders of the urinary tract. However, similar to all fields of diagnostic testing, there is never a shortage of attempts to improve the tools and techniques that have been used in the past.

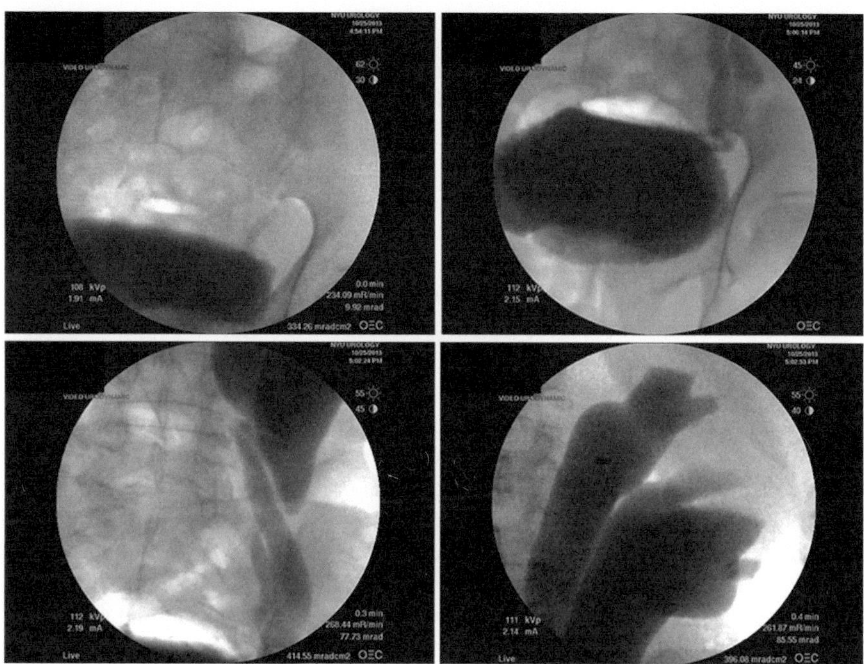

Fig. 1.5 The presence of reflux is noted on this fluoroscopic image obtained during filling CMG. The true bladder compliance may actually be less than what is measured on CMG because of the "pop-off" mechanism provided by the *left upper tract*

Though invasive testing has been shown to be well tolerated [47] newer technology attempts to improve the patient experience and minimize associated morbidity. However, if the technology is going to replace older methods, it must not sacrifice diagnostic ability.

Imaging studies have been investigated in the diagnosis of lower urinary tract disorders. Though not a new concept, researchers continue to look at resistive index from color flow Doppler of the prostate in men with Benign Prostatic Hyperpertrophy to assess bladder outlet obstruction [48]. Many different measurements of the prostate anatomy by ultrasound imaging have also been investigated, but still remain difficult to reproduce and practically apply [49]. Ultrasound technology has also been used in order to determine estimated bladder weight and bladder wall thickness, but has had mixed results [50, 51].

Near infrared spectrometry (NIRS) is another technique that has now been applied to investigate for the presence or absence of bladder outlet obstruction [52]. This is based on the premise that during voiding when bladder outlet obstruction exists, the detrusor contraction will be excessive as compared to unobstructed patients. This increased contraction results in a decrease in total hemoglobin and oxyhemoglobin concentrations. NIRS is able to monitor these changes. This technology is intriguing, but technical limitation and reproducibility remain issues.

UDS in Clinical Practice

Although UDS has been used as part of clinical practice for decades, clear-cut, level 1 evidenced-based "indications" for its use in many conditions are lacking. There are a number of reasons for this lack of evidence. It is difficult to conduct proper randomized controlled trials on UDS for conditions where lesser levels of evidence and expert opinion strongly suggest clinical utility and where "empiric treatment" is potentially harmful or even life-threatening (e.g., neurogenic voiding dysfunction). Additionally, symptoms can be caused by a number of different conditions, and it is difficult to study pure or homogeneous patient populations [53]. Recently the American Urological Association (AUA) and the Society of Urodynamics, Female Pelvic Medicine and Urogenital Reconstruction (SUFU) published the AUA/SUFU Urodynamic Guidelines [5]. The purpose of that guideline was not to present an exhaustive review of the "indications" for UDS, but rather to review the literature regarding urodynamic testing in common lower urinary tract conditions and assist clinicians in the proper selection and application of urodynamic tests, following an appropriate evaluation and symptom characterization. When it comes to "indications" for UDS for any condition, the most important factors are that the clinician has clear-cut reason(s) for performing the study, and that the information obtained will be used to guide treatment of the patient. Therefore it is probably more useful to describe the role of UDS in clinical practice rather than precise "indications" for its use.

In practical terms, UDS is most useful when history, physical exam, and simple tests are not sufficient to make an accurate diagnosis and/or institute treatment [53]. This has clinical applicability in two general scenarios:

1. To obtain information needed to make an accurate diagnosis for what condition(s) is causing symptoms (i.e., lower urinary tract symptoms (LUTS) or incontinence).
2. To determine the impact of a disease that has the potential to cause serious and irreversible damage to the upper and lower urinary tract (i.e., neurological diseases like spinal cord injury and multiple sclerosis, radiation cystitis). Sometimes profound abnormalities can be found in the relative absence of symptoms.

As with most diagnostic studies in medicine, understanding the results of the test is only part of a much broader picture. It is equally important to understand those results in the context of a specific clinical condition or situation. Another important consideration is the understanding of when to order the given test. Indiscriminate testing leads to unnecessary cost, subjects patients to risk, and can even complicate the diagnosis when these results are misinterpreted.

The information that follows is obviously not exhaustive, but begins to explore the process of choosing the "right test." This will be within the framework of the current AUA/SUFU Urodynamic guideline document [5]. These guidelines also include the level of evidence and the strength of the recommendation made by the committee.

Stress Urinary Incontinence

UDS in SUI, like in many other conditions, should be performed if the results will have a significant impact on patient management or counseling. This is most often applicable to pre-surgical UDS testing or cases where the diagnosis of SUI is in doubt or when SUI appears to co-exist with other conditions that could affect management (i.e., detrusor overactivity of bladder outlet obstruction). Recently, a large multi-center randomized controlled trial to determine the value of UDS prior to surgery for women with SUI concluded that UDS is not needed prior to the surgical treatment of women with "straight forward" SUI who have demonstrable clinical SUI with no significant overactive bladder symptoms and normal emptying [54]. We would agree with this for patients and clinicians who would not change the type of surgery based on the results of UDS testing. However some surgeons may alter the type of procedure done based on a measure of urethral resistance, such as ALPP. In such cases, it would seem reasonable for that particular surgeon to consider UDS. It is also important to remember that if one chooses not to do UDS prior to SUI surgery in women it is critical that SUI be demonstrated on physical exam, that storage symptoms are adequately characterized and that emptying is assessed (symptoms and measurement of PVR).

We believe that the recommendations from the AUA/SUFU Guideline for the utility of Urodynamic studies in adult women with SUI and pelvic organ prolapse [5] provide useful information for the clinician. Please note that these "guidelines" do not specifically say when or on whom to perform UDS, but rather provide information based on the literature and expert opinion/clinical principles. Ultimately the decision to perform UDS on a given patient should be based on certainty of diagnosis and whether or not the results will affect treatment or counseling.

Key points from AUA/SUFU Guideline Statements [5]:

1. When diagnosing stress incontinence on UDS, clinicians should assess urethral function.
2. If considering invasive therapy to treat SUI, surgeons should assess PVR urine volume.
3. Multichannel UDS may be performed in patients with both symptoms and physical findings of SUI if considering "invasive, potentially morbid, or irreversible treatments."
4. If SUI is suspected, but not demonstrated on UDS with a catheter in place, repeat stress testing with the urethral catheter removed should be performed.
5. Stress testing with reduction of POP (high-grade) should be performed in women without the symptom of SUI (if the presence of SUI will alter the surgical treatment plan). Multichannel UDS may be used for this assessment of SUI with reduction of prolapse and detrusor dysfunction in women with associated LUTS.

Urgency Urinary Incontinence

Urgency urinary incontinence (UUI) is another common condition that is often evaluated with UDS. For patients with UUI, UDS is most applicable when the diagnosis is in doubt (i.e., when significant portion of incontinence may be caused by urethral insufficiency), when a concomitant problem such as bladder outlet obstruction can co-exist or even be the cause of bladder overactivity, and in certain conditions (neurological conditions, radiation cystitis, or chronic outlet obstruction) where high pressure storage and impaired bladder compliance can co-exist. The recommendations from the AUA/SUFU Guideline for the utility of Urodynamic studies in adults with UUI [5] provide useful information for the clinician and consider all of these possibilities. Again the "guidelines" do not specifically say when or on whom to perform UDS, but rather provide information based on the literature and expert opinion/clinical principles:

1. If it is important to determine if compliance is altered, detrusor overactivity (DO) is present, or other urodynamic abnormalities exist (or not) multichannel filling cystometry may be performed in patients with UUI when considering "invasive, potentially morbid, or irreversible treatments."
2. In patients with UUI after procedures on the bladder outlet, PFS may be performed to evaluate for bladder outlet obstruction.
3. Absence of detrusor overactivity on an urodynamic study does not mean that it may not still be a *causative agent* for symptoms of UUI and mixed urinary incontinence.

Neurogenic Bladder

UDS probably has its most important role in the diagnosis and management of patients with neuropathic voiding dysfunction. This is because certain conditions can have a profound impact on the lower urinary tract that can affect upper tract (kidney) function. In such cases management is not driven by symptoms, but rather by the need to preserve renal function. The term "neurogenic" encompasses a broad spectrum of diseases that can result in bladder storage and bladder-emptying dysfunction. Here too, a clear understanding of the underlying neurogenic process and its effect on the lower urinary tract should help guide appropriate selection of urodynamic testing. Patients who are at risk for upper tract decompensation are those with high storage pressure and incomplete bladder emptying. This most frequently occurs in cases of detrusor-sphincter dyssynergia (suprasacral spinal cord lesions). In such patients VUDS can be particularly useful to evaluate for the presence of vesico-ureteral reflux (see above). For patients with neurological disease not at risk for upper tract decompensation (i.e., women post-cerebral vascular accident) UDS has its greatest utility when patients have failed appropriate empiric therapy. The recommendations from the AUA/SUFU Guideline for the utility of UDS in adults with Neurogenic Bladder [5] *offer appropriate* "guidelines" based on the literature and expert opinion/clinical principles:

1. PVR measurements should be assessed, as part of complete urodynamic study or as a separate test, during evaluation of patients with "relevant neurological disease" (i.e., spinal cord injury, myelomeningocele). The PVR should also be measured in follow-up when appropriate.
2. Complex CMG should be performed during initial urological evaluation of patients with "relevant neurological conditions" regardless of the presence (or absence) of symptoms. Complex CMG should also be performed as part of the continued follow-up in appropriate situations. In the urologic evaluation of patients with other neurologic diseases, CMG may be considered as an option to evaluate LUTS.
3. Pressure-flow analysis should be performed in patients with "relevant neurologic disease" regardless of the presence (or absence) of symptoms. Pressure-flow analysis should also be performed in cases of patients with other neurologic disease that have an elevated PVR or urinary symptoms.
4. Fluoroscopy (if available) may be done at the time of UDS (VUDS) in patients with "relevant neurologic disease at risk for NGB." The same is true for patients with other neurologic disease who have an elevated PVR or urinary symptoms.
5. Clinicians should perform EMG along with CMG and with pressure-flow studies (if performed) in patients with "relevant neurologic disease at risk for NGB." EMG should also be carried out with the aforementioned studies in cases of other neurologic disease where patients have an elevated PVR or urinary symptoms.

Voiding Dysfunction/LUTS

UDS is often used to assist in the evaluation of men and women with storage and voiding LUTS. We have found UDS most useful in patients with LUTS who: have failed empiric treatment; have multiple symptoms that cannot be easily differentiated; have mixed storage and voiding symptoms, especially when surgery for the relief of obstruction is being considered; or have underlying conditions that can affect lower urinary tract function (i.e., prior pelvic surgery or radiation). Often a clinician's own treatment algorithm, comfort with diagnosis, and expertise will determine at what stage UDS are introduced. In many patients with LUTS, a step-wise use of tests seems to be most appropriate. The evaluation of bladder emptying can be of critical importance. Therefore, it is common to utilize non-invasive uroflow and/or PVR determination early in the evaluation. History and physical exam alone or in combination with these simple tests are often all that is needed to initiate therapy. However, when initial therapy fails, or when uroflow and PVR results are concerning, more comprehensive UDS testing may be employed. There is also evidence to support the use of UDS prior to surgical intervention for suspected benign prostatic obstruction with LUTS, to document the presence of obstruction. In women and young men with LUTS and suspected outlet obstruction, we have found VUDS to be particularly helpful in aiding in the diagnosis and localization of obstruction [35, 55]. Again the recommendations from the AUA/SUFU Guideline for the utility of UDS in adults with LUTS [5] provide useful information for the clinician without a presentation of absolute indications for any specific patient.

1. During the initial evaluation (and follow-up) of patients with LUTS measurement of PVR may be used as a "safety measure" to rule out significant retention of urine.
2. During the initial (and follow-up) evaluation of male patients with LUTS that suggest abnormal voiding/emptying, Uroflow may be used.
3. Multichannel filling cystometry may be used if "it is important to determine DO or other abnormalities of bladder filling/urine storage" exist in patients with LUTS. This has may have more importance when "invasive, potentially morbid, or irreversible treatments are considered."
4. If it is "important to determine if urodynamic obstruction is present in men with LUTS" clinicians should perform PFS. This may be particularly important when "invasive, potentially morbid, or irreversible treatments are considered."
5. In female patients if it is "important to determine if obstruction is present," PFS may be performed.
6. VUDS may be carried out in "properly selected patients" where localization of the level of obstruction is particularly important. For example to diagnose PBNO.

Summary

UDS consists of a number of different tests that evaluate lower urinary tract function. These tests can be employed individually or in combination depending on a specific clinical scenario to aid the clinician in diagnosing and treating patients with LUTS other conditions that affect the lower urinary tract function. UDS is most useful when performed for specific reasons to obtain specific information to guide management (treatment or no treatment). We would caution that the indiscriminate use of UDS is not appropriate and can be counterproductive, or even harmful. However, when used appropriately, these tests can be invaluable.

References

1. Davis DM. The hydrodynamics of the upper urinary tract (urodynamics). Ann Surg. 1954;140:839 [Lippincott, Williams, and Wilkins].
2. Brown ET, Krlin RM, Winters JC. Urodynamics: examining the current role of UDS testing. What is the role of urodynamic testing in light of recent AUA urodynamics and overactive bladder guidelines and the VALUE study? Curr Urol Rep. 2013;14:403–8.
3. Abrams P, Blaivas JG, Stanton S, Andersen JT. ICS standardisation of terminology of lower urinary tract function. Scand J Urol Nephrol. 1988;114:5–19.

4. Abrams P, Cardozo L, Fall M, Griffiths D, Rosier P, Ulmsten U, et al. The standardisation of terminology of lower urinary tract function: report from the Standardisation Sub-committee of the International Continence Society. Neurourol Urodyn. 2002;21:167–78.
5. Winters JC, Dmochowski RR, Goldman HB, Herndon CDA, Kobashi KC, Kraus SR, et al. Urodynamic studies in adults: AUA/SUFU guideline. J Urol. 2012;188:2464–72.
6. Nitti VW, Combs AJ. Urodynamics: when, why and how. In: Nitti VW, editor. Practical urodynamics. Philadelphia: W.B. Saunders; 1998. p. 15–25.
7. Schäfer W, Abrams P, Liao L, Mattiasson A, Pesce F, Spangberg A, et al. Good urodynamic practices: uroflowmetry, filling cystometry, and pressure-flow studies. Neurourol Urodyn. 2002;21:261–74.
8. Haylen BT, de Ridder D, Freeman RM, Swift SE, Berghmans B, Lee J, et al. An International Urogynecological Association (IUGA)/International Continence Society (ICS) joint report on the terminology for female pelvic floor dysfunction. Neurourol Urodyn. 2010;29:4–20.
9. Haylen BT, Lee J. The accuracy of post-void residual measurement in women. Int Urogynecol J Pelvic Floor Dysfunct. 2008;19:603–6.
10. Park YH, Ku JH, Oh S-J. Accuracy of post-void residual urine volume measurement using a portable ultrasound bladder scanner with real-time pre-scan imaging. Neurourol Urodyn. 2011;30(3):335–8.
11. Boone TB, Kim YH. Uroflowmetry. In: Nitti VW, editor. Practical urodynamics. Philadephia: W B Saunders; 1998. p. 28–37.
12. Drach GW, Layton TN, Binard WJ. Male peak urinary flow rate: relationships to volume voided and age. J Urol. 1979;122:210–4.
13. Gray M. Traces: making sense of urodynamics testing—part 2: uroflowmetry. Urol Nurs. 2010;30:321–6.
14. Chan C-K, Yip SK-H, Wu IPH, Li M-L, Chan N-H. Evaluation of the clinical value of a simple flowmeter in the management of male lower urinary tract symptoms. BJU Int. 2012;109:1690–6.
15. Abrams P, Blaivas JG, Stanton SL, Andersen DJT. The standardization of terminology of lower urinary tract function recommended by the international continence society. Int Urogynecol J Pelvic Floor Dysfunct. 1990;1:45–58 [Springer].
16. Brucker BM, Fong E, Shah S, Kelly C, Rosenblum N, Nitti VW. Urodynamic differences between dysfunctional voiding and primary bladder neck obstruction in women. Urology. 2012;80:55–60.
17. Barrett DM. Disposable (infant) surface electrocardiogram electrodes in urodynamics: a simultaneous comparative study of electrodes. J Urol. 1980;124:663–5.
18. Sakakibara R, Fowler CJ, Hattori T, Hussain IF, Swinn MJ, Uchiyama T, et al. Pressure-flow study as an evaluating method of neurogenic urethral relaxation failure. J Auton Nerv Syst. 2000;80(1–2):85–8.
19. Wein A, Barrett D. Etiologic possibilities for increased pelvic floor electromyography activity during cystometry. J Urol. 1982;127(5):949–52.
20. Gleason DM, Bottaccini MR, Reilly RJ. Comparison of cystometrograms and urethral profiles with gas and water media. Urology. 1977;9(2):155–60.
21. Gleason D, Reilly B. Gas cystometry. Urol Clin North Am. 1979;6(1):85–8.
22. Godec CJ, Cass AS. Rapid and slow-fill gas cystometry. Influence on bladder capacity and diagnosis of hyperreflexic bladder. Urology. 1979;13(1):109–10.
23. Sorensen S, Gregersen H, Sorensen SM. Long term reproducibility of urodynamic investigations in healthy fertile females. Scand J Urol Nephrol Suppl. 1988;114:35–41.
24. van Waalwijk van Doorn ES, Remmers A, Janknegt RA. Conventional and extramural ambulatory urodynamic testing of the lower urinary tract in female volunteers. J Urol. 1992;147:1319–26.
25. Hosker G. Urodynamics. In: Hillard T, Purdie D, editors. The yearbook of obstetrics and gynaecology. London: RCOG Press; 2004. p. 233–54.
26. Stohrer M, Goepel M, Kondo A, et al. The standardization of terminology in neurogenic lower urinary tract dysfunction with suggestions for diagnostic procedures. Neurourol Urodynn. 1999;18:139–58.

27. McGuire EJ, Woodside JR, Borden TA, Weiss RM. Prognostic value of urodynamic testing in myeloplastic children. J Urol. 1981;126:205–9.
28. McGuire EJ, Fitzpatrick CC, Wan J, et al. Clinical assessment of urethral sphincter function. J Urol. 1993;150:1452–4.
29. Zimmern P, Nager CW, Albo M, FitzGerald MP, McDermott S. Interrater reliability of filling cystometrogram interpretation in a multicenter study. J Urol. 2006;175:2174–7.
30. Nitti VW. Pressure flow urodynamic studies: the gold standard for diagnosing bladder outlet obstruction. Rev Urol. 2005;7 Suppl 6:S14.
31. Gleason DM, Lattimer JK. The pressure-flow study: a method for measuring bladder neck resistance. J Urol. 1962;87:844–52.
32. Abrams PH, Griffiths DJ. The assessment of prostatic obstruction from urodynamic measurements and from residual urine. Br J Urol. 1979;51:129–34.
33. Abrams P. Bladder outlet obstruction index, bladder contractility index and bladder voiding efficiency: three simple indices to define bladder voiding function. BJU Int. 1999;84(1):14–5.
34. Chassagne S, Bernier PA, Haab F, et al. Proposed cutoff values to define bladder outlet obstruction in women. Urology. 1998;51:408–11.
35. Nitti VW, Tu LM, Gitlin J. Diagnosing bladder outlet obstruction in women. J Urol. 1999;161(5):1535–40.
36. Blaivas JG, Groutz A. Bladder outlet obstruction nomogram for women with lower urinary tract symptomatology. Neurourol Urodyn. 2000;19:553–64.
37. Defreitas GA, Zimmern PE, Lemack GE, Shariat SF. Refining diagnosis of anatomic female bladder outlet obstruction: comparison of pressure-flow study parameters in clinically obstructed women with those of normal controls. Urology. 2004;64:675–9.
38. Akikwala TV, Fleischman N, Nitti VW. Comparison of diagnostic criteria for female bladder outlet obstruction. J Urol. 2006;176:2093–7.
39. Brown M, Wickham JEA. The urethral pressure profile. Br J Urol. 1969;41:211–7.
40. Lose G, Griffiths D, Hosker G, et al. Standardisation of urethral pressure measurement: report from the Standardisation Sub-Committee of the International Continence Society. Neurourol Urodyn. 2002;21:258–60.
41. Tanagho EA, Miller ER, Meyers FH, Corbett RK. Observations on the dynamics of the bladder neck. Br J Urol. 1966;38:72–84.
42. Bates CP, Whiteside CG, Turner-Warwick R. Synchronous cine/pressure/flow/cysto-urethrography with special reference to stress and urge incontinence. Br J Urol. 1970;42:714–23.
43. Webster GD, Older RA. Video urodynamics. Urology. 1980;16(1):106–14.
44. Mayo ME, Chapman WH, Shurtleff DB. Bladder function in children with meningomyelocele: comparison of cine-fluoroscopy and urodynamics. J Urol. 1979;121(4):458–61.
45. Kuo HC. Videourodynamic characteristics and lower urinary tract symptoms of female bladder outlet obstruction. Urology. 2005;66(5):1005–9.
46. McGuire EJ, Woodside JR. Diagnostic advantages of fluoroscopic monitoring during urodynamic evaluation. J Urol. 1981;125(6):830–4.
47. Porru D, Madeddu G, Campus G, Montisci I, Scarpa RM, Usai E. Evaluation of morbidity of multi-channel pressure-flow studies. Neurourol Urodyn. 1999;18:647–52.
48. Zhang X, Li G, Wei X, Mo X, Hu L, Zha Y, et al. Resistive index of prostate capsular arteries: a newly identified parameter to diagnose and assess bladder outlet obstruction in patients with benign prostatic hyperplasia. J Urol. 2012;188:881–7.
49. Sahai A, Seth J, Van der Aa F, Panicker J, De Ridder D, Dasgupta P. Current state of the art in non-invasive urodynamics. Curr Bladder Dysfunct Rep. 2013;8:83–91.
50. Huang T, Qi J, Yu YJ, Xu D, Jiao Y, Kang J, et al. Predictive value of resistive index, detrusor wall thickness and ultrasound estimated bladder weight regarding the outcome after transurethral prostatectomy for patients with lower urinary tract symptoms suggestive of benign prostatic obstruction. Int J Urol. 2012;19:343–50.
51. Han DH, Lee HW, Sung HH, Lee HN, Lee Y-S, Lee K-S. The diagnostic efficacy of 3-dimensional ultrasound estimated bladder weight corrected for body surface area as an alternative nonurodynamic parameter of bladder outlet obstruction. J Urol. 2011;185:964–9.

52. Macnab AJ, Stothers L. Near-infrared spectroscopy: validation of bladder-outlet obstruction assessment using non-invasive parameters. Can J Urol. 2008;15:4241–8.
53. Nitti VW. Urodynamic and videourodynamic evaluation of the lower urinary tract. In: Wein A, Kavoussi L, Novick A, Partin A, Peters C, editors. Campbell Walsh urology. 10th ed. Philadelphia: Elsevier Saunders; 2011. p. 1847–70.
54. Nager CW, Brubaker L, Litman HJ, Zyczynski HM, Varner RE, Amundsen C, et al. A randomized trial of urodynamic testing before stress-incontinence surgery. N Engl J Med. 2012;366(21):1987–97.
55. Nitti VW, Lefkowitz G, Ficazzola M, Dixon CM. Lower urinary tract symptoms in young men: videourodynamic findings and correlation with non-invasive measures. J Urol. 2002;168:135–8.

Chapter 2
The 9 "C's" of Pressure-Flow Urodynamics

Kelly C. Johnson and Eric S. Rovner

There exists no generally agreed upon orderly or methodical approach to interpreting pressure-flow urodynamic (PFUD) studies. The amount of information produced during a routine PFUD study can be imposing to fully understand and properly interpret. For a given study, the modern electronic multichannel pressure-flow urodynamic machine produces a large amount of data in a graphical display usually supplemented with other information. The format varies depending on the type of urodynamic equipment, the specific study, and the end-user customization. Nevertheless, in most instances, the various channels on the graph represent a set of continuous variables over time including vesical and abdominal pressure recordings, urine flow rate and volume, infused volume, and potentially other signals as well. An event summary, annotations, nomograms, and other features now commonly found on commercially available urodynamics equipment add to the tremendous set of data available from a routine PFUD study.

In the same manner in which radiologists interpret their imaging studies, it is crucial to be systematic and organized in approaching the PFUD tracing in order to properly and completely distil the optimal amount of information from the study. It is quite possible to overlook salient and relevant features of a PFUD tracing especially in those cases where there exists one single overwhelming abnormality. Like the astute radiologist, the expert urodynamicist will not be dissuaded from completely interpreting the study even in the setting of a distracting feature so that other, subtler findings can be noted as well. Such nuances can be crucial in formulating an accurate interpretation of the study and should not be overlooked. The 9 "C's" of PFUD are a method of organizing and interpreting the PFUD study in a simple, reliable, and practical manner [1]. In doing so, this system minimizes the potential for "missing" an important and relevant finding on the tracing. This framework is easy

K.C. Johnson, MD • E.S. Rovner, MD (✉)
Department of Urology, Medical University of South Carolina,
96 Jonathan Lucas St., CSB 644, Charleston, SC 29425, USA
e-mail: rovnere@musc.edu

© Springer Science+Business Media New York 2015
E.S. Rovner, M.E. Koski (eds.), *Rapid and Practical Interpretation of Urodynamics*, DOI 10.1007/978-1-4939-1764-8_2

Table 2.1 The 9 "C's" of pressure-flow urodynamics

Filling and storage
Contractions (involuntary detrusor)
Compliance
Coarse sensation
Continence
Cystometric capacity
Emptying
Contractility
Complete emptying
Coordination
Clinical obstruction

to understand, remember, and applicable to all PFUD studies for virtually all lower urinary conditions.

The 9 "C's" are listed in Table 2.1. In the functional classification as popularized by Wein [2] the micturition cycle consists of two phases: (1) bladder filling/urinary storage, and (2) bladder emptying. All voiding dysfunctions therefore can be categorized as abnormalities of one or both of these phases. This classification system also provides a useful framework for organizing the 9 "C's". The 9 "C's" represent the nine essential features of the PFUDs tracing that represent a minimum interpretive data set. Each of the features begins with the letter "C." In the filling phase, the "C's" consist of contractions (involuntary), compliance, continence, capacity, and coarse sensation. In the emptying phase contractility, complete emptying, coordination, and clinical obstruction are evaluated.

The "C's" are not specific for all types of urinary dysfunction or all urodynamic abnormalities. Nevertheless, by organizing and interpreting a study within this framework, it provides an organizing thread from which to formulate a diagnosis and begin to assemble a management plan.

Of course all PFUD tracings should be interpreted in the context of the patients history, physical examination, and other relevant studies. Additionally, reproducing the patient's symptoms or at least notating whether this was achieved during the study is also important in order to properly interpret the tracing and any abnormalities seen. Notwithstanding these limitations, it remains that a systematic and organized approach to interpretation of the PFUD tracing is likely to yield the most useful and complete set of data and optimize clinical care and outcomes.

The 5 C's of Filling and Storage

There are five key parts of the filling and storage portion of the PFUD study that should be recorded in the final interpretation of the study. This segment of the PFUD study is sometimes referred to as "filling cystometry." This portion commences with bladder filling and ends with the command "permission to void" [3].

The aims of this part of the study are to assess involuntary detrusor activity, bladder compliance, sensation, capacity and, in the appropriate setting, urethral function.

Contractions refer to the presence or absence of phasic (or terminal) involuntary bladder contractions with respect to detrusor function (specifically during bladder filling only) [3]. Though the actual definition of an involuntary bladder contraction is sometimes debated, the finding of the characteristic wave form, along with whether it is spontaneous or provoked, or phasic or terminal should be recorded. The pressure and volume and amplitude of such a finding may be recorded as well, although the clinical significance of such information is variable and debatable depending on the clinical circumstances of the patient under study. Nevertheless, just as importantly, the absence of such a finding should be recorded as normal.

Compliance is the relationship between the change in bladder pressure and bladder volume during bladder filling. Physiologically, compliance is determined by the innate viscoelastic properties of the bladder. Generally the rise in bladder pressure with filling, in the absence of involuntary bladder contractions, is very small, and frequently imperceptible. Compliance is calculated by dividing the change in bladder volume by the change in bladder pressure at the point in the PFUD study just prior to the command to void, and in the absence of an involuntary bladder contraction [4]. Normative values are not universally agreed upon and compliance is generally recorded as either normal or abnormal. Abnormal bladder compliance is a significant risk factor for upper urinary tract deterioration. Classically, abnormal compliance can be seen in radiation cystitis, neurogenic bladder (especially spina bifida), and denervated bladders following radical pelvic surgery.

Coarse sensation of bladder filling is quite subjective and variable due to the very artificial and non-physiological circumstances under which the PFUD study is performed. Using the term "coarse sensation," though fairly non-descript, is pragmatic and useful. In general, the description of the sensation of bladder filling is very general and abnormalities of sensation may be described as absent, reduced, or increased [3]. Due to the need for urethral catheterization, causing some degree of urethral discomfort and/or pain, as well as the tip of the catheter within the bladder and the non-physiological filling rate, fluid and fluid temperature, the perception of bladder filling can be considerably altered. Furthermore, the patient's ability to perceive sensation and verbally express to the examiner such sensations as the bladder fills are somewhat compromised. The volumes at which the first sensation of bladder filling, first desire to void, normal desire to void, strong desire to void, urgency, and pain are documented. It is essential to note when such sensations correlate with particular urodynamic findings such as bladder overactivity. Normative parameters and assessment methods for bladder sensation have been proposed but none are universally accepted [5].

Continence refers to the presence or absence of urinary leakage during the PFUD study. Urinary incontinence may be due to abnormalities of bladder function (involuntary detrusor contractions, or abnormal compliance), or urethral function, or a combination of both. Incontinence occurring coincident with an involuntary bladder contraction is termed detrusor overactivity incontinence [4]. Stress incontinence, due to diminished sphincter function, may be provoked with cough or Valsalva or other maneuvers. Urethral function during bladder filling may be assessed by abdominal leak point pressure or urethral pressure profilometry. Incontinence recorded during the study may reproduce the patient's symptoms or not. For the patient without a clinical complaint of urinary incontinence, the finding of stress or detrusor overactivity incontinence is often artifactual and of little clinical significance. Alternatively, in the patient with a clinical complaint of urinary incontinence, it is important to make every effort to reproduce the incontinence during the study. For purposes of interpreting the study, it is important to record whether incontinence was noted during the study, the type of incontinence, and whether it reproduced the patient's symptoms. Other parameters specific to the episode(s) of incontinence such as volume infused, bladder pressure, urethral pressure, and sensation at the moment of incontinence should be recorded as well.

Cystometric capacity is the volume contained within the bladder at the point during the filling phase of the PFUD study when the patient cannot tolerate further filling. This is also termed maximum cystometric capacity. This is usually recorded as cc or ml. This volume is often quite different from the functional bladder capacity that is obtained from a voiding diary or frequency/volume chart in combination with a post-void residual. Voiding diaries should be obtained prior to an urodynamic evaluation as they can be useful in determining the clinical relevance of the cystometric bladder capacity. Cystometric capacity is generally smaller than the functional bladder capacity. Normative values for cystometric capacity are widely variable and have been reported between 370 and 540 cc ±100 cc [6].

The 4 C's of Bladder Emptying

The bladder emptying or voiding phase of the PFUD study is sometimes referred to as voiding cystometry. This phase commences with the command "permission to void" and ends when the subject under study considers themselves to have completed micturition [3].

Contractility is the strength of detrusor contraction or force generation during voiding. In order to empty properly, the detrusor must generate a contraction of adequate magnitude and duration to overcome outlet resistance and empty the contents of the bladder satisfactorily. Contractility is related to force generation by the detrusor and overall bladder outlet (urethral) resistance during voiding. However, the assessment of contractility may also be affected by anatomic abnormalities such as bladder diverticula or massive vesicoureteral reflux that result in dissipation of pressure during the contraction. In addition, in some cases contractility may be difficult to assess where urethral resistance is very low or negligible such as in cases of severe stress urinary incontinence. There are various formulae that have been developed in order to assess contractility such as the bladder contractility index (BCI), especially in men; however, these should be interpreted in the context of the clinical situation [7, 8].

Abnormalities of contractility include conditions that result in an inability to obtain, maintain, or sustain an adequate contraction. This may be due to poor detrusor force generation overall (neurogenic or myogenic) or due to inadequate duration of the contraction. Contractility is most often recorded as either normal or abnormal (underactive); however, using the BCI a numerical value may be obtained classifying the contraction as strong, normal, or weak.

Complete emptying indicates the lack of a significant post-void residual (PVR). The precise definition of what constitutes an elevated PVR is not universally agreed upon. PVRs are often assessed twice during the PFUD study. The initial PVR value is obtained by catheterizing the bladder after instructing the patient to void to completion just prior to the start of the PFUD study. The second PVR is obtained at the end of the PFUD study and is calculated by subtracting the voided volume from the infused volume. Incomplete emptying (elevated PVR) is due to either detrusor underactivity or bladder outlet obstruction or a combination of both. Complete emptying may be recorded as normal or abnormal, or as the PVR values obtained.

Coordination refers to the synchronization of the detrusor contraction and the voluntary and involuntary activity of the bladder outlet, including the bladder neck, and smooth and striated sphincters (vesicourethral coordination). Normal voiding commences with the relaxation and opening of the bladder outlet just prior to the detrusor contraction. The coordinated outlet remains open for the duration of the bladder contraction. If all or part of the bladder outlet does not open prior to the onset of a detrusor contraction, or fails to remain open for the duration of the contraction, this is abnormal. Many conditions can lead to a lack of coordination between the bladder and bladder outlet including detrusor striated dyssynergia and dysfunctional voiding ("non-neurogenic neurogenic bladder"). Lack of coordination between the bladder and bladder outlet may result in high pressure voiding, and/or incomplete bladder emptying. For purposes of documentation, vesicourethral coordination is present or absent.

Clinical obstruction, or bladder outlet obstruction is defined by the relationship between bladder pressure and urinary flow. Subjectively, high voiding pressure associated with low urine flow is the definition of bladder outlet obstruction. Objectively, various nomograms and calculations have been devised to more precisely define this dynamic relationship in both men and women but none are universally utilized though the findings between the various methods correlate quite well [9]. Such nomograms categorize individuals as obstructed, equivocal, or unobstructed. Obstruction may occur with or without lower urinary tract symptoms (LUTS). Clinically, LUTS in the presence of obstruction or other negative prognostic signs mandates therapy. In males, obstruction may be secondary to BPH, prostate cancer, urethral stricture, bladder neck contracture, neurological disease, and a variety of other causes. Bladder outlet obstruction in females is less common but may be iatrogenic due to stress incontinence surgery, or due to vaginal prolapse, urethral diverticula, neurological disease, and a variety of other causes. Various nomograms for objectively quantitating female bladder outlet obstruction have likewise been developed but none are universally utilized [10].

The study depicted in Figure 2.1 provides a schema for interpreting a urodynamics study with the context of the "9 C's". This study demonstrates absence of involuntary bladder contractions. The change in Pdet with filling is negligible consistent with normal compliance. There was no incontinence seen during this study. The first sensation of bladder filling occurred at a volume of approximately 100 cc

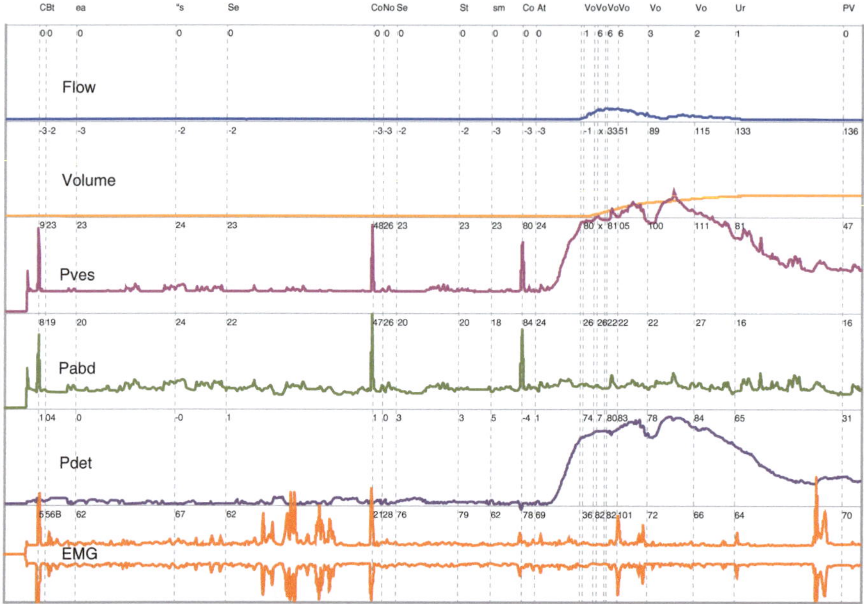

Fig. 2.1 Urodynamic tracing using the "9 C's" organizational schema. This is a 65-year-old male with LUTS. Infused volume (*not shown*) was 230 cc

(Volume infused not shown but is indicated on the tracing by the annotation "Se" just after the 1:00 min mark of the study.) Bladder capacity was 230 cc (infusion volume not shown on this tracing).

Bladder emptying commenced with a volitional detrusor contraction. The command to void was given just prior to the 3:00 min mark and is indicated by the annotation "At." There was no inappropriate activity of the external sphincter as suggested by the EMG during voiding. The bladder did not empty completely as the voided volume was only 136 cc. Detrusor pressure, despite being elevated, was insufficiently sustained to empty the bladder. The voiding pressure in excess of 70 cm H_2O, and the low flow rate ($Q_{max}=6$) is very suggestive of bladder outlet obstruction.

The 9 C's for this study are as follows:

Filling/Storage:

Contractions (involuntary): none
Compliance: normal
Continence: no incontinence demonstrated
Coarse sensation: normal
Capacity: 230 cc

Emptying:

Contractility: abnormal, underactive
Coordination: yes
Complete emptying: no, PVR=94 cc
Clinical obstruction: yes

References

1. Rovner ES, Wein AJ. Practical urodynamics: part I and II. Am Urol Assoc Update Ser. 2002;19:146–59.
2. Wein A. Classification of neurogenic voiding dysfunction. J Urol. 1981;125:605–9.
3. Haylen B, de Ridder D, Freeman RM, Swift SE, Berghmans B, Lee J, Monga A, Petri E, Rizk DE, Sand PK, Schaer GN. An International Urogynecological Association (IUGA)/ International Continence Society (ICS) joint report on the terminology for female pelvic floor dysfunction. Int Urogynecol J. 2010;21:5–26.
4. Abrams P, Cardozo L, Fall M, Griffiths D, Rosier P, Ulmsten U, van Kerrebroeck P, Victor A, Wein A. The standardisation of lower urinary tract function: report from the Standardisation Subcommittee of the International Continence Society. Neurourol Urodyn. 2002;21:167–78.
5. De Wachter S, Smith PP, Tannenbaum C, Van Koeveringe G, Drake M, Wyndaele JJ, Chapple C. How should bladder sensation be measured? ICI-RS 2011. Neurourol Urodyn. 2012;31(3):370–4.
6. Rosier PFWM, Kuo H-C, De Gennaro M. Urodynamic testing. In: Abrams P, Cardozo Khoury A, Wein A, editors. Incontinence. 5th ed. ICUD-EAU Publishing; 2013;429–506.
7. Schafer W. Analysis of bladder outlet function with the linearized passive urethral resistance relation, linPURR, and a disease-specific approach for grading obstruction from complex to simple. World J Urol. 1995;13:47–58.
8. Abrams P. Bladder outlet obstruction index, bladder contractility index and bladder voiding efficiency: three simple indices to define bladder voiding function. BJU Int. 1999;84(1):14–5.
9. Lim CS, Abrams P. The Abrams–Griffiths nomogram. World J Urol. 1995;13:34–9.
10. Akikwala TV, Fleischman N, Nitti VW. Comparison of diagnostic criteria for female bladder outlet obstruction. J Urol. 2006;176:2093–7.

Chapter 3
Urodynamics Equipment: Selection and Training

Alana M. Murphy and Howard B. Goldman

Abbreviations

EMG	Electromyogram
EMR	Electronic medical record
ICS	International Continence Society
LUT	Lower urinary tract
P_{abd}	Intra-abdominal pressure (cm H_2O)
P_{det}	Detrusor pressure (cm H_2O)
P_{ves}	Vesical (bladder) pressure (cm H_2O)
SUFU	Society of Urodynamics, Female Pelvic Medicine, and Urogenital Reconstruction
SUNA	Society of Urologic Nurses and Associates
UDS	Urodynamics
UTI	Urinary tract infection

Urodynamics Manufacturers

The market for Urodynamics (UDS) equipment continues to grow globally. A 2009 report by Global Industry Analysts projected that the global market for UDS equipment and disposables will reach $170 million by 2015 with the United States

A.M. Murphy, MD (✉)
Department of Urology, Thomas Jefferson University, Philadelphia, PA 19107, USA
e-mail: alana.m.murphy.md@gmail.com

H.B. Goldman, MD
Cleveland Clinic, Lerner College of Medicine, Glickman Urologic and Kidney Institute, Cleveland, OH, USA
e-mail: goldmah@ccf.org

© Springer Science+Business Media New York 2015
E.S. Rovner, M.E. Koski (eds.), *Rapid and Practical Interpretation of Urodynamics*, DOI 10.1007/978-1-4939-1764-8_3

Table 3.1 UDS manufacturers

Company	Headquarters
Laborie	Canada
Cooper Surgical	United States
SRS Medical Systems	United States
Dantec	United Kingdom
Mediwatch	United Kingdom
Albyn Medical	United Kingdom, Spain
Medical Measurement Systems [MMS]	United States, Germany, Netherlands
Neomedix	Australia
Shippers	Germany
Andromeda	Germany
Menfis bioMedica	Italy
Mindray Medical International	China

representing the largest market share [1]. A number of UDS equipment manufacturers are available to meet the market's needs. Table 3.1 includes a comprehensive, but not complete list of UDS manufacturers. In January of 2013, the North American market was impacted by the merger of Laborie and Life-Tech. Following Laborie's acquisition of Life-Tech, Life-Tech UDS systems are no longer commercially available. However; Laborie has continued to supply the disposable components for Life-Tech machines.

Choosing the Right System

The International Continence Society (ICS) has published recommendations regarding the minimal equipment requirements and the minimal technical specifications for a UDS system. According to the ICS good UDS practice statement, a UDS system should include the following components [2]:

- Three measurement channels: two for pressure (abdominal pressure [P_{abd}], vesical pressure [P_{ves}]) and one for flow
- Display and secure storage of pressure measurements (P_{abd}, P_{ves}, detrusor pressure [P_{det}]) and flow over time
- Display of infused volume and voided volume either graphically or numerically
- Clear labeling of all axes with no loss of data if tracings go off-scale
- Ability to annotate display with events

According to the technical recommendations, the following specifications should be met [3]:

- Minimum accuracy: ±1 cm H_2O for pressure, ±5 % full scale for flow and volume
- Detection range: 0–250 cm H_2O for pressure, 0–50 mL/s for flow, 1,000 mL for volume

- Frequency: $\geq$10 Hz per channel for pressure and flow; $\geq$20 kHz for electromyogram (EMG)
- Scaling: 50 cm H_2O per cm for pressure, 10 mL/s per cm for flow, 5 s/mm during filling, 2 s/mm during voiding

UDS equipment has advanced considerably since the last publication of the ICS technical recommendations in 1987. An updated ICS guideline on UDS equipment performance will be available in the near future.

A number of other factors should be considered when purchasing a UDS machine (see Table 3.2). Other important factors to consider include clinical needs, the physical

Table 3.2 UDS systems

Manufacturer	UDS system	Wireless	EMR compatible	Number of pressure channels	Description
Laborie [4]	Aquarius TT™	X	X	8	– Compatible with fluoroscopy – Available upgrade for anorectal manometry – High speed EMG sampling (5,000 Hz)
Laborie [4]	Dorado KT	X	X	8	– Compatible with fluoroscopy – 50 Hz EMG
Laborie [4]	Triton™	X		8	– Available EMG upgrade to 3,000 Hz
Laborie [4]	Goby KT	X		4	– Step by step voice commands – Cart option offers in-office portability
Laborie [4]	Delphis/ Delphis KT	X		4	– Cart option offers in-office portability
Laborie [4]	Delphis IP	X		4	– Attaches to an IV pole for easy portability
Laborie [4]	Goby mobile	X	X	4	– Designed for modular use – Allows patients to void in the bathroom – Step by step voice commands
Cooper Surgical [5]	Lumax™ TS Pro Elite		X	4	– Available EMG upgrade – Attaches to IV pole for easy portability
Cooper Surgical [5]	Lumax™ TS Pro Advanced		X	4	– Available EMG upgrade – Attaches to IV pole for easy portability
Cooper Surgical [5]	Lumax™ TS Pro Basic		X	4	– Available EMG upgrade – Attaches to IV pole for easy portability

space available for the UDS machine, and the available budget. Prior to selecting an appropriate UDS system, the clinician should answer a series of questions:

Is there a role for UDS in my practice?
What type of clinical questions can UDS help me answer?
Do I need an electromyogram (EMG)?
Do I need the ability to integrate fluoroscopy with my UDS testing?
Is electronic medical record (EMR) integration necessary?

While a community-based practice may only require the capability to perform multi-channel cystometry, a larger tertiary referral center will require the ability to perform more sophisticated testing and integration of fluoroscopy. A review of health care claims from approximately 30 million individuals in the United States from 2002 to 2007 captured the diversity in current UDS practices [6]. A total of 16,574 UDS procedures were identified: 23 % were cystometrograms, 71 % were cystometrograms with pressure flow studies, and 6 % were fluoroscopic UDS procedures. UDS centers with higher volume (≥ 14 UDS studies in the specified time period) were more likely to perform cystometrograms with pressure flow studies and fluoroscopic UDS. In light of the available UDS systems currently on the market, determining the clinical needs of a practice will help guide the search for an appropriate system.

The physical space allocated to the UDS system is an important factor that will also help determine what type of machine is best suited for a clinical practice. A dedicated UDS room allows for a more elaborate setup, whereas a less sophisticated mobile system is more appropriate if the plan is to move the equipment from room to room. Whether or not the UDS system is stationary or portable, the testing environment should be a private and quiet setting that will minimize unnecessary anxiety for the patient. Providing such an environment will facilitate the reproduction of day to day symptoms. If simultaneous fluoroscopy is desired, then the room must be large enough to accommodate a portable C-arm unit and its attached console (see Fig. 3.1). In addition, provisions must be made to either line the UDS room with lead, a costly endeavor, or ensure that the room is large enough to prevent any significant degree of radiation exposure to other personnel in adjacent rooms. Regulations regarding the use and safety requirements for fluoroscopy vary from state to state in the US. Finally, the room should also be large enough to accommodate wheelchair and stretcher patients. If a significant number of immobile patients are included in the practice, then consideration should also be given to the purchase of a patient lift (e.g., Hoyer lift).

Transducers

A pressure transducer allows conversion of an applied pressure into an electrical signal. Three different types of catheters allow transduction of P_{ves} readings: water-filled catheters, air-filled catheters, and catheters with a small transducer mounted on the tip (microtip catheter). When water-filled catheters are used as a transducer, the measurement of P_{ves} is independent of the position of the catheter tip within the bladder,

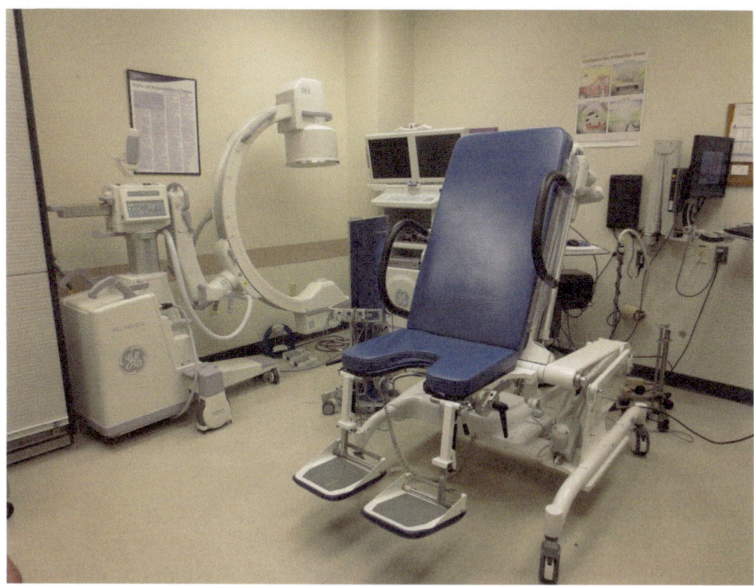

Fig. 3.1 Urodynamic system with fluoroscopic unit and fluoroscopic compatible chair

which facilitates reproducible measurements. In contrast, P_{ves} measurements obtained using air-filled catheters and microtip catheters depend on the location of the catheter tip in the bladder, which may hinder precision. A recent direct comparison of air-filled and water-filled catheters in a laboratory setting determined that the two means of pressure transmission did not lead to inter-changeable results [7]. While air-filled catheters provided overdamped pressure transduction, water-filled catheters provided under-damped pressure transduction and were more susceptible to motion artifact. Although water-filled catheters require a more time intensive setup and are subject to motion artifact when the tubing is manipulated during UDS, the superior degree of reliability led the ICS to recommend the use of water-filled catheters [2].

The majority of P_{ves} catheters are either dual lumen, which allow simultaneous pressure transduction and filling, or triple lumen catheters, which also allow measurement of urethral pressures. The ICS recommends use of a balloon catheter placed in either the rectum or vagina for P_{abd} readings [2]. The balloon should be free of air and filled with fluid to only 10–20 % of its capacity to avoid falsely elevated abdominal pressures.

Cost of Equipment

Commercially available UDS systems provide a variety of options to meet a wide range of budgets. Answering the aforementioned clinical questions will help ensure that the appropriate UDS system is purchased for each clinical practice and avoid

Table 3.3 UDS disposable P_{ves} catheters

Manufacturer	Product	Specifications
Laborie [4]	Water-filled catheter	– Single lumen 6 or 8 Fr – Triple lumen 7 Fr
Laborie [4]	Air-filled catheter (TDOC®)	– 7 Fr – Single or dual sensor
Laborie [4]	Electronic microtip catheter	– Reusable
Cooper Surgical [5]	Lumax™ fiberoptic microtip catheter	– 7 or 10 Fr – Also used for P_{abd} measurement

either unnecessary features or a lack of functionality. The addition of features tends to correlate with an increase in price; however, a more sophisticated machine is not always the right choice for a particular clinical practice. The exact cost of UDS systems is variable and is largely driven by regional market forces and a clinical practice's purchasing power.

In addition to a UDS system, two considerable budget items include a UDS chair and the purchase of a fluoroscopy unit and the necessary accessories (see Fig. 3.1). The type of chair should complement the UDS system. A simple uroflow commode will accommodate most patients undergoing simple cystometry in a community-based setting [5], while a motorized chair with multiple adjustments and radiation compatibility will be more appropriate for a tertiary referral center performing fluoro-scopic UDS testing on patients who may have limited mobility [8]. Most UDS centers utilizing fluoroscopy will invest in a portable C-arm unit, which includes a viewing console and a mobile X-ray source and image intensifier. The use of radiation also requires the purchase of appropriate lead barriers for all medical personnel in the UDS room during active fluoroscopy. Lead aprons provide excellent protection from radia-tion or a portable lead barrier may be more appropriate for the room configuration.

In addition to the base price of the UDS system, one must also consider the cost of the disposable components (see Table 3.3). The most commonly used disposable components include vesical (bladder) pressure catheters, abdominal pressure catheters, EMG patches, and connection tubing. Similar to the cost of the UDS system, the cost of disposable components is variable between suppliers, region, and institution. UDS systems that employ fluoroscopy will also require the purchase of radiopaque contrast. A recent study by Marks and colleagues demon-strated that cost saving can be achieved by utilizing contrast for the first 250 mL of bladder filling and then switching to infused saline without altering the quality or interpretability of fluoroscopic images [9].

UDS Training

A successful UDS practice requires the UDS staff to be familiar with the components of a UDS system, to be knowledgeable about performing a UDS evaluation, and be able to perform basic troubleshooting. In addition to the physician interpreting the

Table 3.4 UDS training courses

Course	Sponsor	Target audience	Duration	Brief description
Comprehensive UDS	Laborie [4]	Physicians, nurses, technicians	2.5 days	– Review of LUT physiology and UDS setup and diagnosis
Hands-on UDS	Laborie [4]	Physicians, nurses, technicians No previous UDS experience required	1 day	– Learn indications for UDS – Review UDS setup and diagnosis
UDS interpretation	Laborie [4]	Physicians	1 day	– Learn to formulate patient-centric UDS objectives and interpret tracings

test, the UDS staff performing the test should be familiar with basic lower urinary tract pathology and concepts that would be tested during UDS. As a rule, UDS is a dynamic test that requires a well-trained team to execute quality studies.

In the United States, there are no specific certification requirements for UDS staff. In addition to the training provided by UDS manufacturers at the time of purchase, several other training options exist for both novice and advanced UDS operators. The ICS has organized certification courses in conjunction with scientific meetings and the Society of Urodynamics, Female Pelvic Medicine and Urogenital Reconstruction (SUFU) website includes an online teaching module that reviews a standardized UDS teaching curriculum for urology residents [10]. Laborie also sponsors a number of training courses that are held at regular intervals for both UDS staff and physicians (see Table 3.4). The Laborie courses address both basic UDS concepts and more advanced interpretation of studies and troubleshooting. For UDS nurses and technicians, the SUNA online store offers two publications focused on UDS training: *Special Series on Urodynamics—Traces: Making Sense of Urodynamics* ($20.00, $8.00 member price) and *A Practical Guide to Performing Urodynamics* ($55.00, $35.00 member price) [11].

Upcoming Technology

In addition to technical refinements, efforts to improve UDS testing should focus on reducing the discomfort associated with UDS, reducing the risk of a urinary tract infection (UTI) by eliminating the urethral catheter, and maximizing the ability of UDS to mimic urinary symptoms experienced at home. Noninvasive UDS was first described by Schafer and colleagues in 1994 [12]. Using this technique, the flow of urine is interrupted and P_{ves} is calculated from the pressure transmitted by the column of fluid from the urethra to the bladder. Although there has been some clinical interest in using noninvasive UDS to evaluate for bladder outlet obstruction, the clinical implementation of this technique is currently limited [13, 14].

References

1. Urodynamics Equipment and Disposables Market to Reach $170 Million by 2015 [Internet] 23 June 2009 [cited 19 September 2013]. http://www.prweb.com/releases/urodynamics_equipment/urodynamics_disposables/prweb2534634.htm.
2. Schafer W, Abrams P, Liao L, Mattiasson A, Pesce F, Spangberg A, Sterling AM, Zinner NR, van Kerrebroeck P. Good urodynamic practices: uroflowmetry, filling cystometry, and pressure-flow studies. Neurourol Urodyn. 2002;21:261–74.
3. Rowan D, James DE, Kramer AEJL, Sterling AM, Suhel PF. Urodynamic equipment: technical aspects. J Med Eng Technol. 1987;11:57–64.
4. Laborie urodynamics [cited 29 September 2013]. http://www.laborie.com/products/urodynamics/.
5. Cooper Surgical urodynamic system [cited 29 September 2013]. http://www.coopersurgical.com/ourproducts/incontinence/urosys/Pages/cslnd.aspx?LC=UrodynamicSystem.
6. Reynolds WS, Dmochowski RR, Lai J, Saigal C, Penson DF. Patterns and predictors of urodynamics use in the United States. J Urol. 2013;189:1791–6.
7. Cooper MA, Fletter PC, Zaszczurynski PJ, Damaser MS. Comparison of air-charged and water-filled urodynamic pressure measurement catheters. Neurourol Urodyn. 2011;30(3):329–34.
8. Stille Sonesta model program [cited 29 September 2013]. http://www.stille.se/sonesta/model-range-summary/.
9. Marks BK, Vasavada SP, Goldman HB. Contrast concentration does not alter fluoro-urodynamic interpretation. Abstract presented at: Annual meeting of the American Urological Association, San Diego, 4–8 May 2013.
10. Urodynamics curriculum for urology residents [cited 5 October 2013]. http://elearning.sufu-org.com/.
11. Society of Urologic Nurses and Associates online store [cited 5 October 2013]. http://www.suna.org/resources/suna-store.
12. Schafer W, Kirschner-Hermans R, Jakse G. Non-invasive pressure/flow measurement for precise grading of bladder outflow obstruction. J Urol. 1994;151(suppl):323A.
13. Losco G, Keedle L, King Q. Non-invasive urodynamics predicts outcome prior to surgery for prostatic obstruction. BJU Int. 2013;112 suppl 2:61–4.
14. Harding C, Robson W, Drinnan M, McIntosh S, Sajeel M, Griffiths C, Pickard R. Predicting the outcome of prostatectomy using noninvasive bladder pressure and urine flow measurements. Eur Urol. 2007;52:186–92.

Chapter 4
Physician Coding and Reimbursement for Urodynamics

David J. Osborn, Denise Lynn Gartin, W. Stuart Reynolds, and Roger R. Dmochowski

Introduction

A significant proportion of health care cost is related to diagnostic evaluation. In the United States, in the year 2000, an estimated 600 million dollars was spent on diagnostic testing related to complaints of overactive bladder [1]. A urodynamic (UDS) evaluation can be an important part of the diagnostic evaluation of certain disease processes. In 2011, the minimum cost billed for urodynamics in women was $500 [2].

Urodynamic testing is both a significant source of income for providers who treat voiding dysfunction and a significant expense for the payers, including government, insurance carriers, and others. In 2010, in an attempt to reduce cost and reimbursement for urodynamics, Centers for Medicare and Medicaid Services (CMS) instituted changes to current procedural terminology (CPT) codes for UDS and bundled several individual codes together, resulting in fewer billable codes. In addition, a greater emphasis has been placed on using an appropriate ICD-9-CM (International Classification of Disease 9th revision, Clinical Modification) diagnosis code with the appropriate CPT codes and modifiers, possibly resulting in more reimbursement denials.

D.J. Osborn, MD (✉) • W.S. Reynolds, MD, MPH • R.R. Dmochowski, MD, MPH
Department of Urology, Vanderbilt University Medical Center,
A1302 Medical Center North, Nashville, TN 37232-2765, USA
e-mail: david.osborn@vanderbilt.edu; william.stuart.reynolds@vanderbilt.edu;
roger.dmochowski@vanderbilt.edu

D.L. Gartin, AAS, CPC
Department of Urology, Vanderbilt University Medical Center,
A1302 Medical Center North, Nashville, TN 37232-2765, USA

Physician Billing Services, Vanderbilt University Medical Center, Nashville, TN, USA
e-mail: denise.coss@vanderbilt.edu

© Springer Science+Business Media New York 2015
E.S. Rovner, M.E. Koski (eds.), *Rapid and Practical Interpretation of Urodynamics*, DOI 10.1007/978-1-4939-1764-8_4

Although the implementation of ICD-10-CM (International Classification of Disease 10th revision, Clinical Modification) has been delayed several times, it is finally supposed to be in operation on October 1st, 2014 [3]. It is believed by the government that ICD-10-CM will be a significant improvement over ICD-9-CM. Specific improvements include: additional information pertaining to ambulatory and managed care encounters, the creation of combination diagnosis/symptom codes that are intended to reduce the number of codes needed to fully describe a condition, and the addition of a sixth and seventh digit to help improve diagnosis code specificity. Overall, coding and reimbursement for urodynamics should not be significantly affected.

Basics of Coding and Reimbursement

CPT Codes

CPT codes are numbers assigned to every task and service a medical provider performs on a patient. For better understanding, CPT codes can be broken down into three different types: E&M (Evaluation and Management) codes, procedural codes, and diagnostic procedural codes. E&M codes pertain to physician–patient encounters that involve discussion with the patient or caretaker, examination and medical decision-making. Typically these take the form of outpatient clinical visits or inpatient evaluations.

The CPT code allows payers such as CMS and insurance companies to value medical services provided and to scale reimbursement. CPT codes are developed and maintained by the American Medical Association (AMA). As medical practice evolves, new codes are added and old codes are discarded. The AMA copyrights CPT codes and controls their publication. The AMA provides an online service to look up individual CPT codes, but because of copyright infringement issues, it can be difficult to search for thorough answers regarding coding and CPT codes on the internet. The AMA prefers that coding material is purchased from them or another company that has a business agreement with the AMA.

Relative Value Units

Relative value units (RVUs) are numbers that are assigned to a specific CPT code to give it value. The range of RVU values for urodynamics is 0.45–10.27. RVUs are used to calculate facility and physician reimbursement for a procedure. For E&M and procedural CPT codes, CMS uses RVUs in the same way. However, for diagnostic CPT codes, CMS uses a slightly different method to calculate reimbursement. The original work with RVUs was started in the 1980s and the value of different CPT codes is continually evolving. Each CPT code is targeted for review every 5 years to determine if the code has become obsolete, redundant or the RVU level of the CPT code has changed. When making changes CMS receives input from the AMA and the Specialty Society Relative Value Scale Update Committee (RUC). The RUC is a 29-member committee composed of people appointed by the different major physician specialty societies.

RVU Use with E&M and Procedural CPT Codes

Under the Medicare physician fee schedule, each E&M and procedural CPT code is assigned four separate RVUs. The four RVUs for physician services are the Work RVU, Facility Practice Expense RVU (Facility PE RVU), Non-Facility PE RVU (Non-Facility PE RVU), and Malpractice RVU (MP RVU). The final compensation level for a particular CPT code is determined by multiplying each of the types of RVU by a Geographical Adjustment (GPCI), adding the three values together and then lastly multiplying this number by a conversion factor (CF, dollar amount). Of note, most coding books will just list total Facility RVU and total Non-Facility RVU values and not the four separate values.

$$\text{Total RVU} = \text{Work RVU} + \text{PE RVU} + \text{MP RVU}$$

$$\text{Facility Payment Amount} =$$
$$\left[\left(\text{Work RVU} \times \text{Work GCPI}\right) + \left(\text{Facility PE RVU} \times \text{PE GCPI}\right) + \left(\text{MP RVU} \times \text{MP GCPI}\right)\right] \times \text{CF}$$

$$\text{Non-Facility Payment Amount} =$$
$$\left[\left(\text{Work RVU} \times \text{Work GCPI}\right) + \left(\text{Non-Facility PE RVU} \times \text{PE GCPI}\right) + \left(\text{MP RVU} \times \text{MP GCPI}\right)\right] \times \text{CF}$$

There are two different practice expense (PE) RVUs for every CPT code because reimbursement depends on whether or not the physician performed the service in a free-standing outpatient clinic or a facility setting. Hospitals, hospital-based clinics, and ambulatory surgery centers (ASC) are considered "facility" settings. Hospital and hospital-based clinics are also referred to as Ambulatory Payment Classification locations (APC). The APC designation pertains to the way the hospital is reimbursed (outpatient and not inpatient reimbursement). In these facility settings, the PE RVU value for the physician reimbursement will be lower. This takes into account some of the services provided by the hospital.

The conversion factor (CF for 2013 was $34.0230) is a simple way for Medicare and the government to control cost by adjusting physician reimbursement [4]. Recently, the implementation of cuts to the conversion factor has been an important topic in the news and medical society communications. Large decreases in the CF have continually been delayed by congress over the past 5 years. Unless it is again delayed, changes to the conversion factor will cut physician reimbursement by 25 % in January 2014.

RVU Use with Diagnostic CPT Codes

For diagnostic CPT codes, the total (global) RVU is a sum of the Professional Component (PC) and Technical Component (TC) RVUs. For a diagnostic test, the PC is similar to the Work RVU and the TC is similar to the PE RVU plus the MP RVU. The global amount paid to a physician who performs a diagnostic test such as urodynamics in the non-facility setting is approximately the sum of the professional component and the technical component payments that are reimbursed for diagnostic procedures performed in a facility.

$$\text{Global Payment Amount} \approx \text{PC Payment Amount} + \text{TC Payment Amount}$$

In the facility setting, the professional component reimburses for the interpretation of a test results and the TC reimburses for the cost of equipment, the technician, and the malpractice expense covered by the hospital.

If a diagnostic test is performed in a facility then only the PC will be used to calculate reimbursement to the physician. However, if a diagnostic test is not being performed in a facility then the physician is reimbursed based on the total Global RVU. It is the authors' opinion that if a physician is performing diagnostic tests in a facility setting, the facility should be paying a portion of the physician's malpractice expenses because the facility is being reimbursed for malpractice coverage by CMS as part of the TC. Of note, there are some CPT codes that are either only PC or only TC. Lastly, the TC payment amount reimbursed to a facility also depends on whether it is a hospital or ambulatory surgery center.

International Classification of Diseases-9th Revision-Clinical Modification Codes

ICD-9-CM Codes are unique numbers assigned to a disease process or diagnosis. They are used as a way for payers to verify that the CPT codes listed are medically necessary. Each CPT code billed should be supported by an ICD-9-CM diagnosis code that substantiates the need for those services provided. In addition, because they also imply the severity of a patient's medical problem, ICD-9-CM codes also limit which CPT codes can be used. Commonly accepted ICD-9-CM codes for urodynamics are listed in Table 4.1.

Proper coding of clinical procedures and diagnoses is dependent on the material documented in the patient's medical record. CMS determines which ICD-9-CM codes are required for a CPT code to be covered or reimbursed. However, because each state has a particular carrier for government Medicare, the required ICD-9-CM codes vary from state to state.

Table 4.1 Appropriate diagnosis ICD-9-CM codes for urodynamics (adapted from Ingenix [5])

ICD-9-CM code with corresponding description			
344.61	Cauda equina syndrome with neurogenic bladder	598.1	Traumatic urethral stricture
595.1	Chronic interstitial cystitis	598.2	Post-operative urethral stricture
595.2	Other chronic cystitis	600.01	BPH with urinary obstruction and LUTS
595.82	Irradiation cystitis	618.01	Cystocele, midline
596.0	Bladder neck obstruction	618.02	Cystocele, lateral
596.1	Intestino-vesical fistula	625.6	Female stress urinary incontinence
596.2	Vesical fistula	753.6	Congenital atresia/stenosis of urethra/ bladder neck
596.3	Bladder diverticulum	788.21	Incomplete bladder emptying
596.4	Bladder atony	788.31	Urgency incontinence
596.51	Bladder hypertonicity	788.32	Male stress incontinence
596.52	Low bladder compliance	788.33	Mixed incontinence (urge and stress) male and female
596.53	Bladder paralysis	788.37	Continuous leakage
596.54	Neurogenic bladder not otherwise specified	788.41	Urinary frequency

Table 4.2 Summary of commonly used modifiers (adapted from: current procedural coding expert by Optum 2012) [6]

Modifier 26	Professional component only of a procedure or service
Modifier 51	Multiple procedures performed at same session by same provider
Modifier 25	Significant, separately identifiable evaluation, and management service by same physician or other qualified health care professional on the same day of procedure or other service
Modifier 59	Distinct procedure, used to identify a procedure not usually reported together but are appropriate under the circumstances
Modifier 58	Staged or related procedure or service by same physician or other qualified health care professional during post-operative period
Modifier 78	Unplanned return to the operating/procedure room by the same physician or other qualified health care professional following initial procedure for a related procedure during the post-operative period
Modifier 79	Unrelated procedure or service by the same physician during the post-operative period

Modifiers

Modifiers are two digit codes that are added to a CPT Procedure code or E&M code in order to clarify the services being billed. The four most commonly used modifiers for urodynamic billing by a physician are the -26, -51, -25, and -59 modifiers. This information is summarized in Table 4.2.

The -26 modifier is used ONLY for diagnostic tests performed in a facility setting where reimbursement is being shared between the facility and the physicians. The -26 modifier designates the professional component of a service provided, such as interpretation of a test results. The -26 modifier tells CMS or other payers that it needs to split reimbursement between the physician and the facility. The physician will receive reimbursement for the Professional Component and the facility receives reimbursement for the Technical Component.

The -51 modifier is used to designate that multiple related procedures were performed on the same patient at the same visit. The first CPT code has the highest RVU value, will not have the modifier appended, and will be reimbursed at 100 % of the allowable reimbursement. All additional codes will have the -51 modifier appended and be reimbursed at 50 % of the allowable reimbursement.

The -25 modifier is used when billing for both an E&M code and a procedure code on the same day. This is often used if the urodynamics are done in the setting of a new patient encounter. The E&M code should be separate, identifiable, and above and beyond what is expected for the procedure/s performed. As long as the visit is properly documented and the modifier is used, billing for a new patient encounter and urodynamics on the same day should not affect reimbursement.

The -59 modifier is used to designate a procedure that is distinct or independent from other services performed on the same day. In the case of urodynamics, this is commonly appended to the cystoscopy CPT code (52000) if a cystoscopy was performed on the same day as urodynamics. The use of this code also does not affect reimbursement.

Three other modifiers that might be used with urodynamic coding are -58, -78, and -79. These modifiers are necessary if the urodynamic test is performed while patient is in a 90-day post-surgery global period. The -58 modifier is used if the urodynamic test is a planned or staged part of the surgery (dictated as part of the plan in the operative note) that created the post-operative global period. The -78 modifier is used when there is an unplanned need for urodynamics during the global post-operative time period because of a medical problem related to the original surgery. The -79 modifier is used when the same physician is performing urodynamics on a patient during the post-operative global time period for a medical condition not related to the original surgery. Of note, when the above three codes are used correctly, reimbursement should not be affected.

Urodynamic Coding Step-by-Step

1. Choose an appropriate ICD-9-CM code (Table 4.1).
2. Choose one primary CPT code from Group A (Table 4.3).
3. Choose one CPT code from Group B and add the -51 modifier (Table 4.3).
4. Choose one CPT code from Group C and add the -51 modifier (Table 4.3).
5. If fluoroscopy was used, choose all three CPT codes in Group D and do NOT add the -51 modifier (Table 4.3).
6. If a urinalysis was performed choose one CPT code from Group E and do NOT add the -51 modifier (Table 4.3).

Table 4.3 CPT codes for urodynamics (adapted from Ingenix [5])

	CPT code	Description	Global RVU
Group A	51725	Simple cystometrogram (CMG)	5.62
	51726	Complex cystometrogram	7.94
	51727	Complex cystometrogram with urethral pressure profile studies	9.47
	51728	Complex cystometrogram with voiding pressure studies and urethral pressure profile studies	9.47
	51729	Complex cystometrogram with voiding pressure studies	10.27
Group B	51736	Simple uroflowmetry (uncommon)	0.45
	51741	Complex uroflowmetry (more common)	0.47
Group C	51784	Electromyography studies (EMG) of anal or urethral sphincter other than needle	5.76
	51792	Stimulus evoked response (e.g., measurement of bulbocavernosus reflex latency time)	7.65
Group D	74430	Contrast, bladder X-ray	1.24
	74455	X-ray, urethra or bladder	2.57
	76000	Fluoroscope examination	1.56
Group E	81002	Urinalysis without microscopy (non-auto)	0
	81000	Urinalysis with microscopy (non-auto)	0
Group F	51797	Measurement of intra-abdominal pressure	3.36
	52000	Diagnostic cystourethroscopy	3.68 or 6.0[a]
	51798	Measurement of PVR bladder scanner	0.58

[a]Facility and non-facility reimbursement

7. If a rectal or vaginal catheter was used to measure intra-abdominal pressure choose 51797 from Group F and do NOT add the -51 modifier (Table 4.3).
8. If a cystoscopy was performed, choose code 52000 from Group F and add the -59 modifier (Table 4.3).
9. If PVR was measured using a PVR scanner, choose 519798 from Group F and add the -51 modifier.
10. If the procedure was performed in a facility setting, the -26 modifier should be added to the UDS and radiology codes.

Three Examples and How They Should Be Billed

1. A 55-year-old patient new to your non-facility clinic and yourself is seen for evaluation of mixed urinary incontinence and pelvic organ prolapse. The patient has the following done (Table 4.4):

   a. Moderately complex history and physical examination.
   b. Urinalysis without microscopy.
   c. Post-void residual measured using a bladder scanner.

Table 4.4 Non-facility, new patient urodynamics

CPT code	Description
99203-25	Moderate complex new patient visit
51729	Complex cystometrogram with voiding pressure studies
51741-51	Complex uroflowmetry (calibrated equipment)
51784-51	Electromyography studies (EMG) of anal or urethral sphincter other than needle
74430	Contrast, bladder X-ray
74455	X-ray, urethra or bladder
76000	Fluoroscope examination
51797	Measurement of intra-abdominal pressure
51798-51	Measurement of PVR bladder scanner
81002	Urinalysis without microscopy (non-auto)
52000-59	Diagnostic cystourethroscopy
51600-51	Instillation of contrast to bladder

Table 4.5 Facility (hospital-based clinic), new patient urodynamics

CPT Code	Description
99203-25	Moderate complex new patient visit
51729-26	Complex cystometrogram with voiding pressure studies
51741-26-51	Complex uroflowmetry (calibrated equipment)
51784-26-51	Electromyography studies (EMG) of anal or urethral sphincter other than needle
51797-26	Measurement of intra-abdominal pressure
51798-51	Measurement of PVR bladder scanner
81000	Urinalysis with microscopy (non-auto)
52000-59	Diagnostic cystourethroscopy

   d. Complex uroflowmetry using calibrated equipment.

   e. Bladder emptied with a catheterization and the PVR is again measured.

   f. Video urodynamics with placement of a pressure transducer catheters in the bladder and vagina.

   g. EKG leads are placed on the perineum to record urethral sphincter activity.

   h. The bladder is filled with contrast.

   i. Fluoroscopy is used to visualize the bladder and urethra.

   j. A standard pressure flow study is performed with voiding pressures.

   k. A PVR is again calculated by subtracting the voided volume from the filled volume.

   l. Cystoscopy with examination of urethra, bladder, and trigone.

2. A 65-year-old male patient new to your hospital-based clinic and yourself is seen for evaluation of post-prostatectomy incontinence. The patient has the following done (Table 4.5):

   a. Moderately complex history and physical examination.

   b. Urinalysis with microscopy.

   c. Post-void residual measured using a bladder scanner.
   d. Complex uroflowmetry using calibrated equipment.
   e. Bladder emptied with a catheterization and the PVR is again measured.
   f. Urodynamics with placement of pressure transducer catheters in the bladder and rectum.
   g. EKG leads are placed in the perineum to record urethral sphincter activity.
   h. The bladder is filled with saline.
   i. A standard pressure flow study is performed with voiding pressures.
   j. A PVR is again calculated by subtracting the voided volume from the filled volume.
   k. Cystoscopy with examination of urethra, bladder, and trigone.

3. A 48-year-old established male patient with a spinal cord injury presents to your non-facility clinic for video urodynamics. The patient has the following done (Table 4.6):

   a. A urinalysis without microscopy.
   b. Post-void residual measured using a bladder scanner.
   c. Complex uroflowmetry using calibrated equipment.
   d. Bladder emptied with a catheterization and the PVR is again measured.
   e. Video urodynamics with placement of pressure transducer catheters in the bladder and rectum.
   f. EKG leads are placed in the perineum to record urethral sphincter activity.
   g. The bladder is filled with contrast.
   h. Fluoroscopy is used to visualize the bladder and urethra and reflux is noted up the ureters into the kidneys on both sides.
   i. A standard pressure flow study is performed with voiding pressures.
   j. A PVR is again calculated by subtracting the voided volume from the filled volume.
   k. Cystoscopy with examination of urethra, bladder, and trigone.

Table 4.6 Non-facility, established patient urodynamics

CPT Code	Description
51729	Complex cystometrogram with voiding pressure studies
51741-51	Complex uroflowmetry (calibrated equipment)
51784-51	Electromyography studies (EMG) of anal or urethral sphincter other than needle
74430	Contrast, bladder X-ray
74455	X-ray, urethra or bladder
76000	Fluoroscope examination
51797	Measurement of intra-abdominal pressure
51798-51	Measurement of PVR bladder scanner
81000	Urinalysis with microscopy (non-auto)
52000-59	Diagnostic cystourethroscopy
51600-51	Instillation of contrast to bladder

And If the Coding Is Done Correctly…

Table 4.7 below displays average national reimbursement for diagnostic tests related to urodynamics performed in multiple settings.

Urodynamic Coding Things to Remember

- If a physician performs more than one urodynamic procedure on a patient on the same day, list the highest RVU value code first and then append additional codes with a -51 modifier.
- The primary procedure is reimbursed at 100 % of the fee schedule or allowable amount and the subsequent procedures will be paid at 50 % of the fee schedule or allowable amount.
- CPT code 51797 is an add-on code and is not subject to the multiple procedure discounts. This code would be reimbursed at 100 % of the fee schedule or allowable amount.
- A cystoscopy (CPT code 52000) performed on the same day is also reimbursed at 100 % of the fee schedule or allowable amount. Remember, this code needs a -59 modifier rather than -51 since it is defined as a separate procedure in CPT.
- When it is appropriate to bill for both an E&M and a procedure code, add a -25 modifier on the E&M code.

Table 4.7 Estimated reimbursement for urodynamics (adapted from Cooper surgical website [7])

CPT code	Non-facility physician receives… ($)	Facility physician receives… ($)	APC hospital receives… ($)	ASC ambulatory surgery center receives… ($)
51725	211	78	221	100
51726	308	89	221	124
51727	306	110	221	124
51728	303	107	221	124
51729	332	129	221	124
51736	35	12	46	17
51741	43	17	77	20
51784	206	79	77	43
51792	233	57	77	43
51797	235	42	140	70

ASC ambulatory surgery center, *APC* ambulatory payment classification

References

1. Hu T-W, Wagner TH, Bentkover JD, et al. Estimated economic costs of overactive bladder in the United States. Urology. 2003;61:1123–8.
2. Ingenix National Fee Analyzer 2011, Charge data for evaluating fees nationally. 2011. Eden Prairie MN. Ingenix. Cited by Smith AL, Wein AJ. Predicting the future of urodynamics. Transl Androl Urol. 2012;1(2):76–7. doi: 10.3978/j.issn.22234683.2012.06.01
3. Pickett D. International classification of diseases. 10th ed. Clinical modification ICD-10-CM. www.cdc.gov. http://www.cdc.gov/nchs/icd/icd10cm.htm. Accessed 14 Nov 2013.
4. Blum J, editor. Letter from director of center for medicare. http://www.cms.gov/Medicare/Medicare-Fee-for-Service-Payment/SustainableGRatesConFact/Downloads/SGR2013-Final-Signed.pdf. Accessed 21 Aug 2013.
5. Ingenix. Coding companion for urology/nephrology. Optum Insight; 2012.
6. IngenixOptumInsight. Current procedural coding expert 2012. OptumInsight Incorporated; 2011.
7. Urodynamics procedures. Cooper surgical. http://www.coopersurgical.com/Documents/Urodynamic%20Reimbursement%202011.pdf. Accessed 12 Aug 2013.

Chapter 5
Conducting the Urodynamic Study

Ahmed El-Zawahry

Introduction

Multichannel urodynamics (UDS) are a group of tests used to measure different dynamic aspects of the lower urinary tract (LUT) during storage (filling) and voiding [1, 2]. The term "urodynamics" was initially employed by Davis [3] in 1954 to describe tests used to evaluate LUT function.

Lower urinary tract symptoms (LUTS) are often overlapping and insufficient to support a diagnosis alone. Bates coined the often-used expression "the bladder is an unreliable witness," in 1970, and it is a maxim that often proves to be true in clinical practice. For this reason, obtaining objective confirmation of the patient's subjective symptoms can be an important element in clarifying complex diagnoses, particularly before proceeding to invasive therapies. However, one should remember that UDS tests do not replace other diagnostic tests such as urinalysis, cystoscopy, or imaging, if needed, and it should be an integral part of the work-up to establish the proper diagnosis, categorize the severity of the condition, and help with choosing treatment options [4].

The main objective of multichannel UDS is to attempt to duplicate the storage and voiding functions of the bladder that are experienced by the patient in daily life to help identify the pathophysiology behind the voiding dysfunction symptoms. There are several key questions that should be kept in mind when thinking about UDS testing.

A. El-Zawahry, MBBCh (✉)
Department of Surgery, Incontinence Center, Southern Illinois University,
301 N. 8th Street, 4th Floor, P.O. Box 19665, Springfield, IL 62711, USA
e-mail: a.elzawahry@gmail.com

© Springer Science+Business Media New York 2015

E.S. Rovner, M.E. Koski (eds.), *Rapid and Practical Interpretation of Urodynamics*, DOI 10.1007/978-1-4939-1764-8_5

When to Consider the UDS Test

Although multichannel UDS is a very helpful test, it has an associated cost. It is an invasive test that is not without discomfort and may carry a risk of infection. It is also expensive. It is therefore imperative that one ask several questions: (1) if the UDS study is needed? (2) what is the information being sought by the exam? and (3) if the information obtained assist with diagnosis and management?

There are several guidelines available to help identify the role of UDS in clinical practice. The American Urological Association (AUA) Urodynamics guideline can be reviewed at the AUA website [5] (http://www.auanet.org/education/guidelines/adult-urodynamics.cfm). A general outline of the proper indications for UDS in clinical practice would include [6]:

1. Characterization of LUT dysfunction and identification of problems associated with LUT dysfunction.
2. Identification of factors causing or contributing to voiding dysfunction.
3. Identification of risk factors associated with LUT dysfunction that can lead to upper tract deterioration.
4. Assessment of the outcome of the anticipated treatment and possible unfavorable side effects.
5. Evaluation for possible reasons of treatment failure and help to plan for future treatment plans and proper patients counseling.

Based on AUA/SUFU guideline statements, the following indications for performing UDS can be summarized [5, 7]:

1. *Indications to perform UDS in patients with stress urinary incontinence (SUI) include*:

    a. When considering invasive surgery, a post-void residual urine (PVR) should be assessed.
    b. Clinician may consider multichannel UDS in patients with both symptoms and clinical findings of SUI before invasive treatments. UDS is considered helpful in patients with complicated history such as previous surgery, mixed storage symptoms, or voiding symptoms.
    c. In patients with high-grade pelvic organ prolapse (POP), UDS should be performed with POP reduction to assess for occult SUI and other detrusor dysfunction issues.

2. *Indications to perform UDS on patients with overactive bladder (OAB), Urgency Urinary Incontinence (UUI), and Mixed Urinary Incontinence (MUI) include*:

    a. When it is important to determine the presence or absence of altered bladder compliance, detrusor overactivity (DO), or other UDS abnormality in patients who are considering invasive or irreversible procedures.
    b. In patients with refractory UUI after bladder outlet procedures, clinicians may perform pressure flow studies to assess for bladder outlet obstruction (BOO).
    c. In women with storage symptoms refractory to treatment following anti-incontinence surgery to identify BOO.

3. *Indications to perform UDS in patients with neurogenic bladder (NGB)*:
   The role of UDS in patients with NGB is to identify patients who are at risk for developing upper tract and renal deterioration associated with storage pressure problems and lower bladder compliance.
4. *Indications to perform UDS in patients with LUTS include*:
   In performing UDS in patients with LUTS, a uroflow, PVR, and a pressure flow study (PFS), or multichannel UDS with or without fluoroscopy can be helpful to diagnose the cause of LUTS.

   a. When an abnormality of voiding/emptying is suggested.
   b. To determine whether DO or other abnormalities of bladder filling/urine storage are present in patients with LUTS particularly when invasive procedures are considered.
   c. When it is important to determine whether urodynamic obstruction is present in men with LUTS especially when invasive or irreversible procedures are being considered.
   d. In women with LUTS when it is important to determine if obstruction is present.
   e. Clinicians may perform video-urodynamics in properly selected patients to localize the level of obstruction, particularly for the diagnosis of primary bladder neck obstruction.

Pretest Questions

Before ordering any test, questions need to be answered and the proper test to answer these questions needs to be identified. As with any diagnostic test, answers that are obtained should help confirm the diagnosis and/or help with the treatment plan. UDS is not different than any other diagnostic test that is used in clinical practice and questions need to be formulated before ordering the test (Table 5.1).

Table 5.1 Questions to think about while thinking about UDS test for patients

Urodynamics	Questions to ask
Pretest	Q1. Does the patient need this test? Q2. What questions do I need to answer? Q3. How should the test be designed to answer the pre-study questions? Q4. What provocative maneuvers if any do I need to perform?
During the test	Q1. Is the study designed appropriately to answer the questions? Q2. Is the study performed appropriately? Q3. Are there any artifacts or technical problems? Q4. Am I able to reproduce the patient's symptoms? Q5. If the patient's symptoms are not reproduced, are there any provocative tests that may reproduce them?
Post-test	Q1. Was the study technically performed well? Q2. Were there any artifacts that needed to be accounted for during interpretation? Q3. Were the patient's symptoms reproduced during the study? Q4. Were the pretest question/s answered?

Before ordering UDS, a physician should have pretest questions formulated in mind with regard to the study objectives:

1. Why do I need to perform this test?
2. What information do I need?
3. What UDS test(s) do I need to perform to understand the patient's problems?
4. Will the information acquired during the study help in diagnosing the problem and the decision-making process for treatment?
5. How can I reproduce the patient's problems during the study?

At the conclusion of the study, the physician asks the questions

"Were the patients' symptoms reproduced during the study?"
"Did the results of the study correlate with the patient symptoms?"

It is important to recognize that a UDS study is most meaningful when the patient's symptoms are reproduced during test. This should be addressed with the patient during and after the study.

UDS Planning

Physicians should consider UDS testing when the clinical data obtained is insufficient to determine the factors contributing to LUTS [8, 9]. Obtaining such knowledge will help to decide the appropriate treatment for the patient [1]. For example, performing multichannel UDS in patients with neurogenic bladder can not only evaluate bladder function but can also help assess risk factors that could lead to upper tract deterioration. It also helps in counseling patients regarding possible therapeutic outcomes and identifying possible causes behind treatment failure.

A working diagnosis is necessary prior to the multichannel UDS study and the test should be individualized to answer questions generated for each patient prior to initiation of the study. The study is most helpful when the clinical symptoms being investigated are reproduced during the study. If the examiner is unable to reproduce the symptoms, then it is essential to consider tailoring the study or changing the environment to reproduce the symptoms to facilitate a successful study [10]. The following questions, considered prior to and during the study, can help define this process.

1. What questions do I need to answer?
2. What symptoms do I need to reproduce?
3. How can I reproduce the symptom while performing the study?
4. What provocative tests do I need to perform to reproduce these symptoms?

Pretest Arrangements

Pretest Counseling

UDS testing is considered a minimally invasive procedure; however, the patient may view it differently. Patients often perceive this test as an intrusion into their privacy and they may experience a great deal of anxiety associated with several aspects of the test including the environment of the test, urethral and rectal catheterization, voiding in front of strangers, and the embarrassment associated with being exposed. Proper patient counseling including a face-to-face explanation of the test as well as supplemental handouts can reduce this anxiety. A variety of online sources are available which patients can use as additional informational resources. Studies [11, 12] have demonstrated that most of the patients who undergo multichannel UDS testing would not object to repeat testing if needed and that the test causes only minimal anxiety and discomfort. However this does not preclude the fact that pretest counseling is important to prepare the patient for the test. It is crucial to explain to the patient about the expectation of catheterization during the study. Physician–patient communication should continue during the study to alleviate any anxiety or concern.

UDS Personnel

The successful UDS study depends on a team effort. Properly trained staff is crucial in order to perform a good quality study. The staff should be familiar with the patient's history, study requirements, the technique, and the machine settings. Proper interpretation of the study also requires the ability to reliably identify artifacts that occurred during the study. This requires a good understanding of the technique and an open communication between the nurse or technician who is performing the test and the physician interpreting the study. The physician or nurse/technician performing the study must carefully record observations that were made during the study [13, 14]. Annotating the graph appropriately noting such activity as changes associated with changes in position, and provocative maneuvers (coughing, straining, command to void, etc.) will aid in accurately interpreting the study. This requires paying attention to fine details while performing the test and the clinical experience to initiate such maneuvers appropriately and record them succinctly on the study graph and/or event summary [15].

Preparing for UDS Evaluation

History

History of Lower Urinary Tract Symptoms

Completing an appropriate and relevant history is an important part of the preparation for UDS testing. History (Table 5.2) should start with a detailed inquiry about the patient's symptoms and analysis of these symptoms (Table 5.3). Symptoms can be quantified with the aid of available validated questionnaires. Examples of such questionnaires include the International Prostate Symptom Score (IPSS), King's Health Questionnaire (ICIQ-LUTSqol), Symptoms Severity Index (SSI), and Urogenital Distress Inventory-6 (UDI-6). LUT symptoms are often quantitated by means of a voiding diary and pad test. It should be clarified if the patients' symptoms are related to lower urinary pathology, patient physiology, or being practiced out of habit/convenience (e.g., increased urinary frequency secondary to increased fluid intake, using pads as precautionary measures for fear of incontinence) or secondary to other comorbidities (e.g., congestive heart failure or sleep apnea). Documentation should include the duration of symptoms, severity and impact of the symptoms [15].

For example, if the patient has urinary incontinence, it should be properly characterized. Is it associated with physical activity (SUI), Urgency Urinary Incontinence (UUI), or other factors? How severe is the leakage? What situations or maneuvers reproduce leakage? How forceful is the urinary stream? Is there any history of treatment or surgery for leakage? Does the patient wear any pads? How many pads? How saturated are the pads? Does the patient wear pads out of convenience for fear of incontinence? Also if the patient has prolapse, does she use any special maneuvers to be able to void such as digital splinting or positioning in order to be able to void [16].

Table 5.2 Pretest evaluation for patients undergoing UDS

History	– History of present illness including using validated questionnaires – Past medical and neurologic history – Drug history – Obstetric history – Past surgical history
Physical examination	– Genitourinary examination – Abdominal examination – Rectal examination – Vaginal examination – Pelvic floor examination – Focused neurological examination
Pretest evaluation	– Pad test – Voiding diary – Post-void residual urine (PVR) – Urinalysis, culture, and sensitivity – Cystoscopy or imaging if indicated

Table 5.3 LUTS based on International Urogynecological Association (IUGA)/International Continence Society (ICS) joint report on the terminology for female pelvic floor dysfunction [20]

Urinary incontinence symptoms	Definition
Continence	The voluntary control of bladder and bowel function
Urinary Incontinence (UI)	Complaint of any involuntary loss of urine
Urgency Urinary Incontinence (UUI)	Complaint of involuntary loss of urine associated with urgency
Stress Urinary Incontinence (SUI)	Complaint of involuntary loss of urine on effort or physical exertion or on sneezing or coughing
Postural (urinary) Incontinence	Complaint of involuntary loss of urine associated with change of body position such as rising from a seated or lying position
Nocturnal enuresis	Complaint of involuntary urinary loss which occurs during sleep
Mixed Urinary Incontinence	Complaint of involuntary loss of urine associated with urgency and also with effort or physical exertion or on sneezing or coughing
Continuous Urinary Incontinence	Complaint of continuous involuntary loss of urine
Insensible Urinary Incontinence	Complaint of urinary loss where the individual is unaware of how it occurred
Coital Incontinence	Complaint of involuntary loss of urine with coitus
Bladder storage symptoms	*Definition*
Increased urinary frequency	Complaint of voiding occurs more frequently during waking hours than previously deemed normal [20] Complaint of voiding too frequent while awake. Eight voids per day or voiding $\leq$2 h [13]
Nocturia	Complain of interruption of sleep one or more times because of the need to micturate. Each void is preceded and followed by sleep [20] It is waking up at night to void. Zero to one episodes in adults <65 years of age or up to 2 in older adults is considered normal [13]
Urgency	A sudden and compelling desire to pass urine that is difficult to defer
Overactive Bladder symptoms (OAB, Urgency)	Urinary urgency, usually accompanied by frequency and nocturia with or without urgency urinary incontinence, in the absence of urinary tract infection (UTI) or other obvious pathology
Voiding symptoms	*Definition*
Hesitancy	Complaint of a delay in initiating micturition
Slow stream	Complaint of a urinary stream perceived as slower compared to previous performance or in comparison with others
Intermittency	Complaint of urine flow that stops and starts on one or more occasions during voiding
Straining to void	Complaint of the need to make an intensive effort (by abdominal straining, Valsalva or suprapubic pressure) to either initiate, maintain, or improve the urinary stream
Spraying (splitting) of urinary stream	Complaint that urine passage is a spray or split rather than a single discrete stream
Feeling of incomplete bladder emptying	Complaint that the bladder does not feel empty after micturition
Need to immediately re-void	Complaint that the bladder does not feel empty after micturition
Position-dependent micturition	Complaint of having to take specific position to be able to micturate spontaneously or to improve bladder emptying
Dysuria	Complaint of burning or other discomfort during micturition, discomfort may be intrinsic to the lower urinary tract or external
Urinary retention	Complaint of the inability to pass urine despite persistent effort
Post-micturition symptoms	*Definition*
Post-micturition leakage	Complaint of a further involuntary passage of urine following the completion of micturition

Past Medical History

The physician should inquire about any other comorbid conditions that can affect the patient's urinary tract. One should specifically ask about any history of any neurological conditions such as lumbosacral intervertebral disc problems, or back/spine surgery, Cerebro-vascular accidents (CVA), Parkinson's disease, and other cerebral abnormalities. In cases of problems with the spinal cord such as spinal cord injuries or spina bifida, the level of the spinal cord lesion should be determined? Other symptoms that may suggest neurological disorders should be kept in mind such as double vision, numbness, or tingling which could be secondary to multiple sclerosis (MS). A history of diabetes and neuropathy is important to elicit, including the duration of the disease. Previous exposure to radiation therapy especially pelvic radiation should be assessed as this could be associated with radiation cystitis, small bladder capacity, and low compliance. It is also important to inquire about a history of constipation as this could affect the bladder function as well as UDS test performance [17]. Any physical or cognitive impairment should be noted as it may require additional arrangements for patient preparation and management during the UDS study [15].

Drug History

Inquiring about drug history is important as some medications can affect the LUT such as narcotics, antihistaminics, antimuscarinics, and sympathomimetics. Also the physician should decide on whether the patient should continue or discontinue any given medication at the time of the study [15]. Discontinuing such medication provides a baseline assessment whereas continuing medications allows an assessment of the patient as they currently exist on the medication.

Obstetric History

It is important to know about the obstetric history including the number of vaginal deliveries, any trauma during delivery, size of the babies, and difficulty during delivery with use of additional equipment (e.g., forceps) to facilitate delivery.

Past Surgical History

It is imperative to obtain the past surgical history as pelvic surgeries could have some effects on bladder function. A prior history of radical hysterectomy or abdomino-perineal resection (APR) could lead to detrusor dysfunction including poor contractility with or without compliance abnormalities. Also a history of prior surgery for prolapse, or incontinence procedures such as slings might suggest alternative diagnoses such as bladder outlet obstruction for which customization of the study would be beneficial. A history of prostate or urethral diseases and/or surgeries in men should be collected as these might suggest difficulties with catheterization for the UDS study.

Physical Examination

Genitourinary Examination

It is important to obtain a good genitourinary (GU) examination prior to the UDS study. The GU examination should include abdominal examination to evaluate for masses, hernia, and/or a distended bladder. The physician can confirm the presence of stress urinary incontinence during the examination by means of a cough stress test. Any urethral abnormalities should be noted. In male patients, a prostate examination should be performed.

Abdominal Examination

The presence of scars from previous surgery especially pelvic surgery is noted. A lower abdominal examination should assess for any evidence of suprapubic fullness indicating a full bladder or urinary retention. Fecal impaction should be noted as this could affect placement of rectal catheters, and in addition, rectal distention due to constipation can significantly affect bladder function [18].

Rectal Examination

Rectal examination is used to assess for anal sphincter tone and strength. It also helps to assess for abnormalities of sacral innervation (S2–S4) via the bulbocavernosus reflex, anal wink, and sensation around the saddle area.

Vaginal Examination

Vaginal examination is extremely important [19] prior to UDS testing. The introitus should be examined for the presence of vaginal atrophy or urethral abnormalities. The presence of vaginal prolapse should be assessed and the degree should be documented. The presence of prolapse can affect LUT function [15, 16] and also may suggest the need to pursue additional maneuvers during UDS testing. For example, if there is significant pelvic organ prolapse, one may choose to reduce it with a pessary during the study in order to assess for occult SUI or alternatively to examine the potential obstructive effects of the prolapse on voiding. The presence of any scar tissue or a urethral abnormality from previous incontinence surgery such as a swan neck deformity should be documented.

Pelvic Floor Muscle

Pelvic floor muscle resting tone and function should be assessed during physical examination and should be noted if it is normal, overactive, underactive, or non-functioning [13, 20, 21].

Focused Neurologic Examination

Neurologic examination should be a part of the evaluation of patients with voiding dysfunction undergoing UDS assessment. The physician should observe for any gait abnormalities and any lower extremity weakness. Sensation of the saddle area and rectal tone is an important part of the neurological examination. Assessment of the sacral is reflexes that should be considered to test for sacral nerve integrity. These reflexes are centrally integrated at S2 to S4. The reflex arc is mediated via afferent and efferent limbs within the pelvic nerves. The reflexes [22] include:

1. The anal wink reflex: this can be elicited by tapping the perianal skin and observing for anal sphincter contraction.
2. The bulbo-cavernosus reflex: this is elicited by digital squeezing of the glans penis (or clitoris), which will result in contraction in the anal sphincter or bulbo-cavernosus muscle [18, 23].

If abnormalities are noted in the neurological examination further evaluation is warranted.

Pretest Evaluation

Post-void Residual Urine

PVR is defined as "the volume of urine left in the bladder at the end of micturition" [13, 20] and is often considered an urodynamic test in isolation. According to the AUA guidelines assessment of PVR should be performed in:

1. Patients with SUI or pelvic organ prolapse who are considering invasive procedures.
2. Patients with neurogenic bladder as a part of their evaluation [5].
3. Patients with LUTS as a part of their evaluation to rule out urinary retention as a cause of their symptoms [5].

There are multiple methods to measure the PVR. These include invasive and non-invasive methods. The invasive approaches can be performed via in-and-out catheterization or endoscopy. Non-invasive means include transabdominal ultrasonography using real-time ultrasound or automated systems. It can also be assessed during IVP, video-urodynamics, or radioisotope studies [6].

Catheterization is the gold standard for measuring PVR. However, it should be noted that proper technique is important to obtain an accurate measurement [24]. Moving the catheter in-and-out and twisting may be important to ensure proper collection of any urinary residual in the bladder [25]. However, this is an invasive procedure that carries some risk of infection and is associated with some discomfort to the patient. Alternatively, portable ultrasound scanners with automated measurement of bladder volume are non-invasive, more comfortable to the patient, and easy to use. They can be used with reasonable accuracy [26].

Based on the 4th International Consultation on Incontinence, ultrasound is the recommended means for measuring PVR as it is the least invasive and is sufficiently accurate for clinical practice [6]. Several measurements should be considered due to intra-individual variability [6, 10, 24, 27]. The PVR reading should be performed as soon as possible after the patient voids to avoid erroneous readings. A delay in performance of the test following a volitional void will result in additional urine accumulation in the bladder which can result in an inaccurate PVR determination. Urine is added to the bladder at a rate of approximately, 1–14 mL/min [28].

There is no standardization on what is considered a normal PVR. Some would argue that less than 50 mL is considered normal in adults [29] and others would consider the upper limit of normal to be 100 mL [28]. However, if the patient is asymptomatic then they may not need treatment even with PVR's in excess of 100 cc depending on the clinical situation and clinical judgment [30]. A consistently elevated PVR is an indication of possibly impaired detrusor contractility or bladder outlet obstruction (or both) and such a finding warrants more in depth investigation.

Voiding Diary (Frequency–Volume Charts)

This is a simple non-invasive test to evaluate patients with LUTS and voiding dysfunction in his/her natural environment and during regular daily activities [31]. The diary evaluation consists of recording the time and volume of each void over 24 h. ICS considers a 24-h properly performed diary as a reasonable evaluation tool for clinical practices [32]. However, a diary for 3 days is preferred for proper assessment and to avoid skewing of the data obtained by spurious behavior on a single day [32]. The diary does not need to be on consecutive days. It is important to note that simply performing the diary may alter the patients' normal behavior.

A voiding diary (frequency–volume charts) should be considered as part of the initial evaluation of patients with LUTS especially those who have frequency and nocturia. The diary helps to establish a quantitative baseline for the symptoms such as frequency and urgency as well as voided volumes and subsequent diaries allow monitoring of sequential therapies over time [27]. Information obtained from a diary includes voiding frequency, nocturia, amount of urine voided in 24 h and overnight, average voided volume, median functional bladder capacity, number and timing of incontinence episodes, and urgency. It is the only tool to diagnose polyuria [20] and nocturnal polyuria (Table 5.3 and 5.4). It is very important to stress to the patient that the diary should be performed on a regular ordinary day that represents their usual routine.

It is very helpful to have the voiding diary prior to performing the multichannel UDS study. This will provide an estimate of the functional bladder capacity, which will allow the UDS to be customized with respect to filling rate and expected bladder capacity. Additional information can be acquired from the diary including the episodes of urgency and urine leakage that could be correlated to involuntary detrusor contractions (IDCs) on the UDS study.

Table 5.4 Information can be obtained from voiding diary and definitions

Information obtained	Definitions
Diurnal frequency	Number of voids during the day (wakeful hours)
Nocturia	Number of times of voids interrupt the sleep and each void is preceded and followed by sleep
24-h urinary frequency	Number of diurnal frequency and nocturia
Maximum voided volume	Maximum voided volume recorded
Average voided volume	The sum of voided volume during 24 h divided by the number of voids
Small voided volumes	Suggest OAB or a pathology results in decrease of bladder volume such as inflammatory process or contracted bladder
Median functional Bladder capacity	Median maximum voided urine in the 24-h activity
Polyuria	Excessive urine production resulting in increased urinary frequency. It is defined as increased urine production more than 40 mL/kg/day. Voiding diary will show increased urine output associated with increased frequency
Nocturnal urine volume	Total volume of urine voided after going to bed for sleeping including the first morning void with intention of rising
Nocturnal polyuria	More than 20–33 % (depending on age) of total urine production is excreted at night

There are multiple voiding diaries available on different websites. Examples of websites containing diary examples include the Society of Urodynamics, Female Pelvic Medicine and Urogenital Reconstruction (SUFU) (http://www.sufuorg.com/docs/patient-resources/SUFU-voiding-diary.aspx), The National Institute of Diabetes and Digestive and Kidney Diseases (NIDDK) (http://kidney.niddk.nih.gov/kudiseases/pubs/diary/diary_508.pdf), and the International Urogynecological Association (IUGA) (http://c.ymcdn.com/sites/www.iuga.org/resource/resmgr/brochures/eng_bladderdiary.pdf). Table 5.5 is the diary used in our institution.

Pad Test

For patients with urinary incontinence, a pad test is an important tool for the detection and quantification of urine loss over a set period of time. It is an objective test that can be performed by the patient and can help to quantitate urine leak. A properly done pad test will enable the physician to have a realistic idea about the severity of incontinence [33]. This also may aid to design and individualize the UDS study [4]. For example, in a patient with a complaint of urinary incontinence as well as incontinence noted on the voiding diary and pad test, every effort should be made to reproduce these symptoms during the UDS study. If a symptom is not reproduced initially during the study, then provocative maneuvers should be performed in order to elicit such a finding.

Table 5.5 Voiding diary adopted in our institution

Name _______________________________

Date _______________________________

Time of Day	Amount of urine Voided (oz or ml)	Amount of Fluid (Drinks) Intake (oz or ml)	Type of Fluid Consumed (water, coffee, soda, beer, etc.)	Urgency Or Pain Before Voiding? (yes or no)	Leakage of Urine (incontinence) at any time prior to Voiding (yes or no)
7am					
8am					
9am					
10am					
11am					
12 noon					
1pm					
2pm					
3pm					
4pm					
5pm					
6pm					
7pm					
8pm					
9pm					
10pm					
11pm					
12 am					
1 am					
2am					
3am					
4am					
5 am					
6am					
Total for24 hours					

Please indicate the time that you went to bed:_______________________

Please indicate the time that you woke up:_______________________

Ideally the pad test should be performed while the patient is performing everyday regular activity. Pad tests have been described for multiple lengths of time from 1 to 24-h and 48-h up to 1 week [16]. The standardized 1-h pad test entails the patient drinks a volume of 500 mL of sodium-free fluid over a short period of time and then engages in a standard set of maneuvers over a 1-h period [4]. The 1-h pad is then collected and weighed. The ICS 1-h pad test upper limit of normal is >1 g [4, 32]. A 24-h pad test is an alternative assessment which offers to be a more practical assessment of patient leakage [4, 33]. The normal upper limit for a 24-h pad test is 4 g [32].

Investigations

Urinalysis

Urine should be tested on the day of the UDS study. If there is evidence of infection, then the UDS test should be postponed. If a patient has a history of repeated urinary tract infection or a high risk of infection, then the appropriate antibiotic coverage should be considered prior to the study [5, 34].

Provided that the patient is asked to void prior to the start of the UDS study, a catheterized urine specimen at the start of the study as the UDS catheters are placed provides an assessment of PVR and a clean urine specimen for testing. Urine can be tested using dipsticks or microscopy. A urine culture is obtained if indicated [4, 15].

Urine Cytology

Cytological studies of urine may be indicated in some patients including those with a history of LUT tumors, or pronounced storage symptoms such as increased urinary frequency, urgency, and hematuria. [20]. In postmenopausal women with LUTS, the hormonal status may affect the vaginal wall and result in LUTS. In such cases, a lateral vaginal wall cytology smear may help to diagnose estrogen deficiency [20].

Imaging

Upper urinary tract imaging is not recommended for patients with LUTS except in certain circumstances. The indications for upper tract imaging as recommended by the 4th International Consultation on Incontinence [6] include

1. Hematuria
2. Neurogenic urinary incontinence
3. Severe pelvic organ prolapse
4. The presence of flank pain
5. Questions about the possible presence of extra-urethral incontinence.
6. Diagnosed low bladder compliance
7. Children with UTI associated with incontinence

Antibiotic Prophylaxis

The risk of developing bacteruria after UDS testing in adults varies from 6.2 to 13.9 % [35, 36] and the incidence of urinary tract infection following multichannel UDS evaluation is rare and varies from 2.1 to 6.9 % [37–39]. Antibiotic prophylaxis helps to reduce bacteruria by 40 % but this is not reflected by a reduced incidence of urinary tract infections [40]. Therefore, routine administration of antibiotic prophylaxis is not recommended. However, it may be reasonable to use in patients with risk factors for bacteruira after UDS testing [41]. These risk factors include recurrent urinary tract infections, diabetes mellitus, neurogenic bladder, and recent history of urologic or urogynecologic surgery [35, 39].

Starting the UDS Study

Patient Positioning During the Study

Multichannel UDS studies may be performed in the seated, standing, or supine position. In performing multichannel UDS, one should consider conducting the study in the position in which the patient usually experiences their symptoms. For example the standing position would be the most likely position to reproduce the patient's symptoms of SUI [4]. Al-Hayek et al. [42] in a meta-analysis found that detrusor overactivity (DO) is elicited at a higher incidence in the vertical position (standing or sitting) or when changing to a vertical position. Performing the study in a supine position would have missed diagnosing DO in 33–100 % of patients.

The International Urogynecological Association (IUGA)/International Continence Society (ICS) joint report recommends performing the UDS study in the sitting position as this will be more provocative to uncover DO than the supine position. They also recommended performing the study at some point with the patient in the standing position [20]. During voiding, the patients should be placed in the usual position that they assume while voiding to simulate ordinary circumstances [18]. Changes in the patient's posture during the study should also be noted as this will result in artifacts which should be accounted for during interpretation [4, 18].

Filling the Bladder

Filling Rate

Bladder filling can be performed using either single lumen catheters or dual lumen catheters. Single lumen catheters may provide a larger caliber lumen for filling. However, such a technique will require insertion of an additional catheter for measuring pressure inside the bladder. Two catheters in the urethra may increase the probability of occluding the urethra and masking some of the UDS findings especially SUI [4]. Dual lumen catheters are recommended by the International Continence Society (ICS) to perform the dual functions of bladder filling and simultaneous recording of intravesical pressure. It is recommended to use the smallest catheter that:

1. Allows an adequate rate of filling.
2. Does not compromise voiding and cause artifact (false obstruction or mask SUI)
3. Does not affect pressure transmission

Filling rates are variable and can be *slow* (10 mL/min), *medium* (10–100 mL/min), or *fast* (>100 mL/min). A medium filling rate is most suitable for most patients. However, faster rates are used as provocative maneuvers to elicit detrusor overactivity (DO) in patients with OAB symptoms. The physiologic rate of filling can be calculated at a rate less than 1/4 of the total body weight in mL/min [43]. At this rate of filling the pressure–volume curve continues to be flat and detrusor pressure changes are related to volume rather than rate [43].

Type of Filling Medium

Fluid medium is preferred over gas and is recommended by ICS for filling [28]. Sterile water, normal saline, or contrast medium can be used for filling [4, 28]. Care should be taken to avoid changing between fluids during the study as calibration will be affected and will result in inaccurate filling volumes. Gas (CO_2) has been used as a filling medium [44], however it does not have the same density as fluid medium. Thus it does not mimic urine which is fluid in nature. Finally, fluid allows for assessment of uroflow during voiding which is not possible with gas.

Temperature of the Medium

Ideally, the temperature of the filling solution should be compatible with body temperature. However, in practice this is often difficult. Infusing fluid at room temperature is appropriate in this setting. On the other hand, cold fluid should be avoided as this can activate aberrant neural pathways and reflexes which may precipitate clinically insignificant IDCs and bladder sensations [4].

Interpretation of UDS Study

Physicians must interpret UDS results in the context of the general assessment of the patient. Interpretation of UDS results should be integrated with and complement all the available information obtained from a complete history, neuro-urological examination, voiding diaries, pad tests, and other work-up deemed clinically relevant. Interpreting a UDS study result out of the context of the clinical scenario could be misleading [10].

Analysis of the UDS test should include not only a full evaluation of the actual graph and images, but also should incorporate observations made during the study [13, 14]. If the physician is not performing the study by himself/herself, such information should be communicated to the physician by the technician performing the study. These observations should reflect any patient behaviors and activities during the study. Any alterations on the graph associated with changes in position, talking, voiding, or pushing to void should be noted and recorded. If these artifacts are not properly labeled and pointed out on the graph, they can be misread and can result in inappropriate and misleading conclusions.

Another important point is that during interpretation, the physician should acknowledge that UDS testing is performed while the patient is in an awkward situation. This is associated with minimal to moderate degrees of anxiety, discomfort, and embarrassment which could result in artifacts during the study [45].

Challenges Facing the Physician During UDS Interpretation

To obtain a meaningful interpretation of the UDS findings, the physician should always recognize the presence of multiple challenges during testing. One should think about factors that can affect the outcome of the study. Such factors should be accounted for while performing and interpreting the UDS study [18]. These factors can be related to place, patient, and/or practitioner.

1. *Place of the study*: It is not always easy to create a suitable and natural environment for the patient during the study, which is by nature an uncomfortable and unnatural situation for the patient. The patient is being exposed in front of strangers and is asked to void, an inherently private bodily function, in front of others, which could be extremely sensitive and could alter their natural behavior leading to potentially abnormal and clinically irrelevant findings [18]. In addition the anxiety produced by this situation can result in an aberrant reaction of the patient resulting in "Shy bladder syndrome" or psychogenic inhibition of voiding, which is associated with social anxiety. [46].
2. *Patient factors:*

    a. *Position of the patient*: Patients are positioned during the study as dictated by the study scenario. However, this is often different from the position wherein the patient ordinarily experiences urinary symptoms. Different positions are associated with pressure changes within the bladder and can alter the bladder behavior unexpectedly during the study. In the setting where the patients symptoms are not reproduced during the UDS study initially, one should consider asking the patient about their position when they usually experience their symptoms and repeat the study in that position.
    b. *Tubes (urethral catheter and rectal transducer)*: Catheters that are used during the multichannel UDS study include, most often, one urethral and the other rectal. Although they are small in diameter they can be painful and bothersome to the patient. Pain may result in external sphincter spasm as well as inhibit the micturition reflex. These effects can result in an artifactual inability to void during the study due to pain, as well as changes in urine flow [47] and mask stress urinary incontinence [9].
    c. *Filling the bladder*: The solution utilized to fill the bladder is not urine and therefore the study is performed with a medium that is non-physiologic in composition, filled at a non-physiologic rate, and most often at a non-physiologic temperature (room temperature). These factors can affect bladder sensation and response during filling [18]. If the patient is showing unexpected findings, these factors should be considered as potential sources for artifact or aberrant findings.

3. *Practitioner interpreting the results*: [48, 49] Identifying artifacts is critical in interpreting multichannel UDS studies accurately. It is imperative to stress the importance of accurately and appropriately labeling events on UDS tracings. Reviewing the UDS tracing and numbers recorded during testing is an important part of interpretation and one should not depend on the computer analysis only to detect artifacts that could occur during the study [10]. It should be kept in mind also while performing the study and during interpretation that the study represents only a momentary glimpse of the patients normal voiding habits and does not reflect the long-term and variable patterns often seen over time in any given individual.

Conclusion

UDS are an important tool in the evaluation of patients with LUTS and voiding dysfunction. UDS provides an objective evaluation of the patient's presenting LUTS which are often "unreliable" in predicting the underlying urodynamic and physiologic findings. UDS are often aimed at the characterization of LUT dysfunction, and assessing risk factors that can lead to kidney deterioration. UDS testing also may help to assess the possible outcomes of expected treatment and possible causes of previous treatment failures. However, the UDS studies do not replace an adequate work-up including proper history, physical examination, and other appropriate tests.

Reliable UDS results depend on the proper design, performance, and interpretation of the study. Patient counseling may help prevent or minimize problems that may arise during the study. Setting up a proper environment and having well-trained and experienced personnel is paramount for an optimal study. Excellent communication between the nurse or technician who is performing the study, and the patient, as well as the physician interpreting the study helps to minimize artifacts during interpretation. It is important to understand that UDS should be utilized and interpreted within the context of the patient's entire clinical picture and should not be isolated from the rest of the evaluation process.

References

1. Nitti VW. Urodynamic evaluation of the lower urinary tract. In: Kavoussi N, Parin P, editors. Campbell-Walsh urology, vol. 3. Philadelphia: Elsevier Saunders; 2012. p. 1847.
2. Abrams P, Blaivas JB, Stanton SL, Andersen JT. The standardization of terminology of lower urinary tract function recommended by the International Continence Society. Int Urogynecol J. 1990;1:45–58.
3. Davis DM. The hydrodynamics of the upper urinary tract (urodynamics). Ann Surg. 1954;140(6):839–49.
4. Chapple C, MacDiarmid S, Patel A. Urodynamics made easy. 3rd ed. Edinburgh: Elsevier Churchill Livingstone; 2009.

5. Winters JC, Dmochowski RR, Goldman HB, Herndon CD, Kobashi KC, Kraus SR, et al. Urodynamic studies in adults: AUA/SUFU guideline. J Urol. 2012;188(6 Suppl):2464–72.

6. Tubaro A, Artibani W, Delancey J, Khullar V, Vierhout M, De Gennaro M, et al. Committee 7 B imaging and other investigations. In: Paul Abrams LC, Saad K, Alan W, editors. Incontinence: 4th international consultation on incontinence. 4th ed. Paris: Health Publication Ltd.; 2009. p. 541.

7. Patel BN, Kobashi KC. Practical use of the new American Urological Association adult urodynamics guidelines. Curr Urol Rep. 2013;14(3):240–6.

8. Byrne DJ, Stewart PA, Gray BK. The role of urodynamics in female urinary stress incontinence. Br J Urol. 1987;59(3):228–9.

9. Summitt Jr RL, Stovall TG, Bent AE, Ostergard DR. Urinary incontinence: correlation of history and brief office evaluation with multichannel urodynamic testing. Am J Obstet Gynecol. 1992;166(6 Pt 1):1835–40. discussion 40–4.

10. Rovner ES, Wein AJ. Practical urodynamics. Part I. Houston: American Urological Association, Inc, Office of Education; 2002.

11. Almallah YZ, Rennie CD, Stone J, Lancashire MJ. Urinary tract infection and patient satisfaction after flexible cystoscopy and urodynamic evaluation. Urology. 2000;56(1):37–9.

12. Yokoyama T, Nozaki K, Nose H, Inoue M, Nishiyama Y, Kumon H. Tolerability and morbidity of urodynamic testing: a questionnaire-based study. Urology. 2005;66(1):74–6.

13. Abrams P, Cardozo L, Fall M, Griffiths D, Rosier P, Ulmsten U, et al. The standardisation of terminology of lower urinary tract function: report from the standardisation Sub-committee of the International Continence Society. Am J Obstet Gynecol. 2002;187(1):116–26.

14. Abrams P, Blaivas JG, Stanton SL, Andersen JT. The standardisation of terminology of lower urinary tract function. The International Continence Society Committee on Standardisation of Terminology. Scand J Urol Nephrol Suppl. 1988;114:5–19.

15. Abrams P, Andersson KE, Birder L, Brubaker L, Cardozo L, Chapple C, et al. Fourth International Consultation on Incontinence Recommendations of the International Scientific Committee: evaluation and treatment of urinary incontinence, pelvic organ prolapse, and fecal incontinence. Neurourol Urodyn. 2010;29(1):213–40.

16. Chaikin D, Romanzi L, Rosenthal J, Weiss J, Blaivas J. The effect of genital prolapse on micturition. Neurourol Urodyn. 1988;17:344.

17. Kaplan S, Dmochowski R, Cash B, Kopp Z, Berriman S, Khullar V. Systematic review of the relationship between bladder and bowel function: implications for patient management. Int J Clin Pract. 2013;67(13):205–16.

18. Abrams P. Urodynamics. 3rd ed. Singapore: Springer; 2006.

19. Blaiva J, Chancellor MB, Weiss J, Verhaaren M. Pre-urodynamic evaluation. In: Jerry B, Chancellor MB, Jeffrey W, Michael V, editors. Atlas of urodynamics. 2nd ed. Malden: Victoria Blackwell Publishing; 2007.

20. Haylen BT, de Ridder D, Freeman RM, Swift SE, Berghmans B, Lee J, et al. An International Urogynecological Association (IUGA)/International Continence Society (ICS) joint report on the terminology for female pelvic floor dysfunction. Neurourol Urodyn. 2010;29(1):4–20.

21. Messelink B, Benson T, Berghmans B, Bo K, Corcos J, Fowler C, et al. Standardization of terminology of pelvic floor muscle function and dysfunction: report from the pelvic floor clinical assessment group of the International Continence Society. Neurourol Urodyn. 2005;24(4):374–80.

22. Vodusek DB. Evoked potential testing. Urol Clin North Am. 1996;23(3):427–46.

23. Blaivas JG, Zayed AA, Labib KB. The bulbocavernosus reflex in urology: a prospective study of 299 patients. J Urol. 1981;126(2):197–9.

24. Stoller ML, Millard RJ. The accuracy of a catheterized residual urine. J Urol. 1989;141(1):15–6.

25. Purkiss SF. Assessment of residual urine in men following catheterisation. Br J Urol. 1990;66(3):279–80.

26. Bano F, Arunkalaivanan AS, Barrington JW. Comparison between bladderscan, real-time ultrasound and suprapubic catheterisation in the measurement of female residual bladder volume. J Obstet Gynaecol. 2004;24(6):694–5.

27. Groutz A, Blaivas JG, Chaikin DC, Resnick NM, Engleman K, Anzalone D, et al. Noninvasive outcome measures of urinary incontinence and lower urinary tract symptoms: a multicenter study of micturition diary and pad tests. J Urol. 2000;164(3 Pt 1):698–701.
28. Haylen BT, Lee J, Logan V, Husselbee S, Zhou J, Law M. Immediate postvoid residual volumes in women with symptoms of pelvic floor dysfunction. Obstet Gynecol. 2008;111(6): 1305–12.
29. Costantini E, Mearini E, Pajoncini C, Biscotto S, Bini V, Porena M. Uroflowmetry in female voiding disturbances. Neurourol Urodyn. 2003;22(6):569–73.
30. Radomski SB. Urodynamics of the female lower urinary tract, resting and stress urethral pressure profiles and leak point pressures. In: Drutz HP, Herschorn S, Diamant NE, editors. Female pelvic medicine and reconstructive pelvic surgery. London: Springer; 2003.
31. Addla S, Adeyouju A, Neilson D. Assessment of reliability of 1-day, 3-day and 7-day frequency volume charts. Eur Urol. 2004;3(2(Suppl)):130.
32. Staskin D, Kelleher C, Bosch R, Coyne K, Cotterill N, Emmanuel A, et al. Initial assessment of urinary and faecal incontinence in adult male and female patients. In: Abrams P, Cardozo L, Khoury S, Wein A, editors. Incontinence. 4th ed. Paris: Health Publication Ltd.; 2009.
33. Siltberg H, Victor A, Larsson G. Pad weighing tests: the best way to quantify urine loss in patients with incontinence. Acta Obstet Gynecol Scand Suppl. 1997;166:28–32.
34. Blaivas J, Chancellor MB, Weiss J, WVerhaaren M. Atlas of urodynamics. Malden: Blackwell Publishing; 2007.
35. Choe JH, Lee JS, Seo JT. Urodynamic studies in women with stress urinary incontinence: significant bacteriuria and risk factors. Neurourol Urodyn. 2007;26(6):847–51.
36. Lowder JL, Burrows LJ, Howden NL, Weber AM. Prophylactic antibiotics after urodynamics in women: a decision analysis. Int Urogynecol J Pelvic Floor Dysfunct. 2007;18(2):159–64.
37. Brostrom S, Jennum P, Lose G. Morbidity of urodynamic investigation in healthy women. Int Urogynecol J Pelvic Floor Dysfunct. 2002;13(3):182–4. discussion 4.
38. Quek P, Tay LH. Morbidity and significant bacteriuria after urodynamic studies. Ann Acad Med Singapore. 2004;33(6):754–7.
39. Pannek J, Nehiba M. Morbidity of urodynamic testing in patients with spinal cord injury: is antibiotic prophylaxis necessary? Spinal Cord. 2007;45(12):771–4.
40. Latthe PM, Foon R, Toozs-Hobson P. Prophylactic antibiotics in urodynamics: a systematic review of effectiveness and safety. Neurourol Urodyn. 2008;27(3):167–73.
41. Gray M. Traces: making sense of urodynamics testing—part 4: preparing the patient for multichannel urodynamics testing. Urol Nurs. 2011;32(2):71–7.
42. Al-Hayek S, Belal M, Abrams P. Does the patient's position influence the detection of detrusor overactivity? Neurourol Urodyn. 2008;27(4):279–86.
43. Klevmark B. Natural pressure–volume curves and conventional cystometry. Scand J Urol Nephrol Suppl. 1999;201:1–4.
44. Merrill DC. The air cystometer: a new instrument for evaluating bladder function. J Urol. 1971;106(6):865–6.
45. Scarpero HM, Padmanabhan P, Xue X, Nitti VW. Patient perception of videourodynamic testing: a questionnaire based study. J Urol. 2005;173(2):555–9.
46. Gray M. Traces: making sense of urodynamics testing. Urol Nurs. 2010;30(5):267–75.
47. Zhang P, Wu ZJ, Gao JZ. Impact of catheter on uroflow rate in pressure-flow study. Chin Med J (Engl). 2004;117(11):1732–4.
48. Mortensen S, Lose G, Thyssen H. Repeatability of cystometry and pressure-flow parameters in female patients. Int Urogynecol J Pelvic Floor Dysfunct. 2002;13(2):72–5.
49. Versi E. Discriminant analysis of urethral pressure profilometry data for the diagnosis of genuine stress incontinence. Br J Obstet Gynaecol. 1990;97(3):251–9.

Chapter 6
Artifact Recognition and Solutions in Urodynamics

Ross Rames and Lara S. MacLachlan

Introduction

Properly performed urodynamics can be an invaluable tool for those charged with the task of caring for patients with complex voiding dysfunction. By capturing specific information regarding a patient's bladder function, these studies can clarify the clinical picture and uncover unexpected issues. The ultimate goal is to use this information to render more effective treatment and relief of symptoms.

Artifacts are observations or findings occurring during urodynamic studies that are not naturally present in the patient's normal micturition process, and are the result of the study itself. They can arise from technical problems with catheters, electrodes, transducers, or other electrical equipment. The unnatural conditions of the urodynamic experience can create problems: the consistency, temperature, and rate of infusion of fluid filling the bladder; the presence of a catheter occupying space in the urethral and bowel lumen; and the socially uncomfortable predicament of genital exposure and bladder filling, followed by voiding in an environment that does not approximate a normal situation in a person's daily routine. When artifacts are present they can obscure the information that is sought. When unrecognized and uncorrected, they may lead to a missed diagnosis, or a misdiagnosis, and result in inappropriate, less effective, or potentially harmful treatment plans.

R. Rames, MD (✉) • L.S. MacLachlan, MD
Department of Urology, Medical University of South Carolina,
96 Jonathan Lucas Street, CSB 644, Charleston, SC 29425, USA
e-mail: ramesr@musc.edu; maclachl@musc.edu

© Springer Science+Business Media New York 2015
E.S. Rovner, M.E. Koski (eds.), *Rapid and Practical Interpretation
of Urodynamics*, DOI 10.1007/978-1-4939-1764-8_6

This chapter will review some of the more common artifacts one may encounter during the performance of urodynamic studies. We will explore the causes of these artifacts and what can be done to mitigate the problems. These technical problems are common, at times frustrating, and possibly overlooked or misinterpreted. It is for this reason that urodynamics should be performed and/or supervised closely by qualified personnel. One should be cautious about accepting the interpretation of studies without a thorough personal review of the actual tracing and any radiographic observations.

Urodynamic Catheters

Catheters used for urodynamic studies have two purposes. The first is the measurement of pressures within a body cavity. The second, in the case of the bladder catheter, is the instillation of fluid, typically saline or a radiographic contrast agent, in order to simulate physiologic bladder filling. This allows a glimpse into the normally unseen world of bladder filling and storage function, and its continence mechanisms, followed by bladder emptying where detrusor contractility and the status of the bladder outlet are investigated.

Currently two types of systems are in common use; fluid charged and air charged. Other systems are available utilizing microtransducer and fiberoptic catheters. Due to practical limitations such as expense, fragility, and the need for sterilization and reuse, these are not often employed clinically.

Water charged catheters transmit pressure from within a body cavity through a continuous fluid medium in the lumen of the catheter to a transducer. The transducer converts pressure changes to electrical signals, which are then recorded. This system depends on an uninterrupted course of fluid for pressure transmission. As such, careful calibration is necessary and technical problems may create artifacts during the study. Common among these would be gas bubbles or kinks in the lines that attenuate pressure changes, and alterations in patient position that could shift pressure readings.

Fluid filled systems are unidirectional, depending on open exposure of the catheter port to the lumen of the body cavity. Occlusion of this port by contact with the wall or debris within the bladder could alter transmission of pressure to the transducer.

Air-charged catheters transmit pressure changes via a small circumferentially positioned balloon through the catheter lumen to an external transducer. In contrast to the unidirectional fluid charged catheter, the sensing membrane of the balloon allows detection of pressure in an omnidirectional manner. This characteristic makes contact with debris or the bladder wall less likely to impair pressure transmission (Fig. 6.1). Additionally, since air is a nearly weightless transmission medium, changes in patient position are less likely to create problematic artifacts such as a shift in baseline pressure. Comparisons of readings obtained from the various systems (air-charged catheters, water-filled catheters, microtip transducers)

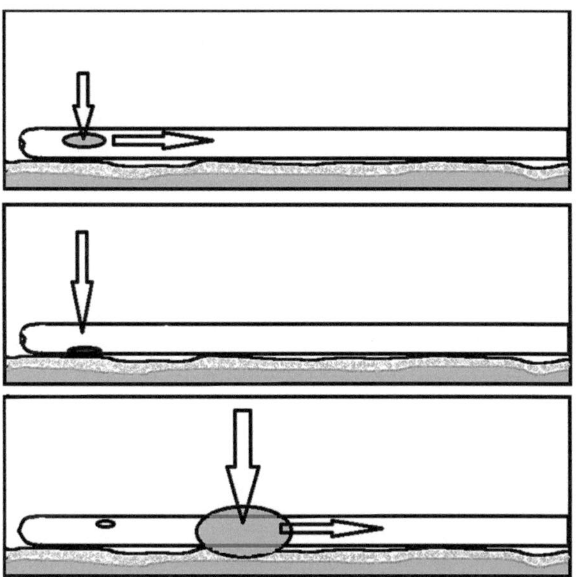

Fig. 6.1 *Top*: Water charged catheter with appropriate orientation of catheter. Lumen transmits pressure to the transducer. *Middle*: Occlusion of the catheter lumen by urothelium precludes pressure transmission. *Bottom*: Air-charged catheter is omnidirectional, transmitting pressure regardless of the balloon orientation with the bladder sidewall

have been shown to quantitatively differ [1, 2]. In addition there appears to be wide variations in the differences between readings produced by the different catheter systems. The clinical significance of this is unknown.

Several parameters are measured during complex cystometry, and all are potential sources of artifacts.

Pves

This is measured via a catheter that is typically inserted per urethra into the bladder and used to infuse fluid into and measure pressure within the bladder during the urodynamic study. The catheter is typically of relatively small diameter, approximately 7 F, to minimize obstruction of the bladder outlet during the voiding phase of the study.

Pabd

This parameter is measured by a catheter that lacks an infusion port and is typically inserted into the rectum to measure abdominal pressures via a fluid filled or air-charged balloon. Some practitioners prefer to insert this into the upper vaginal vault to capture abdominal pressure readings. The International Continence Society recommends use of a rectal balloon catheter with the balloon only filled to 10–20 % of its unstretched capacity [3]. This can help prevent pressure artifacts arising from contact between the catheter opening and the cavity wall. The Pabd catheter measures the total abdominal pressure including that due to intra-abdominal contents.

Pdet

This represents the intrinsic pressure generated by the detrusor, determined by subtracting Pabd from Pves. This value reflects static pressure from the compliance of the bladder wall and contractions of the detrusor muscle.

EMG

Along with pressure readings recorded over time, the electrical activity of the perineal musculature is recorded as a part of most pressure-flow urodynamic studies. This electromyographic, or EMG, portion of the study allows the examiner an insight into the activity of the pelvic floor and striated sphincter during the filling and voiding phases of micturition. While needle electrodes might give a more accurate representation of muscle activity, they are impractical due to invasiveness and patient discomfort. As a rule, patch electrodes are positioned over the perineum to record EMG activity. These surface electrodes are noninvasive, rarely cause any discomfort for the patient, but do introduce sources of artifact.

Uroflowmetry and Voided Volume

Gravimetric uroflow machines utilize a load cell, essentially a scale, or a hydrostatic transducer to record the weight of voided fluid over time and in total. A second type of system utilizes a spinning disc rotated at a constant rate. Flow rates are determined by measuring the increased electrical energy required to maintain the constant rotational velocity of the disc as it is slowed by contact with the voided fluid.

Filling Rate

The rate of filling is usually standardized for each lab. A typical medium filling rate for an adult is around 50–70 mL per minute. Rates for pediatric patients may be based on age and estimated bladder capacity.

Potential Sources of Study Artifacts: Recognition and Trouble-Shooting

Infusion

Typical "medium" and "high" filling rates are usually much higher than what would be considered physiologic, and can lead to changes in bladder behavior manifested by increases in detrusor pressure and sensory sensitivity.

Solutions

When infusion at a standard rate triggers immediate increases in detrusor pressure either due to decreased compliance or detrusor overactivity, a reduction in the filling rate may allow the bladder to accommodate a larger volume. The goal should be to attain a filling volume similar to typical voiding volumes seen in the patient's voiding diary. At times the infusion rate may be adjusted based on the capacity and irritability of the individual's bladder. For instance, when filling a very capacious low-pressure bladder, one may choose to increase infusion to a rapid rate of 100 mL per minute in order to expedite completion of the study.

Mismatch of Signals

One of the more common artifacts seen during performance of urodynamic studies is mismatch of signals. During voluntary abdominal straining or cough maneuvers, both Pves and Pabd should demonstrate nearly mirror-image increases in pressure. If the Pves and Pabd readings do not track each other (Fig. 6.2) the examiner should be alerted that the pressures read by the transducers may not accurately reflect those within the bladder or the abdomen.

One of the more common issues seen with mismatch of signal is catheter misplacement and resultant dampening of the signal from the transducer. A common finding encountered is the placement of the catheter tip against or within a fold of the wall of the bladder. In such a situation, the sensor port or balloon is not exposed to the lumen and therefore will not accurately transmit the lumen pressure. As the bladder fills, distention of the bladder wall may expose the tip of the catheter, suddenly revealing a different pressure or a dramatic change in the sensitivity to variations in pressure.

Stool in the rectal vault may impact readings from the Pabd catheter. This is a common issue in the population undergoing urodynamics due to the prevalence of constipation. Fecal material engulfing the tip of the Pabd catheter may cause considerable signal dampening and thus prevent accurate pressure measurements.

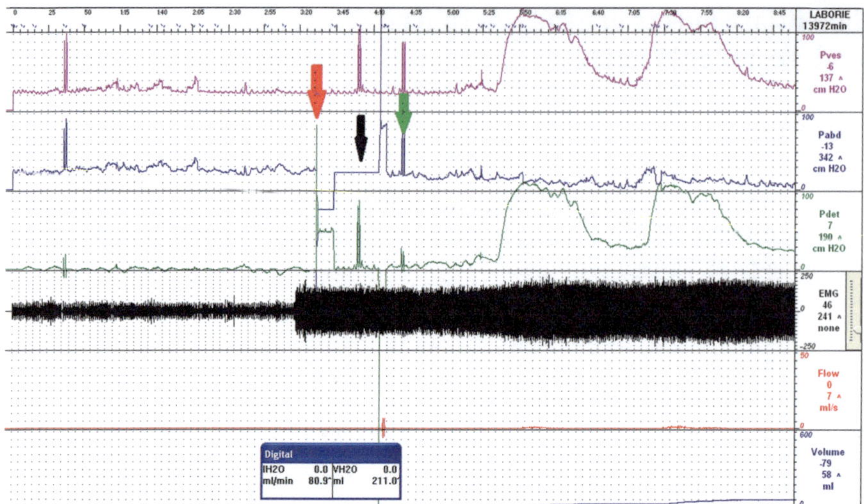

Fig. 6.2 Signal mismatch. The Pabd catheter stops transducing (*red arrow*) and a cough maneuver demonstrates brisk pressure increases in Pves, but not in Pabd (*black arrow*). The Pabd issue is corrected, and repeat cough maneuver demonstrates mirrored pressure increases in Pves and Pabd (*green arrow*)

Likewise, air bubbles or kinks in the tubing, incorrectly positioned stopcocks in the lines of water-filled systems, or failure to charge an air-charged catheter may dampen or obscure the transmission of pressures. At times one may observe decreasing pressures, along with mismatch, raising the possibility of a poor connection and resultant leak somewhere in the system. Observing a gradual increase in resting pressures may suggest migration of a catheter into the region of the urethral or anal sphincter. Should continued catheter migration occur beyond the sphincter, resting pressure may decrease accompanied by pressure transmission attenuation. Rarely one may encounter a catheter with a defect rendering it unusable for a study.

Solutions

Signal transduction should always be confirmed at the start of the pressure-flow urodynamic study by observing symmetric changes in Pves and Pabd with a cough or Valsalva maneuver. Observation of signal mismatch should be followed by a systematic investigation of its cause, correction, and resumption of the study. A thorough check of the tubing, connections, stopcocks, and transducers may reveal the source of the artifact. Air within a line or transducer of a water charged system, or a partially closed stopcock or a loose connection point can drastically alter and dampen transmission of pressure changes. Flushing out the water-filled system and placing all stopcocks fully in the appropriate positions should remedy the situation. Assure tight connections between the catheters and lines, and that the tubing is connected to the correct port of the catheter. Double check that the air-charged catheter is in the charged position.

Once the tubing and connections have been checked, the investigator should consider problems with the position of the catheter. Visual inspection may reveal a catheter that has clearly migrated out of position. If utilizing radiography during the study, this may be an adjunct to establishing catheter position. Excessive advancement of catheters may result in kinking and subsequent obstruction and dampening of pressure transduction. Correction of these issues may be accomplished by gently changing the position of the catheter while monitoring the pressure reading during cough and strain maneuvers. The catheter should be secured when appropriate readings are obtained. The infusion of a small amount of fluid into the bladder may make it easier to attain an interface between the catheter tip and intravesical fluid.

Mismatch caused by advancing the Pabd catheter into a fecal bolus or within a fold in the rectal wall may be remedied by repositioning or fecal evacuation. Asking the patient to attempt to have a bowel movement prior to the study may prevent issues with stool in the rectal vault. Patients on a bowel regimen can time their treatments in order to enter the urodynamics laboratory with an empty rectum. Occasionally more aggressive interventions, such as enemas, laxatives, and manual disimpaction are required.

If all investigations and repositioning attempts are unsuccessful, consideration should be given to replacement of the malfunctioning catheter.

Pabd/Pves Drift

On occasion pressure readings will begin to shift, or "drift," after zeroing as the study ensues. This results in an inaccurate calculation of detrusor pressure (Pdet).

Changes in the pressure within the rectum caused by peristalsis may also cause shifts in Pabd (Fig. 6.3). If the lead was zeroed during a period of increased tone, subsequent relaxation during the study will cause a decrease in Pabd and a corresponding increase in the Pdet reading that does not reflect a true increase in bladder pressure. If Pabd is zeroed at low rectal pressure, a peristaltic increase in rectal pressure during the study results in increased Pabd readings with corresponding spurious decrease in Pdet. Pdet pressure readings therefore may even be deflected into the negative range, which is not physiologically possible.

Connection problems or changes in position of the Pves catheter can cause drifts in the Pves pressure readings. As noted previously, Pves drift may occur when the tip of the Pves catheter is initially against the bladder wall and obscured. As the bladder fills, the sensing portion of the Pves catheter becomes exposed to the lumen resulting in a shift in baseline pressure that may be gradual or dramatic.

During voiding, a decrease in Pabd pressure that is not present in Pves may be seen in approximately 5 % of studies [4]. Pabd readings falling below resting pressure will cause a false increase in Pdet, potentially giving the artifactual appearance of adequate contractility (when it is not present) or even a diagnosis of bladder

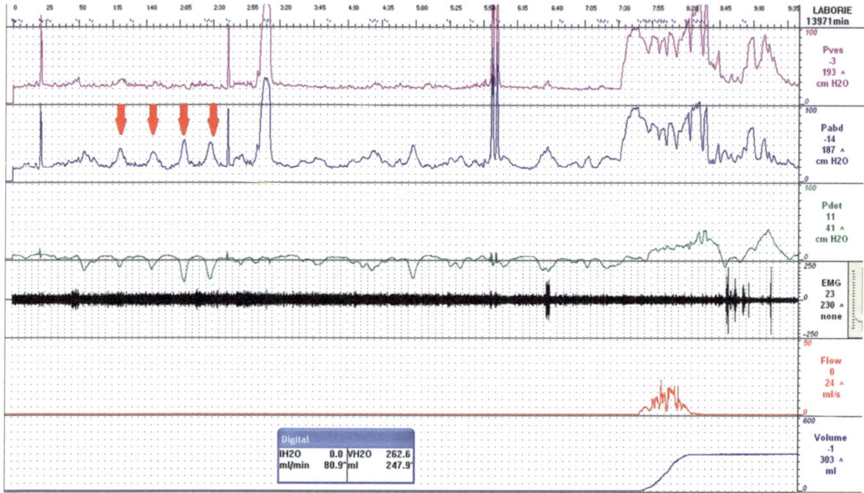

Fig. 6.3 Pabd drift. Rectal contraction (*red arrows*) with resultant artifactual negative deflection of Pdet. Note that Pves remains relatively constant and is not the source of changes in the pressure readings of Pdet

outlet obstruction. Although the mechanism involved is not well defined, this may be caused by relaxation of the pelvic floor. Thus, it is necessary to do a careful examination of all traces emanating from all channels during the voiding portion of the study to avoid misinterpretation.

Solutions

Filling should be stopped and the patient should be queried about any change in sensation, such as an urge to void, passing of flatus, or urgency to have a bowel movement. This should be noted on the tracing. The examiner should compare the Pves to Pdet channel. Observations of increases or decreases in Pdet not associated with a corresponding change in Pves are likely from Pabd "drift." Pressures should be observed for a period of time. Quite often the rectal peristaltic wave will subside, pressure readings will return to baseline, and the study may be resumed. Persistent rectal peristaltic waves may simply have to be carefully taken into account during interpretation of the study.

The catheters should be checked to confirm appropriate positioning and connections. Dislodged catheters may enter the bladder neck or sphincter, with resultant alterations in pressure. If the examiner determines the pressure reading change is due to alterations in the catheter position, they should be repositioned appropriately. Pabd and Pves may then be re-zeroed if necessary when pressures are at baseline and the study completed.

EMG Trouble-shooting

Extraneous electrical activity due to a malfunction in the CMG machine or leads may appear as muscle activity on the EMG. It is not uncommon for an electrode to become wet during a study, or for a patch to lose adherence to the perineal skin. This will result in abnormal activity similar to that demonstrated in Fig. 6.4. This issue occurs more commonly in women due to proximity of the urethral meatus to the patch electrodes in the perineum.

While this artifact is less common in men, it may be encountered. Excess hair, moist skin, or topical agents such as moisturizers or barrier creams at the electrode application site may lead to poor adherence and abnormal EMG tracings.

Similarly, patient movement or abdominal straining may result in increased EMG activity. This can be confusing, particularly when one of the objectives of the study is to evaluate the patient for detrusor external sphincter dyssynergia. Patients should be carefully observed for movement and straining throughout the study and it should be noted on the tracing. Straining during voiding is quite common and may result in a flare of the EMG tracing as seen in Fig. 6.5. This straining pattern is typically marked by an increase in the EMG activity and the pressure in Pabd and Pves. When observed, the patient should be queried if this represents their usual voiding pattern.

Patients undergoing urodynamic evaluation often have complex voiding dysfunction, and may have undergone prior surgical interventions. Neuromodulation therapy, as well as other implanted electrical devices, may produce a distinctive regular pattern on EMG, demonstrated in Fig. 6.6.

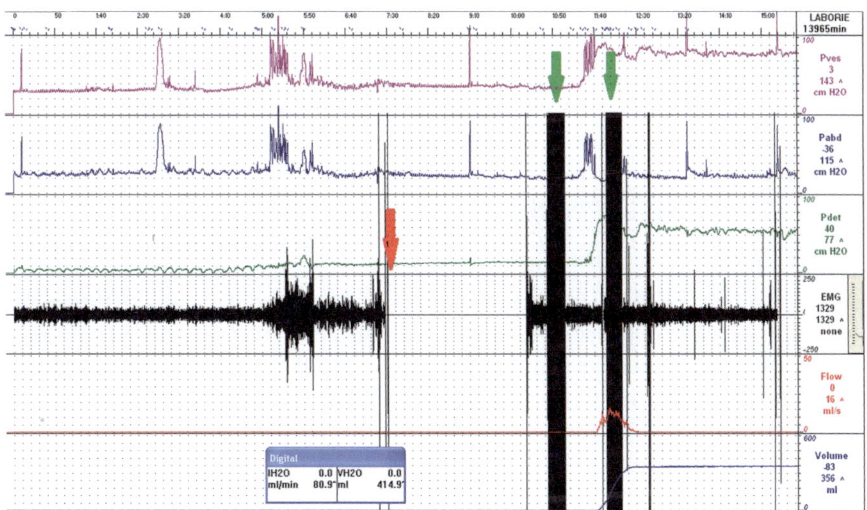

Fig. 6.4 EMG artifact. All of the EMG leads lose contact and stop transducing during the study (*red arrow*). Loss of contact of one of the EMG leads causes flaring not associated with perineal muscular activity (*green arrows*)

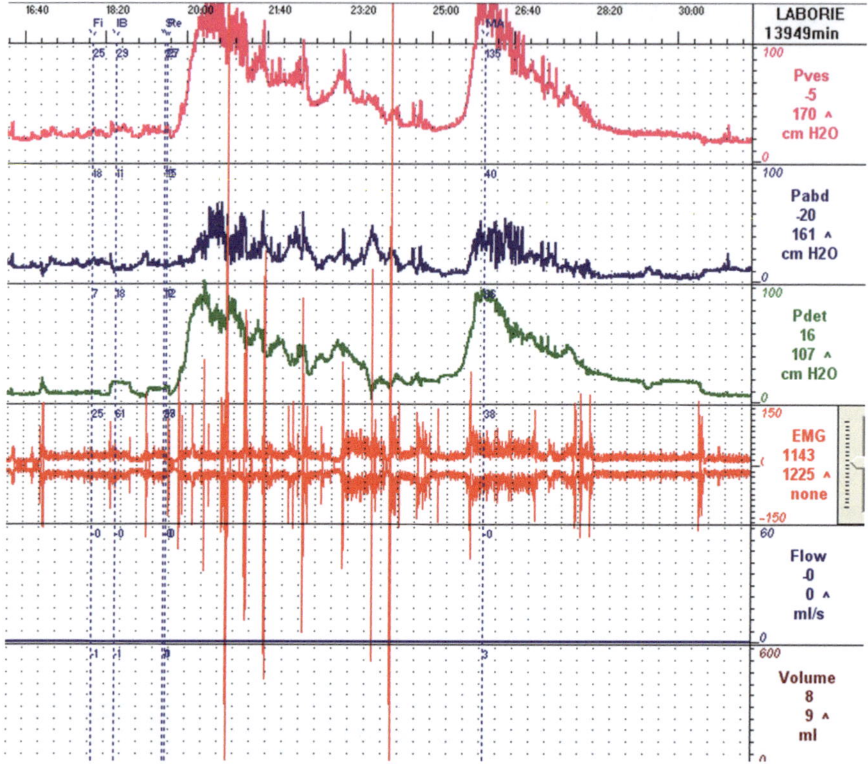

Fig. 6.5 EMG flares as patient strains during voiding attempt

Solutions

EMG patches with shielded cables are preferable to patches with unshielded wires because they avoid potential artifacts when exposed to urinary flow or environmental noise [5]. The application of an occlusive dressing or tape may help solve the problem of dislodged EMG leads. Clipping or shaving excess hair and the removal of topical barrier protectants with a cleanser may be necessary to maintain adequate electrode adherence. Alcohol-based cleansers should be avoided because they paradoxically increase impedance to the EMG signal [5]. History and examination should reveal the presence of an implanted pulse generator. If a regular pulsed pattern is noted on the EMG tracing, sacral neuromodulation may be temporarily stopped to confirm and eliminate this source of potential artifact.

Psychogenic Inhibition

Perhaps one of the most common issues encountered in the urodynamics lab is the inability to void normally during the study. This may be a new issue for the patient, or they may relate a long history of "bashful bladder" with difficulty using public

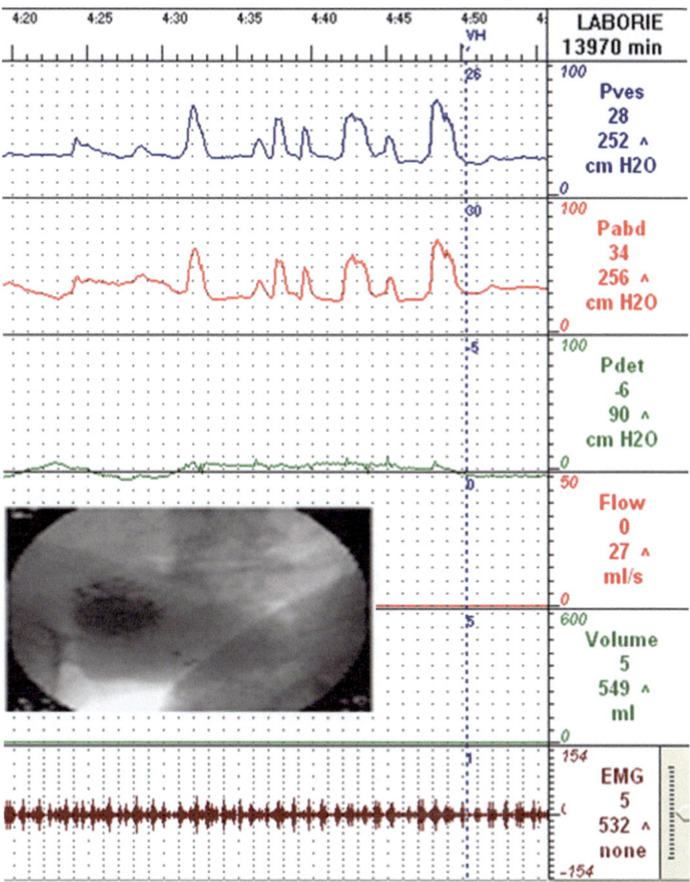

Fig. 6.6 Regular pulsed pattern noted on the EMG with its likely source an implanted pulse generator, seen on fluoroscopy inset

restrooms, or changes in voiding habits associated with stressful situations such as travel or medical visits.

When a patient is unable to void during an urodynamic study, the examiner is unable to definitively determine if the patient has poor detrusor contractility, bladder outlet obstruction, vesicoureteral reflux, or any other voiding dysfunction. Psychogenic inhibition has no specific diagnostic meaning, and patients who are unable to void may have a variety of findings when monitored with ambulatory urodynamics such as concomitant non-relaxation of the urinary sphincter or pelvic floor, bladder outlet obstruction, or normal voiding patterns [6–8]. Most patients who are unable to void during a clinical UDS study are able to mount a detrusor contraction during voiding attempts on ambulatory urodynamics during normal daily life activities [6, 8].

Solutions

Privacy screens, limiting personnel present, and avoiding unnecessary traffic in the urodynamics lab may help the patient feel more relaxed. Using a "white noise" generator or playing relaxing music may cover background clinic sounds and create an environment more conducive to voiding. Running water in the sink and bathing the patient's hands in warm water may help initiate micturition. At times leaving the exam area and monitoring the study remotely, or returning only after the patient has begun voiding, may be enough to capture the sought after information [9].

Common Uroflowmetry Artifacts

Several commonly seen uroflow issues should be recognized and corrected during the performance of urodynamic studies. Inadvertent contact or bumping of the uroflow collection receptacle can cause a spike in the uroflow reading, and subsequent misreporting of urinary flow rates and voided volumes (Fig. 6.7).

A second common source of uroflow artifact results when the urine stream "misses" and is not captured on the study. The flow of urine may arc over the capture funnel, or track down tubing outside of the flow capture zone. In women, voided urine may reflux up into the vagina or seep back down along the drapes and avoid capture on uroflowmetry.

A flow artifact most typically seen with male subjects presents with alternating increases and decreases in the flow rate caused by pinching and occluding, and then releasing the urethra. A second, perhaps more common cause of this flow pattern has been described as "waggling" or "cruising," and is the result of the urinary

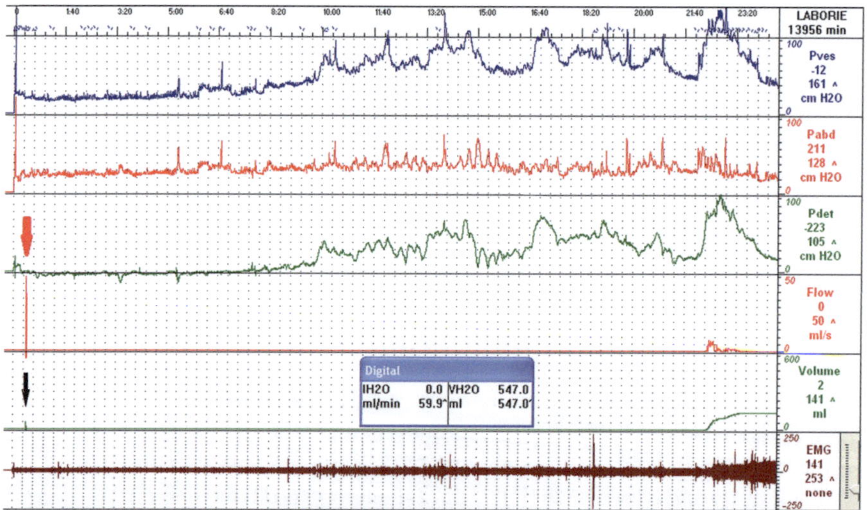

Fig. 6.7 Bumping the uroflow. The uroflowmeter is inadvertently bumped at the beginning of the study. This artifact may alter flow (*red arrow*) and volume (*black arrow*) measurements if not corrected

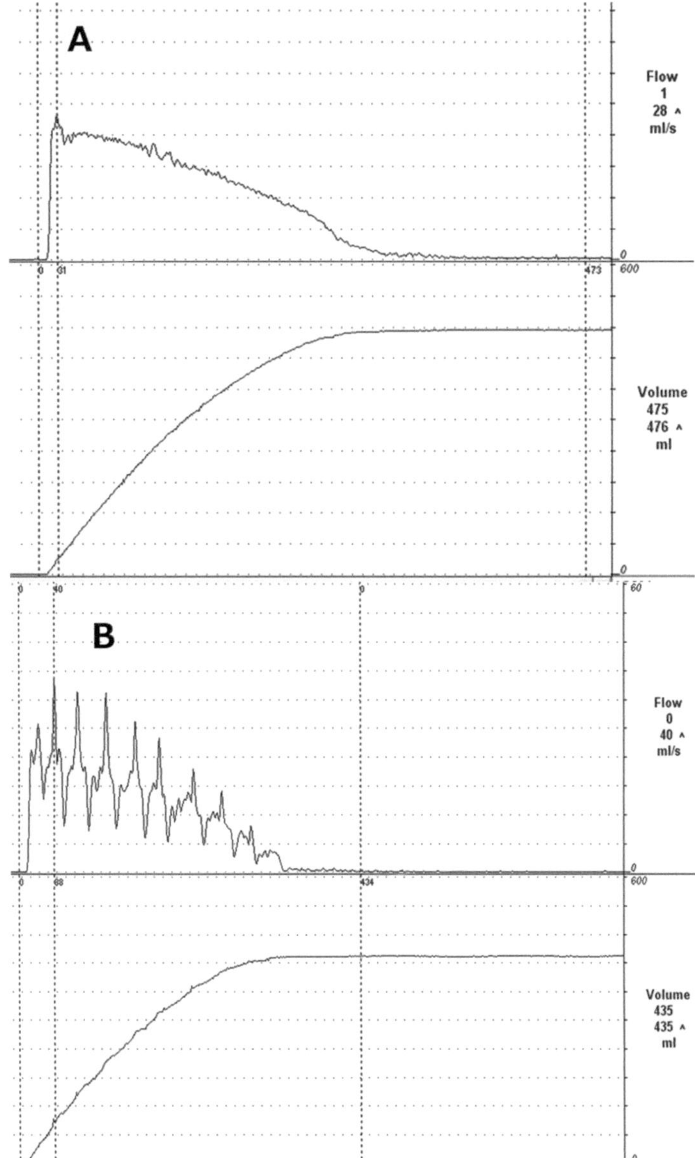

Fig. 6.8 Cruising/waggling uroflow (**a**) Uroflowmetry with stream directed at a single site on the collection funnel. (**b**) Uroflowmetry demonstrates the "cruising" or "waggling" pattern when an identical flow and volume are directed up and down the collection funnel

stream being directed up and down the side of the collection funnel. As the stream is directed toward the upper portion of the funnel, the transit time down to the collection and measurement device increases and results in an apparent and false decrease in flow rate. Movement of the stream impact point toward the center of the funnel has the opposite effect [10]. See Fig. 6.8.

Solutions

Should an inadvertent "bump" of the uroflowmeter occur, the examiner should note this on the tracing, and manually mark initiation of flow, peak flow as well as the termination of voiding. Alternatively, during the study, one may re-zero the flow and voided volume portion of the study.

Complete capture of the urine stream can be enhanced by the use of wide collection funnels, draping the tubing into the funnel and improvised deflection screens to channel urine flow to the collection unit. Capture devices create a slight delay in the recording of urine flow as the urine works its way down to its intended destination. While this delay is not usually clinically significant, the examiner may wish to mark the exact time that urine flow begins during the study.

Patients should be directed to refrain from manually occluding their urethras, and to direct their streams to a single spot on the collection funnel to avoid the "waggling" or "cruising" artifact.

Fixed Restrictions

Lesions such as urethral strictures and bladder neck contractures may create annular restrictions in the normally distensible urinary outlet. Here the presence of the small diameter Pves catheter can create obstruction, decrease urinary flow rates, and increase voiding pressures. What appears to be a significant obstruction, may in fact be an artifact, and not reflecting the true status of the urinary outlet in the absence of the urodynamics catheter [9].

Solutions

Uroflowmetry performed prior to placement of Pves should be used as a baseline. When significantly different from the observed pressure-flow study, further investigation should be considered. Cystoscopy or urography may reveal the underlying source of this finding, such as a fixed obstruction.

Infusion Errors

Pumps used to infuse fluid into the bladder may employ various mechanisms. One common form is the use of a roller to sequentially compress a malleable portion of tubing to move the infusing fluid along in a calibrated fashion. Trouble may arise from errors in calibration, obstruction of tubing, incorrect placement of tubing within the infusion pump, or leaks in the tubing.

Solutions

Calibration according to manufacturer's recommendations should be performed regularly and when a problem is suspected. During the study, visual monitoring should confirm that infusion is occurring by observing the drip chamber. Clamped, kinked, or reversed tubing in the pump can result in impeded flow or even withdrawal of fluid from the bladder. A visual inspection of the entire length of tubing will often reveal the issue.

During the study the examiner should monitor the markings on the bottle or bag of infusing fluid to confirm that the volumes approximate the readings recorded on the CMG tracing. Finally, a direct measure of the voided volume in the collection beaker should be compared to the infused volume on the study. Lack of concordance may indicate missed flow, the need for calibration, or other issues such as diuresis or post-void residual urine.

Conclusions

Complex urodynamics are, by their nature, prone to significant artifacts owing to the difficult task of examining a human subject using invasive, sophisticated, and complicated equipment. Erroneous input can be entered at multiple points, and the readings obtained on the CMG can also be adversely impacted by technical and human factors. The key to obtaining accurate and informative studies lies first in the performance of the study, and then in the careful interpretation. Artifacts detected during the performance of the examination can often be corrected prior to the completion of the study. Those recognized after completion can be taken into account in order to arrive at more meaningful conclusions. In some cases the investigator may conclude that the study should be repeated. All of these efforts are necessary to afford our patients the best possible treatment and outcomes.

References

1. Digesu GA, Derpapas A, Robshaw P, Vijaya G, Hendricken C, Khullar V. Are the measurements of water-filled and air-charged catheters the same in urodynamics? Int Urogynecol J. 2014;25(1):123–30.
2. Hundley AF, Brown MB, Brubaker L, Cundiff GW, Kreder K, Lotze P, et al. A multicentered comparison of measurements obtained with microtip and external water pressure transducers. Int Urogynecol J Pelvic Floor Dysfunct. 2006;17(4):400–6.
3. Schafer W, Abrams P, Liao L, Mattiasson A, Pesce F, Spangberg A, et al. Good urodynamic practices: uroflowmetry, filling cystometry, and pressure-flow studies. Neurourol Urodyn. 2002;21(3):261–74.
4. Hogan S, Gammie A, Abrams P. Urodynamic features and artefacts. Neurourol Urodyn. 2012;31(7):1104–17.

5. Gray M. Traces: making sense of urodynamics testing—part 3: electromyography of the pelvic floor muscles. Urol Nurs. 2011;31(1):31–8.
6. van Koeveringe GA, Rahnama'i MS, Berghmans BC. The additional value of ambulatory urodynamic measurements compared with conventional urodynamic measurements. BJU Int. 2010;105(4):508–13.
7. van Waalwijk van Doorn E, Anders K, Khullar V, Kulseng-Hanssen S, Pesce F, Robertson A, et al. Standardisation of ambulatory urodynamic monitoring: report of the Standardisation Sub-Committee of the International Continence Society for ambulatory urodynamic studies. Neurourol Urodyn. 2000;19(2):113–25.
8. Rosario DJ, Chapple CR, Tophill PR, Woo HH. Urodynamic assessment of the bashful bladder. J Urol. 2000;163(1):215–20.
9. Gray M. Traces: making sense of urodynamics testing—part 10: evaluation of micturition via the voiding pressure-flow study. Urol Nurs. 2012;32(2):71–8.
10. Addla SK, Marri RR, Daayana SL, Irwin P. Avoid cruising on the uroflowmeter: evaluation of cruising artifact on spinning disc flowmeters in an experimental setup. Neurourol Urodyn. 2010;29(7):1301–5.

Chapter 7
Optimizing the Study

Lynette E. Franklin

Comprehensive guidelines for good urodynamic practices have been developed and reviewed by experts within the International Continence Society [1]. These expert guidelines are best translated into a clinically effective study when combined with practical clinical knowledge that helps identify and resolve any barriers to performing a high quality study. Pressure-flow urodynamics are, in general, a nonphysiological test: the study involves rapid filling, with room temperature fluid, which is NOT urine, conducted in a clinical setting without privacy. Advance planning and real time trouble-shooting of issues such as patient factors, laboratory environment, and other challenges in performing this test can improve the patient experience and clinical utility, as well as the resultant treatment outcomes of urodynamics. This chapter will outline some methods to optimize this study under these difficult conditions.

Patient Factors Prior to the Start of the Study

Ultimately, the clinician conducting the test needs to be able to fulfill the aim of the study, which is to reproduce the symptoms or assess the lower urinary tract condition that the patient experiences outside the clinic, and to accomplish these goals in an artificial laboratory setting. Appropriate clinical questions must be asked prior to, during, and at the completion of the study to direct effective performance of the study. Complete assessment of the patient's chief complaint and other signs and symptoms are gathered by oral report, physical exam, pad test, and voiding and/or catheterization diaries. A thorough understanding of the patient's clinical condition will allow comparison of pre-study findings with those demonstrated during the

L.E. Franklin, MSN, APRN-BC, CWOCN-AP, CFCN (✉)
Wound Ostomy & Continence Nursing Education, Emory University,
1762 Clifton Road, NE, Suite 2200, J205, Atlanta, GA 30322-4001, USA
email: lynette.franklin@emory.edu

© Springer Science+Business Media New York 2015
E.S. Rovner, M.E. Koski (eds.), *Rapid and Practical Interpretation of Urodynamics*, DOI 10.1007/978-1-4939-1764-8_7

urodynamic examination, which will allow the practitioner to gauge the reliability of the study data and to help guide the reproduction of key symptoms.

Patient factors such as embarrassment, anxiety, and pain must be carefully considered. Pressure-flow urodynamics are invasive studies that are done with a lack of privacy, however the expectation is to reproduce functions that are not typically a public occurrence. An initial discussion with the patient about the study and its expectations may overcome one of the first obstacles to eliciting good results by establishing open communication and stating the basics of the test. Simply identifying that this is an anxiety producing situation may be beneficial. Additionally, consideration of alternative therapies to reduce anxiety may be beneficial to the study outcomes. One such intervention might be playing appropriate, low level music, or attention to patient gowning in the laboratory. One study has shown that simple measures such as music or attention to gowning may significantly reduce anxiety during gynecologic exams. Considering that the gynecological exam is an experience in some ways similar to that of urodynamics, such measures, or other comforting measures, may translate into reducing anxiety in the urodynamic laboratory as well [2].

Improving Diagnostic Utility

Room Preparation

It is important to prepare an urodynamic room that will provide a setting that conveys privacy, warmth, and economy of movement to the best possible extent. The exam room area should include a private changing space as well as toileting facilities. An ergonomic design facilitates patient movement, especially for those with mobility limitations, which are common in the patient population undergoing urodynamic studies.

Urodynamics are often performed in individuals with significant mobility limitations. Because of this fact, consideration should be given for adequate space in the room to accommodate the transfer of the patient who is dependent on a wheelchair, scooter, or stretcher such that a minimum of movement of the urodynamic and radiology equipment will be needed to position the patient and perform the study. This care will help ensure dignity to the patient who is unable to move independently while decreasing the potential for damage to the urodynamics equipment. In addition, patient transfer lifts, boards and slides should be readily available, and the staff should be well trained in the mechanics needed to provide safe and efficient patient movement and positioning in the urodynamics room. Training with a physical therapist, practice demonstrations, and competency testing will ensure that the staff have confidence in their skills with dependent patient transfer.

Strategically placed curtains at door entrances help to provide a room that is more private and secure. The room should be set up so that supplies are easily available throughout the study without the need to leave the patient unattended. Surplus supplies can be housed in fixed cupboards or shelving in the room, but routine testing supplies and extras should be available on a rolling cart within close proximity to the exam table, which will assist in timely preparation of the patient for the study.

Room temperature should be ambient, as beyond first consideration of patient comfort, excessively cold temperature may suppress the ability to void. The temperature should be a balance between enough warmth for the minimally clothed patient while maintaining an environment cool enough for the proper function and maintenance of the mechanical equipment needed for urodynamic testing. Checking with the manufacturer of the urodynamic and radiology equipment for ideal operational temperatures is advised.

A well stocked urodynamics room includes a variety of adjunctive supplies necessary for a well done, expedient, and efficient study. Such supplies include the following. (1) A pessary fitting kit that will aid in reduction of pelvic organ prolapse (POP), (2) Penile clamps and urethral plugs for patients who have intractable stress urinary incontinence (SUI) such that an assessment of bladder capacity can be made. (3) Various tape selections to help secure tubes while providing for patients who may have adhesive allergies. (4) Ostomy supplies for intubation of ostomy pouches, and ability to change the appliance if needed. (5) A variety of catheters (see later discussion). (6) Lubrication supplies. (7) Sterile catheterization kits. (8) Drapes. (9) Extra UDS transducers, EMG pads, and leads, etc.

Reproduction of Symptoms

Education regarding the performance of the study and patient experience/expectations of the study should be communicated prior to, during and after testing. Written instructions at a grade four to six reading level in black print on a white surface are ideal. The patient education should be succinct, providing key information to help complete the study successfully. This education should include:

- a brief overview of the study
- expectations of the time required for the study
- how the study is performed including key portions of the study such as the need for urethral and rectal catheters
- the information that will be obtained from the study and how such information may benefit the patient
- patient responsibilities prior to study:

  - pad test
  - voiding diary
  - need and directions for prophylactic premedication (for example prophylaxis for contrast dye allergy in video urodynamic studies or antibiotics in certain populations)

- patient responsibilities during the study:

  - communicate if study is reproducing home symptoms
  - notification of first sensation, desire to void, attempt to void when directed, pain, strong desire to void
  - to ask questions if unclear of instructions

- patient responsibilities after the study:
  - take prophylactic antibiotic as directed
  - to call healthcare provider for unexpected signs and symptoms (fever, dysuria, hematuria, etc.)
  - schedule follow-up with provider to discuss study and treatment plan

Orally communicating these same teaching points with the patient will help to reinforce the concepts with the patient. Cues in the exam room will also reinforce the data needed to help optimize the study. Large plain cards, with written cues, fastened to the wall in front of the patient will remind the patient throughout the study using visual stimuli.

Examples of visual cue cards to be posted in the room include:

1. "Goal of study: to reproduce your voiding symptoms as if you are at home"
2. "First sensation: any feeling of something in your bladder once test is started: wet, cold, pressure or pain, etc"
3. "First desire to void: when you feel you need to void (pee) 'If you were driving in a car, you would ask to stop at the next rest area' or 'You would get up at the next commercial if watching television'"
4. "Strong desire to void 'If you were driving down the road you would ask to pull over to void (pee) behind a bush/tree' 'Can't hold one more drop'"
5. "Do not attempt to void until you are told to do so"

For some patients reproducing symptoms can be challenging. For example, the demonstration of urodynamic SUI can be difficult in some individuals. The urodynamics testing environment may create anxiety or pain in these individuals resulting in pelvic floor spasm and a situationally increased urethral resistance which may mask SUI. The AUA/SUFU UDS Guidelines state that when evaluating such a patient with symptomatic SUI in whom a leak point pressure cannot be demonstrated, that the clinician can repeat the study with the urethral catheter removed. This may permit the demonstration of SUI and an assessment of the abdominal leak point pressure using the Pabd transducer. For other patients with symptomatic SUI in whom the condition has not been demonstrated even with the urethral catheter removed, it can be helpful to reposition the patient into a standing position during the urodynamic study. Attempting to place the patient in the position that most commonly elicits leakage (which would be the standing position for most patients with SUI) will aid in reproducing the home symptoms. Finally, reduction of a high grade POP and testing for SUI may be beneficial in diagnosing obstruction, occult SUI, and/or detrusor overactivity in some women with LUTS. Reduction of the prolapse can be done with a pessary from a pessary fitting kit, and/or a lubricated gauze roll. If using a gauze roll, the examiner must account for the potential of urethral obstruction as well as wicking of the fluid onto the gauze during voiding, which may or may not compromise the quality of voiding images under fluoroscopy while performing video urodynamics [3].

Table 7.1 Facilitation of voiding

• Running water: either by physically turning a tap on in the room producing an audible sound in the sink or playing a recording of a similar sound
• Hand warming and watering: Submerging the patient's fingers in a bucket with warm water and encouraging a relaxed approach to voiding
• Repositioning: Positioning the patient into the same voiding position that they use when in the non-laboratory setting. For example, some individuals may universally void in the standing or seated position. Accommodation should be available for repositioning of these patients in the urodynamics room. Nevertheless, when such accommodations are made, it is important that the patient is safely able to void without disrupting the wires, urodynamic, or radiographic equipment.
• Physically leaving the room: Some individuals will have great difficulty initiating voiding in the presence of others. Sometimes called "bashful bladder," voiding can be facilitated in these patients by simply leaving the room. The patient should be reassured that they will be safe alone in the room during this period of time. Use of a remote control marker will allow continued monitoring and recording of events even if not at the urodynamics computer.
• Guided imagery: verbally walking the patient through the scenario of voiding can be helpful in initiating urination.

Difficulty with the initiation of voiding is another common problem in the urodynamics room. Volitional urination is a complex phenomenon involving the integration of neurological, muscular, pharmacological, and psychological factors among others. Difficulty with initiation of voiding may be caused by the testing environment, obstruction or pain from the urethral catheter, or a number of other issues. Psychogenic inhibition during the voiding phase is common. The practitioner can help facilitate voiding by initiating one or more of the following practices as seen in Table 7.1.

Urge Suppression Techniques

During the study, the goal is to reproduce the symptoms experienced by the patient as at home. By comparing the presentation of the symptoms in the lab with the objective data recorded in a voiding and/or catheterization diary, the clinician can direct the study in order to reproduce symptoms. With the introduction of catheters and an un-physiologic filling rate, the patient may experience multiple involuntary bladder contractions (IBCs) that do not correlate with physiologic capacity and/or their normal sensations of urgency.

An important point is that directing the patient to attempt to suppress incidental detrusor contractions may afford the clinician with important data which is not only diagnostic, but potentially therapeutic. The sensation of urgency is annotated on the tracing and, if coincident with an IBC, this is recorded as well. The clinician then can ask the patient to suppress the urge as they would at home and label this event on the tracing. This maneuver will help to evaluate if the patient can inhibit the involuntary contraction, which can serve as a future basis for therapeutic pelvic floor muscle training with the goal of urge suppression. In addition, if the patient inappropriately recruits abdominal muscles during attempted suppression, as indicated by a rise in the abdominal pressure recording, then they can be educated, using this biofeedback technique, in the proper performance of pelvic floor muscle isolation and recruitment. The EMG activity seen coincidently with the proper performance of a pelvic floor contraction can aid in teaching the patient about their pelvic floor as an additional form of biofeedback. In the event the patient is unable to suppress the IBC, the clinician can teach the patient various urge suppression techniques. One such technique is to instruct the patient to "squeeze the pelvic floor as if they were trying to prevent passing gas". An alternative maneuver for the patient who is unable to isolate the pelvic floor muscle is the "heel click" maneuver. In order to do this action, the patient is instructed to click the heels in place while keeping the feet planted on the floor. This action, when done correctly, will elicit a rise in the EMG recording without a rise in the abdominal pressure lead. This phenomenon is demonstrated in Fig. 7.1.

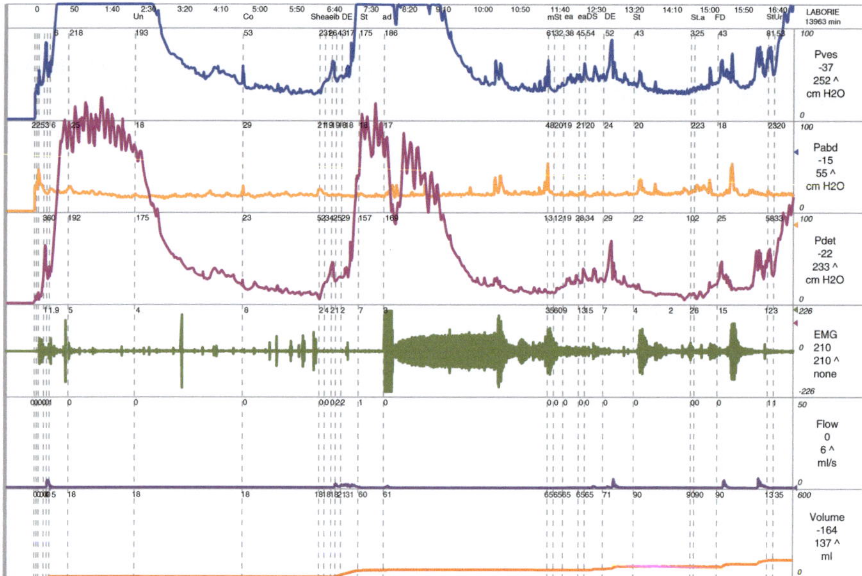

Fig. 7.1 This pressure-flow urodynamic tracing demonstrates involuntary bladder contraction. The patient then attempted a long sustain pelvic floor contraction, but then was taught how to do heel clicks to suppress subsequent contractions

Finally, it is important to periodically reassess the signal quality of the UDS equipment during the study. This can be done by having the patient perform a stress maneuver such as a valsalva, or cough, and compare the expected changes in the vesical, abdominal, and EMG leads to that at rest.

Medication Management

Antibiotic Prophylaxis

The American Urological Association has issued a Best Practice Policy statement for antimicrobial prophylaxis [4]. This evidence-based document reviews surgical antimicrobial prophylaxis for a variety of urological procedures and states that *"An important change in antimicrobial prophylaxis pertaining to urologists is that antimicrobials are no longer recommended by the American Heart Association in association with genitourinary procedures solely to prevent infectious endocarditis [4]."* The panel reviewed current research and recommended that antimicrobial prophylaxis for urodynamic studies is not necessary if the urine culture prior to the procedure is negative. If coverage is indicated for individualized clinical scenarios (i.e., the severely immunosuppressed patient), the drug of choice is a fluoroquinolone or trimethoprim-sulfamethoxazole for a 24 h duration. Positive cultures should be treated with appropriate antibiotic coverage. Of note, the US Food and Drug administration (FDA) has released a statement that patients should be notified about the possible risk of permanent peripheral neuropathy associated with the oral or intravenous use of fluoroquinolones [4]. The principle of not treating urine unless there is growth noted on culture also applies for the removal of an external urinary catheter and for the patient undergoing clean intermittent catheterization, which also may apply to this population. Urine culture and appropriate antibiotic coverage is recommended prior to study if infection is suspected in this population.

Other "Premedications"

Patients undergoing video urodynamics are infused with a contrast agent. Such agents are associated with allergic reactions, and anaphylaxis in a small number of individuals when infused intravenously or when these agents gain access to the systemic circulation. Whether allergic reactions are relevant to bladder filling during video urodynamics is unclear in the absence of a traumatic catheterization. In patients with a shellfish allergy, iodine allergy, or a known contrast allergy, video urodynamics should be done with caution and with appropriate preparation. When possible, the use of non-ionic contrast agents, and a prophylactic steroid and antihistamine regimen starting 24 h prior to the study may reduce or eliminate systemic reactions.

Premedication for neurogenic patients and potential autonomic dysreflexia is discussed in Chap. 9: Special Considerations in the Neurogenic Patient.

Other Challenging Situations Related to UDS Testing

Catheterization

Difficult catheterization can impede the study from the beginning. It is important to recognize that many individuals presenting for UDS have an anatomically abnormal lower urinary tract such as that due to stricture or contracture. This may result from prior surgery, trauma, infection, or other urological conditions. Other individuals are simply very anxious and will volitionally contract the external sphincter either in response to the anticipation or pain of urethral manipulation making catheterization increasingly difficult. Interventions for these situations are varied and although the first catheterization to empty the bladder is often successful, subsequent catheterization with the smaller urodynamics catheters for the pressure-flow study may be difficult.

At times, the use of urethral anesthetics, such as lidocaine infused lubrication gel, prior to catheterization may be beneficial and provide some comfort to both men and women during the catheterization process. Siderias et al. [5] conducted a randomized controlled trial of males in the emergency department and concluded that topical lidocaine gel reduced pain as compared to topical non-medicated lubricants during urethral catheterization. A similar study was also conducted comparing water-based lubricating gels with lignocaine gel in the female population requiring catheterization in the emergency department. This randomized controlled trial found that the lignocaine gel reduced procedural pain for urethral catheterization [6]. Although these studies are not directly related to the traditionally non-emergent setting of urodynamics, the use of anesthetic gels may provide a less painful catheterization. Gels also provide gentle atraumatic dilation of the urethral lumen, which may ease subsequent catheterization.

Other interventions to assist in easing the catheter into the bladder include:

1. For male difficult catheterization: initial catheterization with 16–18 French coude tip catheter followed by attempt with a 12 French silicone catheter. For difficult passage of an urodynamics catheter, use of a 0.035 coated guide wire may be feasible, if the urodynamic catheters can be threaded over a wire [7]. If not, use of flexible cystoscopy and passage of the urodynamics catheters alongside the scope may facilitate introduction into the bladder. This may require movement of equipment between rooms and staff flexibility to change procedures as indicated by patient need.

2. Piggy-backing the air charged catheter on an intermittent straight catheter. By placing the air charged (AC) catheter tip into the eyelet of the larger, firmer straight catheter, both catheters can be introduced into the bladder. Then the practitioner uses a quick flick of the AC catheter to dislodge it from the straight catheter. The straight catheter is then removed from the urinary system, and the AC catheter is in place and ready to be charged for the test.

3. A well stocked urodynamic supply closet will facilitate locating appropriate supplies. Supplies should include an assortment of urinary catheters with various tips.

These catheters should include coude tip, council tip, olive tip, and straight catheters ranging in size from 12 to 18 F. Hydrophilic catheters may also aid in difficult situations.

4. Strategies to aid in passing a catheter include providing a quiet, secure, and private setting that allows for the patient to relax during the procedure [8]. Currently, the literature lacks research based techniques. Anecdotal techniques include urging the patient to attempt to void, without straining, while the catheter is passed. "Wiggling toes" will promote relaxation of the pelvic floor to aid in passing the catheter into the bladder. If the patient already self-catheterizes without difficulty, he/she may be offered to place the catheters for the procedure.

5. As noted above, intraurethral injection of 10–20 cc lubricant with or without lidocaine can greatly ease placement of urethral catheters

Surgically Implanted Hardware

Typical hardware that may be encountered in urodynamic preparation is artificial urinary sphincters, implanted neuromodulation devices for bladder and bowel control, spinal and pelvic orthopedic implants and/or penile prosthesis. Careful history taking will identify such individuals. Staff should be educated to ask about implanted devices so that traumatic catheterizations especially in the setting of an artificial urinary sphincter can be avoided when catheterizing the patient. For example, the artificial urinary sphincter should be deactivated for catheterization, and catheterization performed only by the clinician or highly trained staff. Also positioning the c-arm throughout the study may be necessary to maximize visualization of urinary tract structures (see Fig. 7.2a, b).

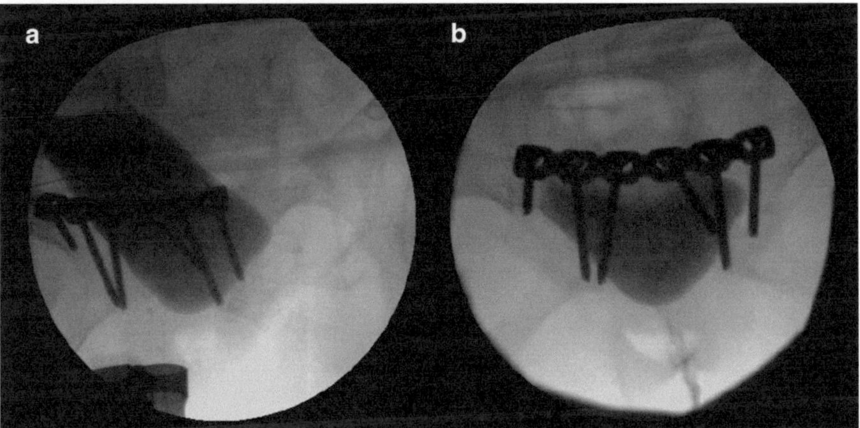

Fig. 7.2 (a) *Left*. Orthopedic hardware in pelvis. In *bottom corner* the top of the table hardware will obstruct the urethral images. (b) *Right*. But with positioning of the c-arm, the urethra can be seen without obstruction

Positioning

Positioning the patient on the UDS table can sometimes be challenging due to surgery (recent or prior) or orthopedic, neurological or cognitive difficulties. For example, patients with neurologic conditions may experience muscular spasms that impair optimal positioning. (see Fig. 7.3a, b) Using soft sheets and padding, patients can be positioned in such a way to provide access to their perineum for catheterization, and, if applicable, allow for the radiologic equipment to be placed around them for video urodynamics (see Fig. 7.3a) Use of funnels and tubing strategically taped in place can direct the urine toward the collection containers and flow transducers. (Fig. 7.3a, b) Devices such as head padding, arm rests, and low positioning tables will help maintain a safe environment that is comfortable for the patient during this sometimes awkward positioning. As noted previously, the use of physical therapy aids such as slide boards and patient lifts helps caregivers move dependent patients from their wheelchairs to the exam table. Ambulatory patients are also positioned with these concepts in mind. Strategically placed funnels and tubing direct drainage into the uroflow equipment (see Fig. 7.4).

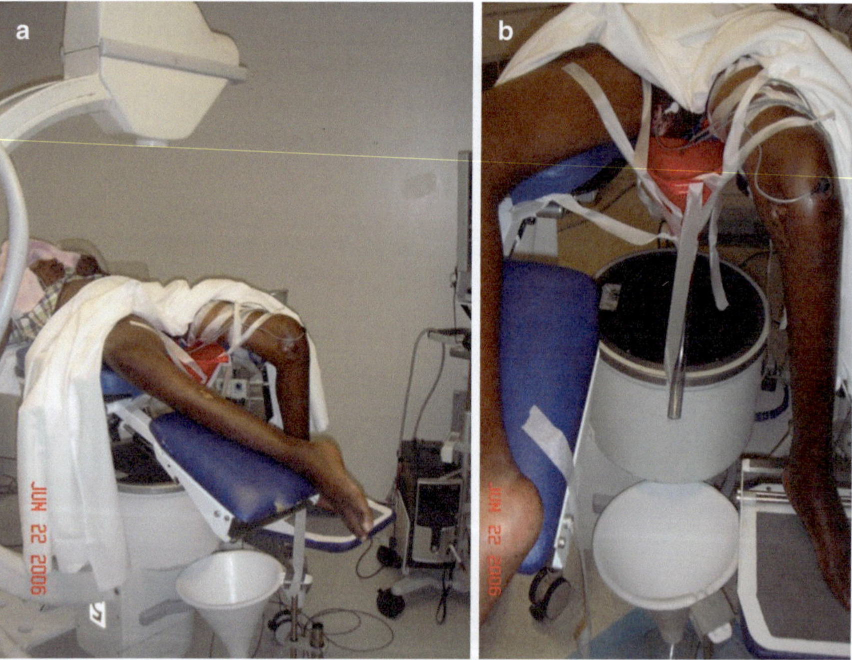

Fig. 7.3 (**a**) *Left*. (**b**) *Right*. This patient, who is wheelchair dependent, was unable to do the testing in the seated position secondary to leg spasms. Her right leg was supported the chair leg rest, while her left leg spasmed less in the seated position. Careful positioning of the funnel provided visualization of the voided stream without spillage on the c-arm of radio-contrast dye

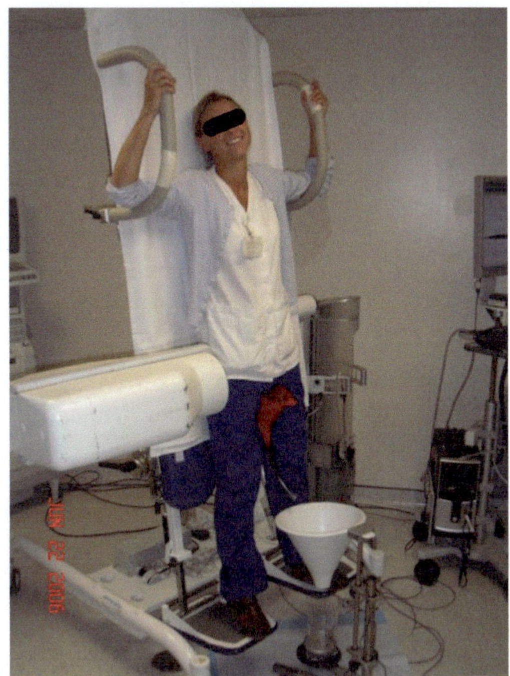

Fig. 7.4 Ambulatory patients who are able to stand are positioned with a funnel and tubing situated to drain into the uroflow machine. *Note*: arm grabs for balance. The hand controls and staff training need to be in place to emergently flatten the bed in the event of patient need

Syncope

Avoidance of syncope during the UDS study and protection of the patient in the event of syncope is imperative. Informing patients prior to the study that fasting is not necessary, and is in fact discouraged, will help to curb syncopal episodes related to hypoglycemia and dehydration. The clinic should have drinking water, candy, juice, and small snacks to use as needed. Certain populations are more predisposed to fainting, such as young men with primary bladder neck obstruction [9].

Safety is paramount for both the patient and the staff. Staff should be trained to efficiently move equipment in order to get the patient in a supine position in the event of syncope. Emergency equipment such as ammonia smelling salts, blood pressure cuff, and resuscitation equipment should be readily available. Safety equipment such as seat belts, transfer aids and hand bars will also aid in providing security for patients while being evaluated. Prevention and anticipation of syncope may be the best measure to prevent this side effect of an invasive study.

Documentation

The study, as a completed document, should include notations on the tracing to provide a succinct account of the study so as to be read and interpreted in the absence of the oral report from the clinicians present during its execution. A brief history including relevant surgical, obstetrical, and medical events should be included in the history along with a statement regarding the rationale or indications for conducting the study. A catheterized post void residual prior to initiation of the study should be included. Throughout the study, annotations, such as position change, pain, and reproduction of home symptoms on the tracing will cue future readers as to the relevant events that occurred during the study.

Staff Training

Competently trained staff will aid the clinician in producing an optimal study.

Initial training of staff may be offered by the company supplying the urodynamic equipment used in the clinic. Staff training should include information on general maintenance of the equipment including calibration checks, cleaning, moving, and general trouble-shooting. Contracts for service and technical support should be established for long-term assistance. Consideration for continued training, especially with staff turnover and annual competencies, needs to be negotiated with the urodynamics company to ensure the long-term needs are met during the life of the equipment. Outside of industry, there are many professional organizations and publications available to provide training and ongoing education for the various staff involved in the performance of urodynamics.

These organizations include:

– American Urological Association www.auanet.org
– International Continence Society www.ics.org
– Society of Urodynamics, Female Pelvic Medicine & Urogenital Reconstruction www.sufuorg.com
– Society of Urologic Nurses and Associates www.suna.org
– Wound Ostomy & Continence Nurse Society www.wocn.org

Conclusion

Understanding the complexities of reproducing a real world experience in the laboratory, while also considering the unique and complex needs of individuals requiring urodynamic testing, will be a benefit to clinicians in optimizing a study that is relevant and useful.

References

1. Schafer W, Abrams P, Liao L, Mattisasson A, Pesce A, Spangberg A, Sterling A, Zinner N, van Kerrebroeck P. Good urodynamic practices: urofolowmetry, filling cystometry, and pressure-flow studies. Neurourol Urodyn. 2002;21:261–74.
2. Kocabas P, Khorshid L. A comparison of special gynaecological garment and music in reducing the anxiety related to gynaecological examination. J Clin Nurs. 2011;21:791–9.

3. Winters C, Dmochowski R, Goldman H, Hendron C, Kobeski K, Kraus S, Lemacks G, Nitti V, Rovner E, Wein A. Urodynamic studies in adults: AUA/SUFU guideline. J Urol. 2012;188(6): 2464–72.
4. Wolf JS, Bennett C, Dmochowski R, Hollenbeck B, Pearle M, Schaeffer A. Best practice policy statement on urologic surgery antimicrobial prophylaxis. 2008. Available from the American Urological Association Education and Research with full text: http://www.auanet.org/common/pdf/education/clinical-guidance/Antimicrobial-Prophylaxis.pdf
5. Siderias J, Guadio F, Singer AJ. Comparison of topical anesthetic and lubricants prior to urethral catheterization in males: a randomized controlled trial. Acad Emerg Med. 2004;11(6): 703–6.
6. Chung C, Chu M, Paoloni R, O'Brien M, Demel T. Comparison of lignocaine and water-based lubricating gels for female urethral catheterization: a randomized control trial. Emerg Med Australas. 2007;19(4):315–9.
7. Villanueva C, Hemstreet G. The approach to difficult urethral catheterization among urology residents in the United States. Int Braz J Urol. 2010;36(6):710–7.
8. Newman D, Wilson MM. Review of intermittent catheterization and current best practices. Urol Nurs. 2011;31(1):12–48.
9. Neurogenic bladder discussion, SUFU Winter meeting, Las Vegas, 2012.

Chapter 8
Special Considerations in the Pediatric Patient

J. Todd Purves and Andrew A. Stec

Abbreviations

ALARA	As low as reasonably achievable
CMG	Cystometrogram
DSD	Detrusor sphincter dysynergia
FR	French
ICCS	International Children's Continence Society
LUTS	Lower urinary tract symptoms
OAB	Overactive bladder
PUV	Posterior urethral valves
SFU	Society for Fetal Urology
UDS	Urodynamics
UTI	Urinary tract infection

Introduction

The management of children presenting with lower urinary tract symptoms (LUTS) depends on an accurate diagnosis of the underlying etiology, just as it does in the adult population. Children present a unique challenge to this endeavor in that they can be at any point along the spectrum of maturation; developing from an infantile voiding physiology to that of an adult. In addition, cognitive and emotional immaturity of the patient can make accurate history taking difficult. Even with more

J.T. Purves, MD, PhD (✉) • A.A. Stec, MD
Department of Urology, The Medical University of South Carolina,
96 Jonathan Lucas Drive, CSB 644, Charleston, SC 29425, USA
e-mail: purves@musc.edu; stec@musc.edu

© Springer Science+Business Media New York 2015
E.S. Rovner, M.E. Koski (eds.), *Rapid and Practical Interpretation of Urodynamics*, DOI 10.1007/978-1-4939-1764-8_8

mature children and unusually attentive parents, the clinician can rarely obtain the intimate details of voiding and bowel habits that can be provided by adult patients. Therefore, UDS studies that provide quantitative measurements of bladder function can be of critical importance in identifying which of the myriad causes of pediatric voiding pathology may be affecting a particular patient.

UDS provides a rich source of information that can help the clinician optimize treatment for any particular patient but these studies can be quite invasive and traumatic to children even under the best of circumstances. Therefore, providers should make an effort to preferentially utilize the least invasive techniques, such as complex uroflowmetry and real time ultrasonography, when these are adequate for designing a treatment plan while avoiding invasive multichannel UDS. In many cases, however, formal video UDS are the only viable means to obtain necessary information and the clinician must be willing and prepared to perform this testing as accurately and as comfortably as possible. UDS should be a component of a comprehensive protocol in the diagnosis and management of children with LUTS to ensure that children who can benefit from testing receive it, while minimizing its use in children where less invasive testing will suffice.

The most frequent use of UDS in pediatrics is in the management of children with chronic conditions, including neurogenic disorders and anatomic outlet anomalies, which affect voiding physiology. These patients often require testing to define their baseline functioning and then later to assess treatment results and follow changes that occur with maturation. Assurance of safe urinary storage pressures is essential to protect renal function and information necessary to achieve and maintain continence necessitates formal UDS studies. In anatomically normal children with LUTS, the role of UDS is more controversial and often plays a role in patients who do not respond well to either empiric treatment or that based on less invasive studies.

Indications for UDS in Pediatrics

A UDS procedure in a child can be invasive or traumatic and thus understanding the proper indications for such testing is imperative. UDS are used in two patient populations in pediatric urology: (1) the child with bladder dysfunction that is neurogenic in origin and, (2) those that have non-neurogenic bladder dysfunction. The indications for each patient population are different.

Non-neurogenic Bladder Dysfunction in Children

Children with non-neurogenic bladder dysfunction generally present after toilet-training with a clinical presentation that may include the following: incontinence, dysuria, recurrent urinary tract infection (UTI), urinary retention, urinary hesitancy, abnormal voiding patterns, or pelvic floor dysfunction. The majority of these complaints can be evaluated with non-invasive testing and do not require UDS.

Basic work-up includes a physical examination, history, and comprehensive voiding diary, then progressing onto non-invasive tests such as post-void residual measurement, ultrasonography, and complex uroflowmetry with evaluation of the pelvic floor. These are the primary tools in the armamentarium for evaluation of the non-neurogenic child with LUTS. The results of these tests may lead a provider to directed behavioral and pharmacotherapy that may alleviate some or all of the child's symptoms and reassure the family that there is no greater problem [1].

Progressing to a UDS study for the non-neurogenic patient requires specific goals or questions that the provider should establish before undertaking the procedure. UDS in the non-neurogenic child is controversial as studies have shown that UDS in many cases does not alter treatment therapies that were based on data from non-invasive studies [2, 3]. In 2008, a prospective European study published results showing that improved treatment outcomes in children with urinary urgency and dysfunctional voiding did not correlate with UDS findings [4]. This starkly contrasts with a comprehensive retrospective review of 89 UDS procedures performed in children with refractory non-neurogenic voiding dysfunction that demonstrated that 37 % of studies were normal, while 63 % of UDS studies were abnormal. In the abnormal patients, UDS demonstrated clinically significant findings that allowed for targeted therapy to the specific issue afflicting the child. The predominant findings were storage abnormalities in 66 %, involuntary detrusor contractions in 55 %, and emptying abnormalities in 34 % of patients [5]. Despite varied opinions and data, the generally accepted premise amongst pediatric urologists is to reserve UDS in the non-neurogenic pediatric population for those patients who have refractory symptoms or who have failed initial therapies based on non-invasive testing.

Potential diagnoses evaluated with UDS in the non-neurogenic patient include bladder outlet obstruction, voiding postponement, underactive bladder, dysfunctional voiding, overactive bladder (OAB), and detrusor overactivity [6]. According to the International Children's Continence Society (ICCS) guidelines OAB is a clinical diagnosis defined primarily as urinary urgency with or without incontinence or urinary frequency. Detrusor overactivity can only be diagnosed with a cystometric evaluation as part of a UDS study.

Urinary urgency is the sudden onset of the sensation to void. This term is generally applied only after the child has attained complete bladder control (typically around age 5). UDS is useful in children with urinary urgency to assess for the presence of involuntary detrusor contractions as well as to elucidate potential issues with bladder sensation and filling. Dysfunctional voiding is a diagnosis that is sometimes widely applied, but specifically refers to a child who contracts the pelvic floor muscular complex or external urethral sphincter during the act of volitional voiding [7]. Dysfunctional voiding can be diagnosed typically on complex uroflowmetry with cystometrogram (CMG) patch electrodes and does not require UDS as a formal part of the investigation [8]. However in the cases of severe dysfunctional voiding, such as Hinman-Allen Syndrome ("non-neurogenic neurogenic bladder"), UDS are indicated to assess for elevated detrusor storage pressures in children at risk, as well as use the video component of the UDS study to assess for the presence of vesicoureteral reflux, and evaluate the urinary sphincter mechanism during active voiding [9]. OAB in children may be associated with involuntary detrusor contractions and smaller than expected bladder capacity, based on the patient's age. These findings can only be diagnosed on a multichannel UDS study. However studies have shown that clinical urge symptoms do not always correlate with detrusor overactivity and studies have not shown that UDS findings improve overall treatment outcomes for OAB [4].

In summary, for the child with non-neurogenic bladder dysfunction, the primary testing required to evaluate the bladder and lower urinary tract are non-invasive measures such as history, physical examination, voiding diary, ultrasonography, and complex uroflowmetry with CMG. Although controversial in this patient population, select patients with refractory symptoms, those who fail initial behavioral and pharmacotherapies, or those who are at high risk for elevated bladder pressures are potential candidates for UDS studies when a directed goal-oriented evaluation is performed.

Neurogenic Bladder Dysfunction

UDS is a cornerstone in the initial evaluation and long term follow-up for children with neurogenic compromise of the lower urinary tract. UDS allows a provider to confirm the diagnosis of neurogenic bladder in a child as well as provide a means to characterize the particular components of the dysfunction. The specific components evaluated are bladder capacity, bladder compliance, storage pressure, emptying pressures, ability of the bladder to contract, assessment and determination of the cause of incontinence as well as vesicoureteral reflux, and external urethral sphincteric function. While UDS does provide sound clinical information on the condition of the lower urinary tract in a child, it does not always provide an absolute measure of when to intervene or treat the child, therefore the providers must use the study combined with a complete clinical understanding of the patient to direct therapy for the lower urinary tract. UDS is indicated as part of the initial work-up in a child with suspected neurogenic bladder, however when and how often to repeat the testing is the source of debate and differing expert opinion. UDS has been shown to benefit children at high risk for urinary tract deterioration in planning aggressive early treatment of these patients. In the neurogenic population, the focus of treatment centers on prevention of progression of urinary tract deterioration, and secondarily assists with improving symptoms such as incontinence and detrusor overactivity [10, 11]. The primary underlying diagnoses for children presenting with neurogenic bladder dysfunction include spinal cord disorders (myelomeningocele, tethered cord, sacral agenesis, cloacal malformations, and spinal cord injury), posterior urethral valves (PUV), anorectal malformations, and CNS disorders.

Spinal Cord Disorders

The most commonly recognized open spinal cord disorder is myelomeningocele, accounting for approximately 90 % of the cases. Myelomeningocele will typically present in neonates and is generally diagnosed by physical examination similar to most cloacal malformations. Tethered cord, sacral agenesis, spina bifida occulta, and CNS disorders may present in a delayed fashion at any point during development; spinal cord trauma presents sporadically due to external blunt or penetrating injury. UDS is recommended in these children after the initial insult has been addressed and after spinal shock has resolved. Children with spinal cord disorders typically demonstrate one of three generalizable findings on UDS: (1) complete denervation of the lower urinary tract with detrusor areflexia, (2) detrusor overactivity with synergic detrusor muscle and urethral sphincter, or (3) detrusor overactivity with dyssynergic detrusor muscle and external sphincter with or without poor bladder compliance. The most deleterious pattern observed for children with spinal cord disorders is detrusor sphincter dysynergia (DSD) and elevated bladder pressures (>40 cm H_2O before expected bladder capacity, or >80–100 cm H_2O with voiding/leaking) [11]. This increased intravesical pressure puts both the detrusor muscle and renal units at risk for progressive damage and deterioration. Early identification of DSD and elevated bladder pressures in pediatric patients facilitates early intervention with a subsequent reduction in detrusor decompensation, renal deterioration, as well as decreasing the incidence of hydroureteronephrosis and vesicoureteral reflux [12].

UDS is indicated in patients with known or suspected spinal cord disorders in order to characterize the physiology of the lower urinary tract as well as direct therapy. Performing follow-up UDS studies is discretionary with most providers tailoring the studies to changes in the clinical picture of the patient. A child with a spinal cord disorder found to have bladder filling pressures ≥40 cm H_2O, voiding or leaking pressures of ≥80–100 cm H_2O, or DSD with a poorly compliant bladder is considered high risk for progressive bladder and renal deterioration. In these high risk children, 3–12 months after institution of directed therapy, a repeat UDS should be strongly considered to confirm whether the therapy is improving the hostile physiologic parameters noted on the initial study. Additionally, interval UDS studies are indicated in the neurogenic pediatric population when a provider notes: (1) a change in the child's neurologic symptoms/exam, (2) 3 months after a spine or spinal cord procedure is performed, (3) newly discovered hydronephrosis or hydroureteronephrosis on ultrasound, (4) recurrent UTIs, (5) a change or increase in the child's degree of incontinence, or (6) increasing urinary difficulty or elevated postvoid residual in a child who has a neurogenic bladder who volitionally voids [6, 13].

Posterior Urethral Valves

PUV represent the most common form of congenital obstruction of the lower urinary tract in infant males. While there is a wide array of management and treatment strategies in children with PUV, UDS testing is a generally accepted mainstay in bladder evaluation in this patient population. The most commonly identified UDS patterns in these children are detrusor overactivity, loss of bladder compliance, myogenic failure, and impaired pelvic floor activity [14, 15]. In up to 80 % of children with PUV, UDS will demonstrate abnormalities in bladder physiology [16]. In at least 15 % of these patients, a progressive phenomenon known as "valve bladder syndrome" may occur [17]. Valve bladder syndrome is a progressive deterioration of the intrinsic ability of the detrusor muscle to function, thereby leading to high detrusor pressures, deterioration of the upper urinary tract and incontinence.

The authors currently employ UDS between 9 and 12 months of age in children with PUV valves that were ablated during infancy as an initial test to evaluate bladder physiology. Interval UDS testing is performed if there is a change in the child's urinary symptoms, recurrent UTI, elevated post-void residual, or new onset/worsening hydroureteronephrosis. Interval UDS testing allows for reassurance that the employed bladder management therapy is working appropriately, while also monitoring for progressive deterioration in detrusor function as well as increased bladder pressures [18]. As opposed to children with neurogenic bladder dysfunction, these children are sensate per urethra and interval UDS testing is minimized unless indicated by non-invasive testing such as ultrasonography or complex uroflowmetry with CMG.

Anorectal Malformations

Neurogenic bladder dysfunction is commonly seen in children with anorectal malformations as there is an increased incidence of intraspinal pathology such as tethered cord and sacral malformations. Additionally, with the extensive malformation in the sacral and pelvic floor areas associated with these conditions, the possibility of neurogenic bladder dysfunction is present at baseline [19]. Subsequently, the radical reconstruction required to repair anorectal malformations can lead to denervation, as well as DSD and neurogenic bladder dysfunction in these patients [20].

Reports suggest that initial UDS prior to radical repair of the anorectal malformation should be undertaken to uncover any underlying bladder pathology and direct treatment. Additionally the study should be repeated 3 months following any spinal cord procedure or radical pelvic procedure to evaluate for any alteration in bladder function [13, 19, 21]. These patients should subsequently be monitored as they develop with aging, and a repeat study is indicated if there is any change in bowel or bladder symptoms, or in ultrasonographic appearance of the bladder, ureter, or kidney occur [6].

Differences Between Pediatric and Adult UDS

While the overall UDS study is performed in the same manner for both children and adults, there are differences in the filling, storage, and voiding physiology in the infant and childhood bladder that are important to keep in mind when performing and interpreting the study. The principle of having a directed study that is tailored to the individual patient and clinical question to be answered is the cornerstone of a quality pediatric UDS study.

Differences in the Setup of the UDS System

As children are frequently active and can exhibit artifactual movement during a study, a CMG sensor system with a sampling rate of 1,000 Hz is recommended. This facilitates the examiners ability to differentiate DSD and motion artifact in the child. While in many cases the standard adult 8 Fr double lumen urethral UDS catheter and 10 French (Fr) rectal catheter can be used in older children, smaller versions for younger children and infants with 6 Fr dual lumen urethral catheter, and 8 Fr rectal catheters are available for use. Routine monitoring of urethral pressures is not generally done during a pediatric study as there is inherent unreliability in the measurement due to frequent motion by children [2]. Appropriate monitoring and notation during the study of an active child with good rectal probe security assist the examiner in determining motion, talking, or crying artifact as a cause of changing abdominal pressures during a study [22]. Sensate children from approximately 10–12 months of age up to 5–6 years of age may require special care prior to starting a study. Dedicated nursing or child-life support may be required to work with and convince a child to accept application of CMG electrodes and placement of urethral and rectal catheters. Needle electrodes for CMG are not recommended in pediatric studies. In some select cases children may also require mild sedation to facilitate the study.

Differences in the Filling and Storage Component of the Study

Bladder filling in most pediatric UDS studies is accomplished in a retrograde fashion through the urethral UDS catheter. Standard pediatric bladder capacity is accomplished via one of several accepted formulas. In infants, bladder capacity is estimated by the formula: $38 + (2.5 \times \text{age in months}) = \text{bladder capacity in mL}$ [23]. In older children (>2 years of age) a widely used formula is $30 \times (\text{age in years} + 2) = \text{bladder capacity in mL}$ with the second most commonly utilized formula being $30 + (\text{age in years} \times 30) = \text{bladder capacity in mL}$ [24–26]. Normal saline or radiographic contrast that is warmed is used for bladder instillation as cold solutions can provoke detrusor contractions; the saline is preferably additive free. The fill rate is calculated as rate $(\text{mL/min}) = 10\ \%$ of the calculated expected bladder capacity. When poor compliance or early involuntary contractions/detrusor overactivity are noted in the study, the rate should be slowed down to less than 10 mL/min.

During filling, any detrusor activity in infants and children should be considered a significant finding on the study when it does not occur during the act of voiding. In some cases detrusor overactivity may be present during the first filling cycle but absent during subsequent fillings. Additionally the initial bladder capacity noted on filling may be small due to patient discomfort or anxiety, and the measurement should be repeated. For both of these reasons, multiple cycles of filling are recommended in children.

Bladder sensation is often an unreliable measure in young children and is only reliable in children who are completely cooperative, have mastered volitional voiding, and can verbalize their first desire to void. In infants or younger children, visual cues such as fidgeting or curling of the toes may be present as a sign that voiding is about to occur, however this is a subjective measure as seen by the examiner [27]. Impaired bladder sensation is defined as the lack of urgency to void after the bladder has been filled beyond the age-appropriate bladder capacity (approximately 150 % of maximum capacity); this is sometimes accompanied by the child developing abdominal pain instead of manifesting the urge to void [6].

Bladder compliance calculations are a dynamic measurement in the pediatric population that are calculated similar to that in adult studies by dividing the change in volume by the change in detrusor pressure at maximal capacity. The generally accepted normal compliance in children is defined by a less than 10 cm H_2O pressure rise in the resting detrusor pressure at the expected age-based bladder capacity [7]. More specifically this can be calculated as 5 % of the any individual patients normal bladder capacity per cm H_2O [28]. When elevated bladder pressures are noted, the shape of the curve during the rise in pressure should be evaluated as to whether it is an exponential increase in pressure around maximum bladder capacity or a linear increase in pressure as filling progresses; the latter implies severely impaired compliance of the bladder. Care should be taken when considering the fill rate on a UDS study in the pediatric population. Studies comparing a natural filling cystometry and saline filling cystometry in pediatric patients with neurogenic bladder dysfunction have demonstrated that the more rapid artificial fill rate can be associated with an elevated bladder capacity measurement, and an elevated intravesicular pressure rise during filling; this may lead to readings suggesting false increases in bladder pressure and artifactually worsened compliance measurements in this population [29]. Resting detrusor pressures exceeding 30 cm H_2O during the storage phase of UDS investigation are considered high and may represent conditions hostile to the upper urinary tract in children [30].

Differences in the Emptying Component of the Study

Normal voiding pressures range from 55 to 80 cm H_2O in boys and from 30 to 65 cm H_2O in girls. Due to the presence of the urethral catheter, infants may have higher voiding pressures than older children. If voiding pressure in infants rise above a mean of 118 cm H_2O in boys or 75 cm H_2O in girls, a urethral obstruction or abnormality should be suspected [31, 32]. When it is difficult to get children to micturate during a UDS study, time and patience are required to obtain the data in this important phase of the study. High voiding pressures with low flow rates may be indicative of lower urinary tract obstruction. Table 8.1 demonstrates mean voiding flow rates in the pediatric population, note both are both age and gender dependent [33]. Fluoroscopy is indicated when obstruction is suspected to better define urethral

Table 8.1 Mean normal maximum voided flow rates (Qmax) in mL/s for healthy children [33]

Qmax	Age (5–10 years) (mL/s)	Age (11–15 years) (mL/s)
Boys	15.2±4.5	22.5±7.2
Girls	17.9±6.0	27.1±9.3

abnormalities and the location of obstruction as the visualization of pelvic floor or sphincteric contractions can be combined with pressure measurements, flow rate, and CMG activity to better understand the clinical scenario for the child [34]. The urethral closure mechanism should also be evaluated during the UDS study as DSD may be noted and sphincter paralysis can occur in the neurogenic bladder dysfunction population [35, 36]. In order to validate the emptying phase of the study, overall voided volumes in children should be at a minimum of 100 mL in older children or greater than 50 % of the expected age weighted bladder capacity [27].

Using Fluoroscopy in Children During a UDS Study

Ionizing radiation exposure has potentially lifelong effects, and its use should be minimized in the pediatric population when possible. The generally accepted premise is to have strict adherence to the "as low as reasonably achievable" (ALARA) principle when performing studies [37]. The fluoroscopic component of a UDS study provides valuable insight in many procedures, as mentioned earlier. In pediatric UDS procedures, the use of fluoroscopy should be directed at answering a specific question with the minimum radiation required, in adherence with the ALARA principle. Video UDS studies have been reported with a range of radiation exposure from an average of 2 mGy (less than an average VCUG) to 10 mGy [38, 39]. Factors that increase radiation exposure during a UDS study are providers who use longer fluoroscopy times, higher body mass index, and larger bladder capacity. Overall recommendations are to use fluoroscopy when required to answer a clinical question, but attempt to minimize radiation exposure in the child.

Pain, Artifact, and Emotional Overlay

Urodynamics (UDS) is a powerful tool that provides objective information about a patient's particular bladder physiology but it can be rendered essentially useless by artifacts that result from fear, pain, and the patient's inability to focus and cooperate with the testing procedure. In pediatrics, the challenge is often greater than in the adult population because children are less likely to understand the test, appreciate the reasons for obtaining it, and they are more likely to respond to fear, pain, and disinterest in ways that disrupt the study. Therefore, one must address these issues prior to, and during the test so that the diagnostic goals of UDS are achievable.

In a study of the adult female population, Ellerkman and colleagues found that the level at which patients anticipated pain with UDS was significantly greater than the actual pain that they reported experiencing during the procedure [40]. This suggests that steps can be taken prior to the visit and at the initiation of the procedure to minimize the major component of psychological trauma associated with UDS. In pediatrics, it is critical to address the fears of both the patient and the parents, as the latter are critically important in influencing how the child perceives the test and they can be very helpful in reducing anxiety [41]. Prior to ordering UDS testing, it is wise to have a clear discussion of what the diagnostic goals are and how the child will be helped by this additional information. This should be followed by a full description of the procedure itself to eliminate any fear of the unknown. Participation by the child depends considerably on his or her age and maturity level but the clinician should make every effort to explain as much of the procedure as possible in an age-appropriate manner. Patients who are familiar with intermittent catheterization are generally more accepting of the catheters used during testing but those who are not may need more explicit instructions on how the catheters work and how they will be inserted. Child-life specialists can be very helpful especially for younger children who may benefit from a demonstration of catheterization using anatomically correct dolls constructed for this purpose. In addition to face to face instruction in the clinic visit, most practitioners provide an easy to understand handout of the procedure with helpful illustrations that describe the technical details as well as the goals and possible morbidities. Many children's hospitals have posted their UDS handouts online and these can be a good reference if one wishes to custom design a packet for use in their practice. After a discussion in the clinic and dissemination of informational materials, patients and parents should be encouraged to contact the provider for any questions or concerns that they may have regarding the study.

Despite optimal preparation of the patient and parents prior to the study, UDS is still an invasive procedure that is associated with pain, embarrassment, and loss of privacy. The procedure clinic should be structured to allow for the test to be conducted privately and include only those staff who are responsible for performance of the study. Outside traffic should be eliminated or minimized as much as possible with respect to the privacy of the patient. With regards to the test itself, pain will be diminished by selecting the smallest catheters possible. Viscous lidocaine should be introduced into the urethra 10–15 min prior to catheterization to provide lubrication and analgesia although children who catheterize regularly may be able to proceed with minimal or no wait time. Positioning of the patient in a comfortable fashion is necessary to minimize motion artifact during the study and since many of these patients have neurological co-morbidities, care must be taken to cushion pressure points that are susceptible to formation of decubitus ulcers. Most studies can be conducted effectively in either the sitting or supine position, depending on the preference of the child. Once the catheters are placed and the patient is in a comfortable position, most studies can be performed with minimal additional discomfort. Before instillation of the contrast or saline, the patient should be told that bladder fullness may be noted, and should be reported to the clinician, but significant pain is not part of the normal study. If the patient notes acute pain during the study, the inflow should be paused and the source of the pain should be identified and corrected.

The vast majority of patients can undergo UDS testing with minimal discomfort and with avoidance of artifacts that make interpretation of results difficult or even impossible. Some children, particularly those who are sensate, may simply not be able to handle the fear and pain without some form of sedation. Sweeney et al. conducted a study to identify which children would require sedation for completion of UDS and found that the most important factor was patient age between 3 and 7 years [42]. In addition to objective parameters, the ordering physician should observe how the child behaves in a non-threatening medical setting, such as a clinic visit, which may suggest how he or she may respond in the UDS suite. Also, parents may have useful information from prior studies that the child may have experienced to help decide when any particular child would best be served with a sedated procedure.

Benzodiazepines are the mainstay of sedative agents for invasive procedures because they are safe, effective, and easy to administer orally, intranasally or intravenously. Bozkurt and colleagues demonstrated that a 0.5 mg/kg dose of midazolam administered intranasally allowed all of their patients to successfully complete meaningful urodynamic studies [43]. They also showed that a single dose of medication did not alter the urodynamic parameters observed, including the maximum cystometric capacity, contractility, compliance, intravesical pressure, maximum flow rate, detrusor pressure at maximum flow, and post-void residual. A recent investigation by Theravaja compared the relative efficacy of midazolam versus ketamine when each was given IV as a loading dose followed by a continuous infusion during the procedure [44]. They found that both agents were equally effective in providing adequate sedation but the ketamine group showed lower reactivity to placement of rectal and urethral catheters. By comparison to historical patient data, they showed that neither agent impacted any of the urodynamic parameters measured. No specific agent has demonstrated clear superiority in the setting of pediatric UDS and so the choice of agent can be made on the basis of physician preference in deference to the setting in which these drugs are used.

With the administration of any sedative, patient safety is a primary concern and institutional guidelines regarding monitoring, equipment, nursing and specialist involvement should be devised and strictly followed. Providing sedation requires regular observation of the patient's blood pressure, oxygen saturation, and sedation level and this must be done by a credentialed individual who remains attentive during the entire procedure and afterwards in recovery. Since the urodynamic study itself demands the full attention of the urology staff, many institutions have created sedation teams to provide this service so that specific team members can focus on the safety and well-being of the patient while others can focus on the performance of the testing itself [42]. While the infrastructure and staffing requirements to provide sedated pediatric UDS may not be attainable in all facilities, they should be considered standard in all major children's healthcare centers with a pediatric urology program.

Under the best of circumstances, pediatric urodynamic studies can be fraught with motion artifacts. Therefore, it is ideal to have the interpreting provider present at the time of the study so that these artifacts do not confuse the analysis of the results. A reasonable alternative would be to have an experienced physician extender (NP, PA) who performs the study carefully documenting the time and source of any activity or phenomena that occur during the test. Notation of artifacts, for example a rise in abdominal and bladder pressure as the child grasps for a toy, should be documented electronically in the official UDS record. Older equipment may not permit this, in which case the artifact and source should be handwritten on the printed copy of the raw data so that urologists consulting the record in the future can accurately interpret the results.

Tips for Conduction of a Good Pediatric Study

Pediatric urodynamic studies are most efficiently and effectively performed in a dedicated pediatric procedure center where staff is dedicated to and comfortable with caring for children. Waiting rooms should be constructed to provide a relaxing family atmosphere as the patient will often be accompanied by multiple family members including siblings. Age-appropriate furniture, décor, and toys/games can help reduce stress prior to the procedure, which makes it easier to acclimate the child and parents before going into the UDS suite. Efficient patient flow strategies minimize aggravating delays that can introduce unnecessary stressors which can manifest in difficult behavior on the part of the child.

A significant percentage of children undergoing UDS testing have neurogenic bowel and will present with large amounts of hard stool in the rectum. Since this can make rectal catheter placement difficult and also introduce instability to the readings from that channel, many providers utilize a bowel washout prior to the procedure. A study by deKort showed that children undergoing colonic irrigation did not appear to have any noticeable change in the results of their UDS studies and there is no literature to support or dissuade the use of a pre-procedural bowel regimen [45]. Nonetheless, administration of an enema the morning of, and in some cases several days preceding the study can help with cleanliness and ease of catheter insertion. Practitioners may set a standard institutional protocol for the use of enemas, suppositories and/or oral laxatives, or custom tailor the regimen to individual patients who are at risk of impacted stools.

The decision as to whether or not parents should be present for the test is controversial and there is certainly a great deal of discretion to be exercised by the provider, based on the social situation and interfamily relationships of individual patients. However, as part of an effort to provide patient and family centered care, the American Academy of Pediatrics endorses the practice of allowing parents to be present for invasive procedures [46]. While UDS testing was not specifically mentioned in the guidelines, it stands to reason that parental presence as a comfort measure is beneficial to the well-being of the patient and the integrity of the test.

Equipment requirements for pediatric UDS testing are similar to that which is necessary for adult testing with the exception of the specific parameters of the bladder and rectal catheters. The effect of catheter size with regards to urodynamic results has not been formally studied in children but has been shown to be an influential factor in men with obstructive urinary conditions [47]. A large catheter, particularly in small boys, has the potential of obstructing the bladder outlet and urethra which can lead to a decrease in measured flow rates and increase in measured leak point pressures. Therefore, the smallest catheter available, usually a 6 Fr dual lumen catheter, is optimal for measurement accuracy.

Even children who are able to tolerate catheter placement and the bladder filling can have difficulties remaining still and focused for the duration of the study and this can introduce troublesome artifacts. Age-appropriate entertainment such as blowing bubbles and visually attractive toys are often effective in calming and settling infants while videos, electronic games, or reading materials are excellent means to maintain focus in older children. A child-life specialist can be a valuable team member, providing suggestions for specific interventions and assistance during the exam by gentle interaction with the child and accompanying parent.

Once the test is complete, it is best to have the child dress and accompany the parent to a separate room or location that provides privacy and comfort so that post-procedural counseling can occur away from the distracting and often crowded space in the UDS suite. This gives both the parent and child an opportunity to settle down and better comprehend the discussion of test results with the provider. A light snack or beverage for the patient may be beneficial for the patient to understand that the invasive procedures are complete and impart a sense of safety.

Congenital Anomalies with Radiographic and Urodynamic Examples

Videourodynamics for Pre/Post-operative Management of Neurogenic Incontinence

Figure 8.1a shows the urodynamic tracing of a 6-year-old girl with neurogenic bladder secondary to spina bifida. She had been managed for several years on a q2h CIC regimen and anticholinergic medication. Despite this, she constantly leaked between catheterizations and she suffered from approximately six breakthrough UTIs while on prophylactic nitrofurantoin. Renal ultrasounds demonstrated left hydronephrosis alternating between SFU (Society for Fetal Urology) grade 3 and 4. From the tracing and cystogram, it is apparent that the bladder is very small, trabeculated, and poorly compliant. Bilateral vesicoureteral reflux is noted with severity of grade 4 on the left and grade 1 on the right. With a capacity of 98 mL (estimated capacity of 180 mL) and a detrusor leak point pressure of 61 cm H_2O (annotated on the tracing as "leak"), it was felt that the patient's bladder was sufficiently hostile to cause renal deterioration over time. The decision to perform an outlet procedure concomitantly with the augmentation is not one that can be based solely on UDS data at this time. Rather, sphincteric incompetency must be suspected when the child has wetting episodes shortly after being catheterized and when videourodynamics shows that the bladder neck appears open during filling and when a low abdominal leak point pressure is noted. Based on the videourodynamics testing and on the clinical presentation, the patient was scheduled for a bilateral ureteral reimplantation, bladder augmentation, and a Pippi-Salle bladder neck reconstruction.

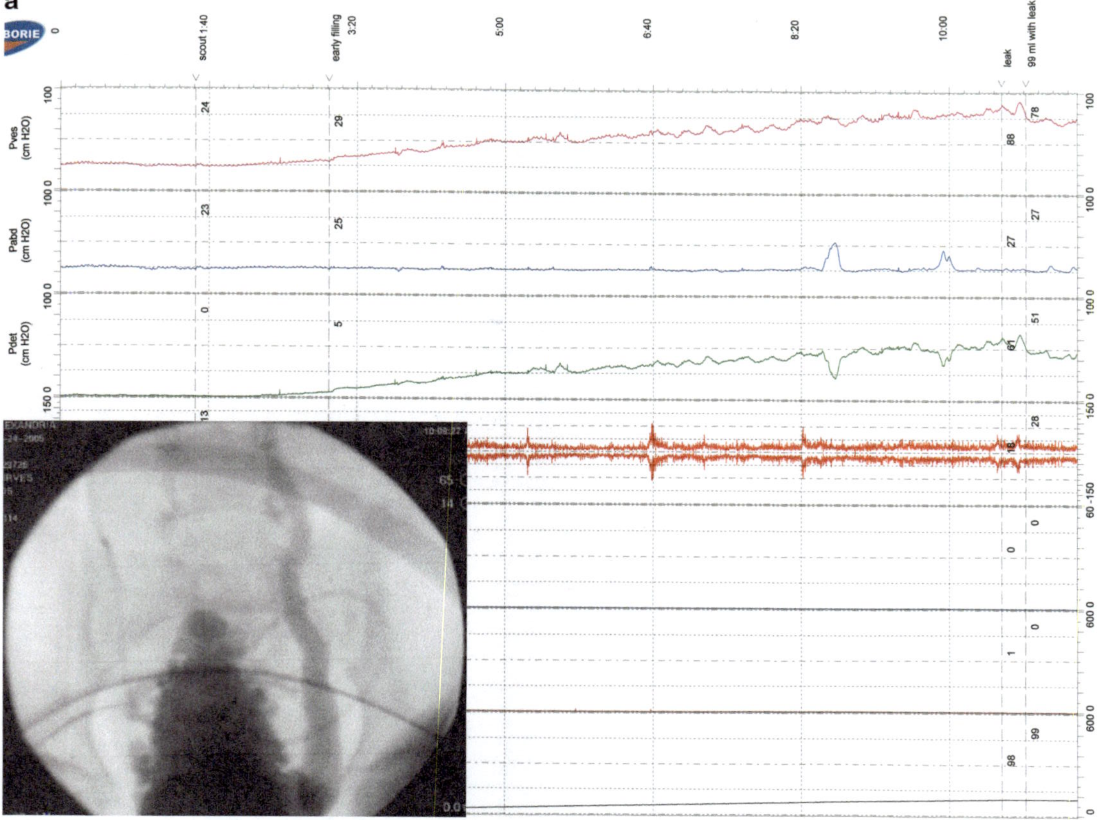

Fig. 8.1 (**a**) Pre-operative urodynamic study for 6-year-old with neurogenic bladder secondary to spina bifida. *Pves* bladder pressure, *Pabd* abdominal pressure, *Pdet* detrusor pressure, *EMG* pelvic floor electromyography. *Inset*: Cystogram at bladder capacity of 98 mL. (**b**) Post-operative urodynamic study for 6-year-old with neurogenic bladder secondary to spina bifida. *Pves* bladder pressure, *Pabd* abdominal pressure, *Pdet* detrusor pressure, *EMG* pelvic floor electromyography. *Inset*: Cystogram at bladder capacity of 286 mL

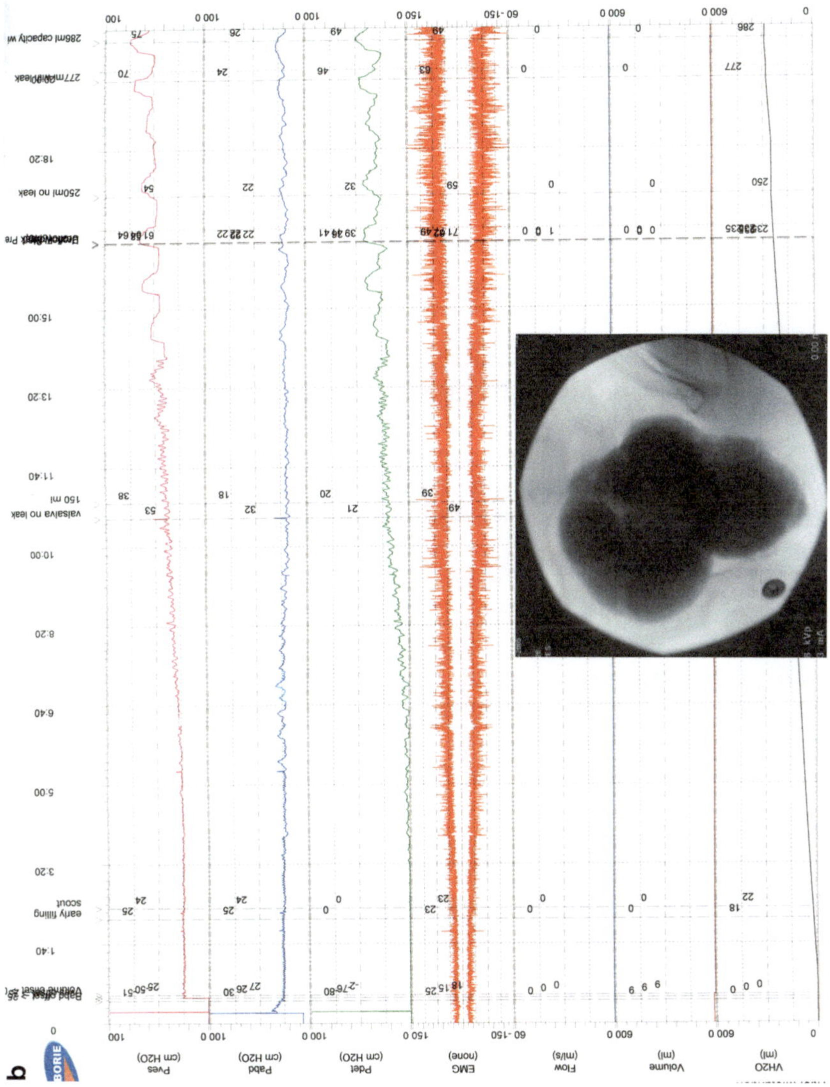

Fig. 8.1 (continued)

Twelve months after surgery, the patient was continent during the day so long as she did not wait more than 4 h between catheterizations. She did not report any UTIs in the 6 months prior to the post-operative follow-up videourodynamic study. In Fig. 8.1b, the post-operative changes are evident with an increase in bladder capacity from 98 to 286 mL and cessation of her bilateral vesicoureteral reflux. Bladder compliance was significantly improved and her storage pressure only reached 25 cm H_2O at capacity before leakage occurred. Detrusor overactivity was noted at the later stages of filling and this has prompted us to re-initiate anticholinergic therapy. However, the study confirms the successful clinical outcomes and assures us that her urine is being stored at sufficiently low pressures to prevent renal deterioration in the future.

Videourodynamics for Diagnosis and Management of Incontinence in a Child with PUV

Figure 8.2 shows the urodynamic tracing and cystogram of an 8-year-old boy who was referred to our institution for ongoing day and nighttime urinary incontinence as well as worsening left hydronephrosis. He had a history of PUV that had been ablated twice before he was a year of age and he had a history of left vesicoureteral reflux that was treated surgically with ureteral reimplantation soon after his first birthday. On the tracing, detrusor overactivity is noted to start when the bladder is filled to 89 mL and it becomes more regular and forceful as the bladder volume approaches 150 mL. None of the involuntary contractions caused leakage but they were associated with urinary urgency as reported by the patient. It is quite possible that during these contractions, the urethral catheter was significantly large enough to obstruct the urethra and prevent urine from escaping. The patient reported severe urgency at 221 mL which is much less than the expected bladder capacity of 300 mL derived from his age and the aforementioned formula. He was instructed to void and did so with a voiding pressure well over 100 cm H_2O and a poor, dribbling stream that left over 50 mL as a post-void residual. The cystogram showed an obvious obstruction in the urethra with a dilated posterior urethra and no evidence of vesicoureteral reflux. Based on this study and the patient's clinical history, it was recommended that he undergo a repeat cystoscopy to diagnose and treat the urethral obstruction that was thought to be due to residual urethral valves or due to scarring from prior surgical attempts at ablation.

In the operating room, cystoscopic examination demonstrated classic appearing PUV and a dilated prostatic urethra. The valves were ablated with hook electrocautery and a 12 Fr Foley catheter was left in place for one day post-operatively. One month after the procedure, the patient and his parents report a decrease in the frequency and volume of urinary accidents during the day. He is being managed conservatively with timed voiding and a good bowel regimen but no medications or other interventions. If his bladder function fails to improve, a repeat videourodynamic test will be indicated to confirm a patent bladder outlet and urethra as well as investigate the persistence of involuntary detrusor contractions that may respond to anticholinergic therapy.

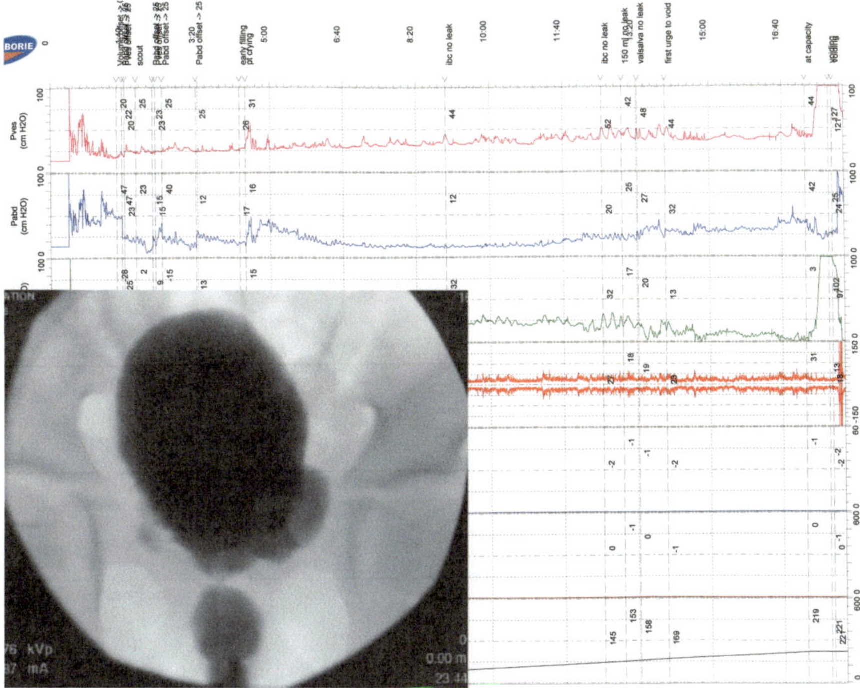

Fig. 8.2 Urodynamic study of 8-year-old boy with posterior urethral valves. *Pves* bladder pressure, *Pabd* abdominal pressure, *Pdet* detrusor pressure, *EMG* pelvic floor electromyography. *Inset*: Cystogram at bladder capacity of 221 mL

Videourodynamics for Diagnosis and Management of Hinman's Syndrome

Figure 8.3 shows the urodynamic tracing and concurrent cystogram of a 14-year-old boy who was initially referred for hydronephrosis that was discovered during a work-up for recurrent UTIs. The child reported that he only typically voided 2 or 3 times maximum during the course of a normal day and only had one bowel movement per week. Videourodynamics was indicated after it was discovered that the patient had underlying renal insufficiency and a complex uroflowmetry demonstrating poor flow and a high post-void residual. The most striking feature of the study is that the patient did not have any sensation to void prior to reaching a bladder volume of 700 mL. During filling, the bladder was stable but he reached a threshold filling pressure of 40 cm H_2O at only 520 mL. The cystogram showed a very large, smooth walled bladder with no evidence of reflux or urethral obstruction. He was able to void volitionally with good pressure generated from the bladder, but there was also evidence of significant sphincter activity during micturition and the patient was left with a post-void residual of 300 mL. Given his high pressure storage, inability to adequately empty his bladder, and worsening hydronephrosis and renal

J.T. Purves and A.A. Stec

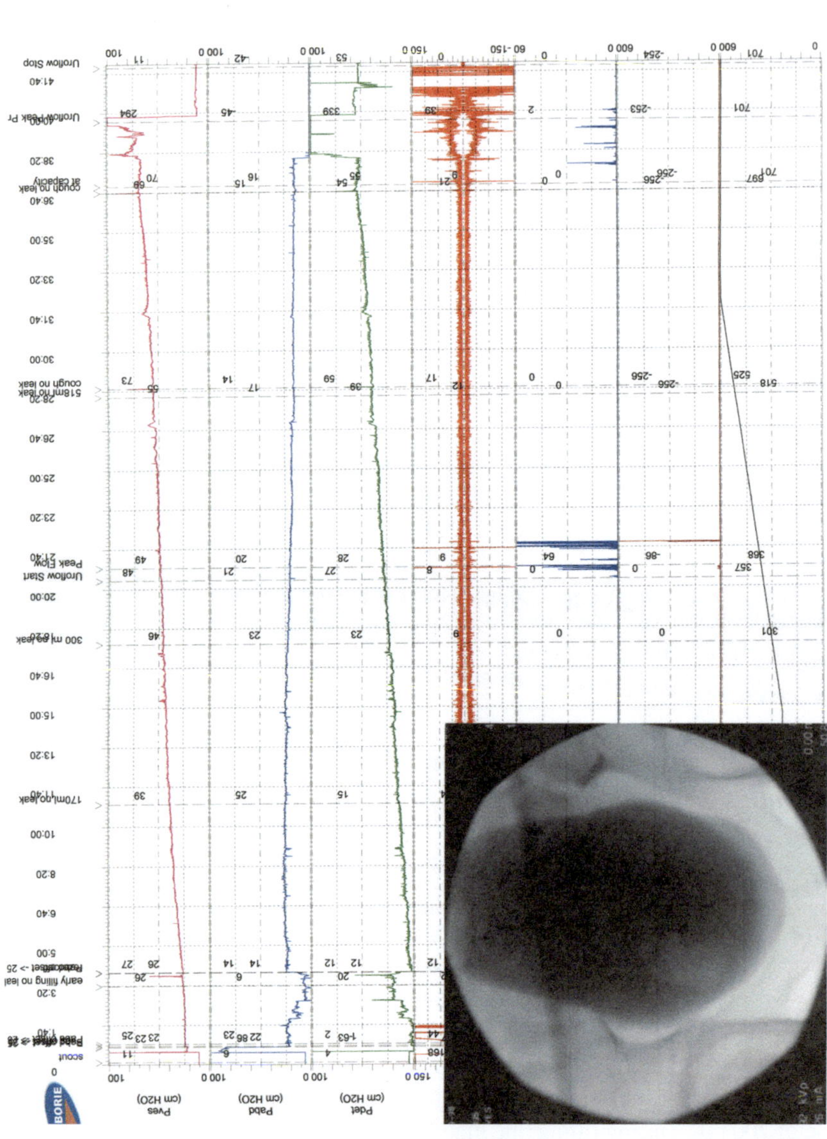

Fig. 8.3 Urodynamic study of 14-year-old boy with Hinman's syndrome. *Pves* bladder pressure, *Pabd* abdominal pressure, *Pdet* detrusor pressure, *EMG* pelvic floor electromyography. *Inset:* Voiding cystogram from bladder capacity of 701 mL

function, the child was started on a q4hr intermittent catheterization schedule. An extensive neurological work-up has not uncovered any underlying pathology to the patient's dysfunctional voiding. He is therefore classified as having Hinman's syndrome which is defined as a functional bladder outlet obstruction in the absence of neurological defects.

Videourodynamic Assessment of Bladder Function in a Pediatric Renal Transplant Candidate

Figure 8.4 depicts the urodynamic tracing and cystogram of a 7-year-old boy in end stage renal failure with Trisomy 18 (Edward's Syndrome). He had experienced several febrile UTIs as an infant and a voiding cystourethrogram done at the time showed severe left reflux and a trabeculated bladder. In the years preceding referral, the patient voided into a diaper and did not have any UTIs despite not being on prophylactic antibiotics. He had been started on dialysis 6 months prior to his visit, after he had presented to an emergency room with vomiting and had been found to be hypertensive and in renal failure. UDS was indicated to investigate whether or not the bladder was a suitable reservoir for a renal transplant. The tracing shows episodic, spontaneous bladder contractions during filling that result in leakage at 40–50 cm H_2O. However, storage pressure remained close to zero and this is partially explained by the findings on the cystograms taken early in the study and again during a bladder contraction at maximum capacity. The cystogram demonstrates severe left vesicoureteral reflux seen in the latter radiograph providing a pressure sink or "functional augmentation" or "pop-off". It was felt that the volume and compliance of the bladder combined with the dilated upper urinary tract were acceptable to support renal transplantation. The study, however, also showed that the patient was unable to efficiently empty his bladder, which could put him at risk for UTIs in post-transplant, immune-compromised state. Since the parents did not feel that the patient would tolerate intermittent catheterization, the family and treating team chose to perform a vesicostomy prior to transplant. When the parents feel that the child is accepting of a catheterization regimen, he will undergo a takedown of the vesicostomy and construction of a continent catheterizable channel.

Conclusion

Current trends in medicine, and particularly in pediatrics, have focused on minimizing the invasiveness of diagnostic and therapeutic procedures. As a result, methods with an inherent level of morbidity, such as UDS, have come under increased scrutiny. Pediatric urologists must address this going forward by defining exactly who benefits from these studies, thereby limiting their performance to the smallest

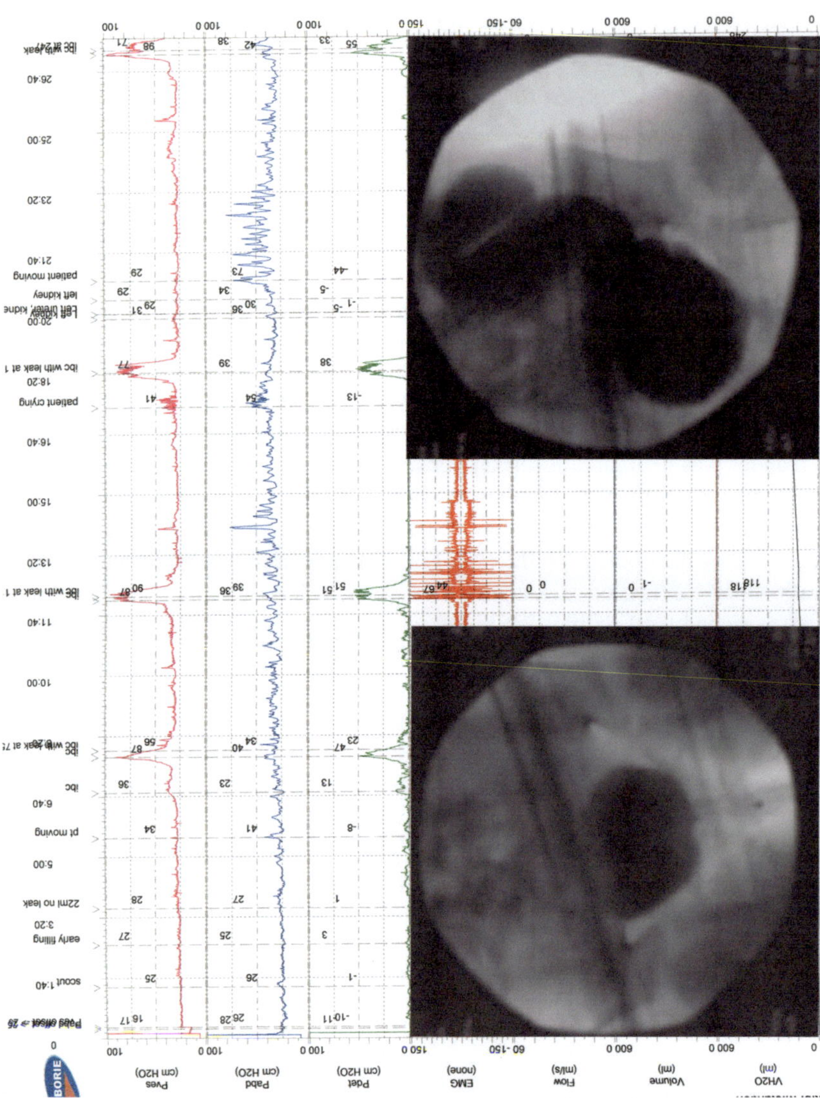

Fig. 8.4 Urodynamic study of a 7 year old boy with end stage renal failure due to reflux nephropathy. *Pves* bladder pressure, *Pabd* abdominal pressure, *Pdet* detrusor pressure, *EMG* pelvic floor electromyography. *Inset*: Cystogram with bladder volume of 22 mL (*left*), and cystogram at bladder capacity of 248 mL (*right*) showing grade 5 vesicoureteral reflux on the *left*

number possible. All steps should be taken to minimize the trauma of the testing and we should be cognizant of the technological advances, such as remote sensing, that are truly necessary to bring UDS into the twenty-first century. However, the value of UDS in diagnosing and formulating treatment for children with voiding pathologies is sufficiently high that we cannot allow the abandonment or serious discouragement of these techniques.

References

1. Koff SA. Evaluation and management of voiding disorders in children. Urol Clin North Am. 1988;15(4):769–75. Epub 1988/11/01.
2. Hoebeke P, Van Laecke E, Van Camp C, Raes A, Van De Walle J. One thousand video-urodynamic studies in children with non-neurogenic bladder sphincter dysfunction. BJU Int. 2001;87(6):575–80. Epub 2001/04/12.
3. Soygur T, Arikan N, Tokatli Z, Karaboga R. The role of video-urodynamic studies in managing non-neurogenic voiding dysfunction in children. BJU Int. 2004;93(6):841–3. Epub 2004/03/31.
4. Bael A, Lax H, de Jong TP, Hoebeke P, Nijman RJ, Sixt R, et al. The relevance of urodynamic studies for urge syndrome and dysfunctional voiding: a multicenter controlled trial in children. J Urol. 2008;180(4):1486–93; discussion 94–5. Epub 2008/08/20.
5. Kaufman MR, DeMarco RT, Pope 4th JC, Scarpero HM, Adams MC, Trusler LA, et al. High yield of urodynamics performed for refractory nonneurogenic dysfunctional voiding in the pediatric population. J Urol. 2006;176(4 Pt 2):1835–7. Epub 2006/09/02.
6. Drzewiecki BA, Bauer SB. Urodynamic testing in children: indications, technique, interpretation and significance. J Urol. 2011;186(4):1190–7. Epub 2011/08/19.
7. Neveus T, von Gontard A, Hoebeke P, Hjalmas K, Bauer S, Bower W, et al. The standardization of terminology of lower urinary tract function in children and adolescents: report from the Standardisation Committee of the International Children's Continence Society. J Urol. 2006;176(1):314–24. Epub 2006/06/07.
8. Hoebeke P, Bower W, Combs A, De Jong T, Yang S. Diagnostic evaluation of children with daytime incontinence. J Urol. 2010;183(2):699–703. Epub 2009/12/22.
9. Acar B, Arikan FI, Germiyanoglu C, Dallar Y. Influence of high bladder pressure on vesico-ureteral reflux and its resolution. Urol Int. 2009;82(1):77–80. Epub 2009/01/28.
10. Bauer SB, Neveus T, von Gontard A, Hoebeke P, Bower W, Jorgensen TM, et al. Standardizing terminology in pediatric urology. J Pediatr Urol. 2007;3(2):163. Epub 2008/10/25.
11. Edelstein RA, Bauer SB, Kelly MD, Darbey MM, Peters CA, Atala A, et al. The long-term urological response of neonates with myelodysplasia treated proactively with intermittent catheterization and anticholinergic therapy. J Urol. 1995;154(4):1500–4. Epub 1995/10/01.
12. Dik P, Klijn AJ, van Gool JD, de Jong-de Vos van Steenwijk CC, de Jong TP. Early start to therapy preserves kidney function in spina bifida patients. Eur Urol. 2006;49(5):908–13. Epub 2006/02/07.
13. Bauer SB. Neurogenic bladder: etiology and assessment. Pediatr Nephrol. 2008;23(4):541–51. Epub 2008/02/14.
14. Peters CA, Bolkier M, Bauer SB, Hendren WH, Colodny AH, Mandell J, et al. The urodynamic consequences of posterior urethral valves. J Urol. 1990;144(1):122–6. Epub 1990/07/01.
15. Bauer S, Labib KB, Dieppa RA, Retik AB. Urodynamic evaluation of boys with myelodysplasia and incontinence. Urology. 1977;10:354.
16. Ghanem MA, Wolffenbuttel KP, De Vylder A, Nijman RJ. Long-term bladder dysfunction and renal function in boys with posterior urethral valves based on urodynamic findings. J Urol. 2004;171(6 Pt 1):2409–12. Epub 2004/05/06.

17. Podesta ML, Ruarte A, Gargiulo C, Medel R, Castera R. Urodynamic findings in boys with posterior urethral valves after treatment with primary valve ablation or vesicostomy and delayed ablation. J Urol. 2000;164(1):139–44. Epub 2000/06/07.

18. Holmdahl G, Sillen U, Hanson E, Hermansson G, Hjalmas K. Bladder dysfunction in boys with posterior urethral valves before and after puberty. J Urol. 1996;155(2):694–8. Epub 1996/02/01.

19. Boemers TM, Beek FJ, van Gool JD, de Jong TP, Bax KM. Urologic problems in anorectal malformations. Part 1: urodynamic findings and significance of sacral anomalies. J Pediatr Surg. 1996;31(3):407–10.

20. Boemers TM, de Jong TP, van Gool JD, Bax KM. Urologic problems in anorectal malformations. Part 2: functional urologic sequelae. J Pediatr Surg. 1996;31(5):634–7.

21. Taskinen S, Valanne L, Rintala R. Effect of spinal cord abnormalities on the function of the lower urinary tract in patients with anorectal abnormalities. J Urol. 2002;168(3):1147–9. Epub 2002/08/21.

22. Schafer W, Abrams P, Liao L, Mattiasson A, Pesce F, Spangberg A, et al. Good urodynamic practices: uroflowmetry, filling cystometry, and pressure-flow studies. Neurourol Urodyn. 2002;21(3):261–74. Epub 2002/04/12.

23. Holmdahl G, Hanson E, Hanson M, Hellstrom AL, Hjalmas K, Sillen U. Four-hour voiding observation in healthy infants. J Urol. 1996;156(5):1809–12. Epub 1996/11/01.

24. Koff SA. Estimating bladder capacity in children. Urology. 1983;21(3):248. Epub 1983/03/01.

25. Hjalmas K. Urodynamics in normal infants and children. Scand J Urol Nephrol Suppl. 1988;114:20–7. Epub 1988/01/01.

26. Hjalmas K. Micturition in infants and children with normal lower urinary tract. A urodynamic study. Scand J Urol Nephrol. 1976;Suppl 37:1–106. Epub 1976/01/01.

27. De Jong T, Klijn AJ. Urodynamic studies in pediatric urology. Nat Rev Urol. 2009;6:585.

28. Nijman RJ, Bower W, Butler U. Diagnosis and management of urinary incontinence and encopresis in childhood. In: Abrams P, Cardozo L, Khoury S, editors. 3rd international consulation on incontinence. Paris: Health Publications Ltd.; 2005. p. 967–1057.

29. Yeung CK, Godley ML, Duffy PG, Ransley PG. Natural filling cystometry in infants and children. Br J Urol. 1995;75(4):531–7. Epub 1995/04/01.

30. Ghobish AG. Storage detrusor pressure in bilateral hydroureteronephrosis. Eur Urol. 2001;39(5):571–4. Epub 2001/07/21.

31. Sillen U. Bladder function in infants. Scand J Urol Nephrol Suppl. 2004;215:69–74. Epub 2004/11/17.

32. Yeung CK, Godley ML, Ho CK, Ransley PG, Duffy PG, Chen CN, et al. Some new insights into bladder function in infancy. Br J Urol. 1995;76(2):235–40. Epub 1995/08/01.

33. Gupta DK, Sankhwar SN, Goel A. Uroflowmetry nomograms for healthy children 5 to 15 years old. J Urol. 2013;190(3):1008–13. Epub 2013/03/30.

34. Glazier DB, Murphy DP, Fleisher MH, Cummings KB, Barone JG. Evaluation of the utility of video-urodynamics in children with urinary tract infection and voiding dysfunction. Br J Urol. 1997;80(5):806–8. Epub 1997/12/11.

35. Vereecken RL, Proesmans W. Urethral instability as an important element of dysfunctional voiding. J Urol. 2000;163(2):585–8. Epub 2000/01/27.

36. McCormack M, Pike J, Kiruluta G. Leak point of incontinence: a measure of the interaction between outlet resistance and bladder capacity. J Urol. 1993;150(1):162–4. Epub 1993/07/01.

37. Furlow B. Radiation protection in pediatric imaging. Radiol Technol. 2011;82(5):421–39. Epub 2011/05/17.

38. Ngo TC, Clark CJ, Wynne C, Kennedy 2nd WA. Radiation exposure during pediatric videourodynamics. J Urol. 2011;186(4 Suppl):1672–6. Epub 2011/08/25.

39. Hsi RS, Dearn J, Dean M, Zamora DA, Kanal KM, Harper JD, et al. Effective and organ specific radiation doses from videourodynamics in children. J Urol. 2013;190(4):1364–9. Epub 2013/05/28.

40. Ellerkmann RM, McBride AW, Dunn JS, Bent AE, Blomquist J, Kummer L, et al. A comparison of anticipatory and postprocedure pain perception in patients who undergo urodynamic procedures. Am J Ob Gyn. 2004;190:1034–8.

41. Kleiber C, McCarthy AM. Parent behavior and child distress during urethral catheterization. J Soc Pediatr Nurs. 1999;4:95–104.
42. Sweeney H, Marai S, Kim C, Ferrer F. Creating a sedation service for pediatric urodynamics: our experience. Urol Nurs. 2008;28(4):273–8.
43. Bozkurt P, Killic N, Kaya G, Yeker Y, Elicevik M, Soylet Y. The effects of intranasal midazolam on urodynamic studies in children. Br J Urol. 1996;78(2):282–6.
44. Theravaja A, Batra Y, Rao K, Chhabra M, Aggarwal M. Comparison of low-dose ketamine to midazolam for sedation during pediatric urodynamic study. Paediatr Anaesth. 2013;23(5): 415–21.
45. de Kort L, Nesselaar C, van Gool J, de Jong T. The influence of colonic enema irrigation on urodynamic findings in patients with neurogenic bladder dysfunction. Br J Urol. 1997;80(5): 731–3.
46. Pediatrics AAO. Patient- and family- centered care and the pediatrician's role. Pediatrics. 2012;129(2):394–404.
47. Smith A, Ferlise V, Wein A, Ramchandani P, Rovner E. Effect of A 7-F transurethral catheter on abdominal leak point pressure measurement in men with post-prostatectomy incontinence. Urology. 2011;77(5):1188–93.

Chapter 9
Special Considerations in the Neurogenic Patient

Teresa L. Danforth and David Ginsberg

Abbreviations

NGB   Neurogenic bladder
UDS   Urodynamics
AD   Autonomic dysreflexia
BP   Blood pressure
VUR   Vesicoureteral reflux
SCI   Spinal cord injury
UTI   Urinary tract infection
FUDS   Fluorourodynamics
CFU   Colony forming units
BPE   Benign prostatic hypertrophy
DESD   Detrusor external sphincter dyssynergia
EMG   Electromyelography
NDO   Neurogenic detrusor overactivity

T.L. Danforth, MD (✉)
Department of Urology, SUNY Buffalo School of Medicine and Biomedical Sciences,
Buffalo General Hospital, 100 High Street, Suite B280, Buffalo, NY 14203, USA

Department of Urology, Keck School of Medicine of USC, University of Southern California,
1441 Eastlake Avenue, Suite 7416, Los Angeles, CA 90089-9178, USA
e-mail: danforth@buffalo.edu

D. Ginsberg, MD, DSc
Department of Urology, Keck School of Medicine of USC, University of Southern California,
1441 Eastlake Avenue, Suite 7416, Los Angeles, CA 90089-9178, USA
e-mail: ginsberg@med.usc.edu

© Springer Science+Business Media New York 2015
E.S. Rovner, M.E. Koski (eds.), *Rapid and Practical Interpretation
of Urodynamics*, DOI 10.1007/978-1-4939-1764-8_9

Introduction

There are various goals in treatment of any patient with neurogenic bladder (NGB) which are outlined in Table 9.1, with the primary goal being preservation of renal function, which is maintained by storage of urine at low detrusor pressure [1, 2]. Urodynamics (UDS) are essential in evaluating the efficacy of treatment regimens for patients with NGB. Current guidelines address the need for urodynamic studies in the initial evaluation of the neurogenic patient; however, there are no guidelines for physicians for following them long-term. This chapter will focus on special considerations for UDS in the neurogenic patient.

Challenges in Reproducing Symptoms in NGB

A significant challenge when performing UDS in patients with NGB is the reproduction of their clinical symptoms during the study. For many NGB patients there is an inherent lack of symptomatology due to impaired bladder sensation. In addition, the degree of symptomatology does not necessarily correlate with findings on UDS, even in the neurologically intact patient. For neurogenic patients, not only this is true, but the degree of symptomatology also does not necessarily correlate with the magnitude of their disease affecting the urinary tract. Many patients may be at risk for upper tract disease but are entirely asymptomatic. Patients also may not be fully aware of symptoms and therefore cannot describe whether their leakage is associated with urinary urgency or stress maneuvers such as transfers. They may have altered bladder sensation or no bladder sensation at all. All of these factors make it more challenging to reproduce symptoms in patients with NGB.

According to Good Urodynamic Practice Guidelines, repeat UDS studies are recommended if "the initial test suggests an abnormality, leaves cause of troublesome lower urinary tract symptoms unresolved, or if there are technical problems preventing proper analysis" [3]. If these guidelines are to be followed, all NGB patients would require repeated studies.

Bellucci et al. [4] addressed this in a prospective study of 226 NGB patients who underwent same session repeat UDS, looking at repeatability based on 95 % limits

Table 9.1 Goals of management of neurogenic bladder dysfunction [1]	
	Upper urinary tract preservation or improvement
	Absence or control of infection
	Low storage pressures with adequate bladder capacity
	Low voiding pressures with adequate emptying ability if not performing intermittent cath
	Minimal or no incontinence
	Avoidance of indwelling catheter or stoma
	Social acceptability and adaptability of bladder management
	Vocational acceptability and adaptability of bladder management

of agreement. The only measure found to have good repeatability was detrusor overactivity. The other measures including maximum cystometric capacity, compliance, maximum detrusor storage pressure, detrusor leak point pressure, and voiding parameters (in the 88 patients who were able to void spontaneously) were not consistent between studies. The authors suggest that the clinical decision-making not be based on one UDS filling, but should base it on multiple cycles and concentrate on the results that cause concern. Another study by Ockrim et al. [5] confirmed that detrusor overactivity is repeatable in patients with NGB, but not necessarily repeatable for men with LUTS. This study did not comment on other urodynamic parameters in spinal cord injury (SCI) patients.

Ambulatory UDS has been used to mimic a more physiologic filling of the bladder. Virseda et al. [6] looked at the test-retest repeatability of two ambulatory UDS 24 h apart in 66 patients with SCI. They found no significant differences between the two studies for bladder capacity, maximum detrusor pressure during a detrusor contraction, and post-void residual. However, they found that filling pressure was not reproducible, which is concerning as the filling pressure is directly related to upper tract damage.

This reinforces the importance of looking at the entire clinical picture in the neurogenic patient. It is also often helpful to obtain history from family members or caretakers as they can give insight into bladder behavior that the patient might be unaware of.

Role of Prognosis in UDS Studies in NGB

As previously stated, there are no current guidelines on how often UDS should be repeated in the NGB population. The real question would be to ask how often do UDS change a patient's bladder management. Nossier et al. [7] performed a retrospective review of 80 SCI patients who underwent UDS once a year for at least 5 years to determine how often treatment is modified based on UDS results. They defined treatment success as detrusor pressure <40 cm of water during filling and <90 cm of water during voiding as well as absence of AD, <3 urinary tract infections (UTIs) per year, one continence pad per day, and no hydronephrosis or scarring on renal ultrasound. With a mean follow-up of 67.3 months, no patient had signs of renal damage and 77 of 80 patients ultimately required treatment modification based on urodynamic findings during the study period. Of patients who were symptomatic at time of UDS, all of them had abnormalities on UDS. More importantly, 68 % of clinical failures would have been undetected based on symptoms alone.

As UDS are time consuming and expensive, attempts at using other clinical tools to assess a patient's need for UDS have been explored. Pannek et al. [8] looked at the use of detrusor wall thickness at various bladder volumes and its correlation to favorable urodynamic results and found that it was sensitive to determine the patients with no risk factors for renal damage; however, clinical parameters such as detrusor overactivity and incontinence could not be evaluated and may require further evaluation with UDS regardless of risk of renal damage.

Preparing for UDS

Many NGB patients also have neurogenic bowel and most have a home bowel regimen. If patients are not on a bowel regimen, it may necessitate bowel evacuation prior to the study to allow accurate rectal catheter pressure readings [9]. If patients are already on a bowel program, rectal suppositories or enemas should be administered with enough time prior to the study to allow the medication to take effect and avoid bowel movements during the procedure.

UDS can be performed in the supine, sitting, standing positions, or even while ambulating [10]. Many patients with NGB have significant limitations in their mobility that do not allow them to sit on or stand at a commode like a typical patient. Keeping in mind that many patients do not void into a toilet, it is perfectly acceptable for neurogenic patients to be in the supine position for urodynamic testing. It is important that they are comfortable and that excess pressure on any limbs is avoided as this may lead to skin breakdown or even autonomic dysreflexia (AD). If performing a study with fluoroscopy (FUDS), it is ideal for patients to be placed in an oblique position to allow for better visualization of the bladder neck. In this case, voided urine may be collected in a wide-bore drainpipe with length to reach the flowmeter. When possible, patients who volitionally void may be able to sit on a commode more easily which would allow for measurement of pressure-flow. Patients might require study repetition in multiple positions, especially if expected results are not achieved in the supine position.

AD: Recognition and Management

The first case of autonomic dysreflexia (AD) was first described as hot flushes in a C5 SCI patient by Hilton in 1960 [11]. Subsequent reports included patients with a variety of symptoms including hot flushes, sweating with bradycardia, and an increase in blood pressure (BP) associated with a distended bladder [12, 13]. In 1947 Guttman and Whitteridge then more fully described the autonomic response after distension of the abdominal viscera leading to effects on cardiovascular activity in SCI patients [14].

AD occurs in approximately 60 % of cervical and 20 % of thoracic SCI patients. The most common etiology is bladder or rectal distension, either spontaneous or by instrumentation. Other etiologies include plugged catheters, urinary tract stones, long bone fracture, decubitus ulcers, or even electroejaculation.

Classic signs of AD include an increase in BP with bradycardia, although true bradycardia is only seen in approximately 10 % of patients. In fact, tachycardia or no significant change in heart rate is more common in patients with AD. Other signs may include cardiac arrhythmias, changes in skin temperatures (vasodilation above the lesion, vasoconstriction below the lesion), or changes in mentation.

Common symptoms include sweating above the lesion, pounding headache, hot flushes, piloerection, nasal congestion, dyspnea, and anxiety. Although we think of

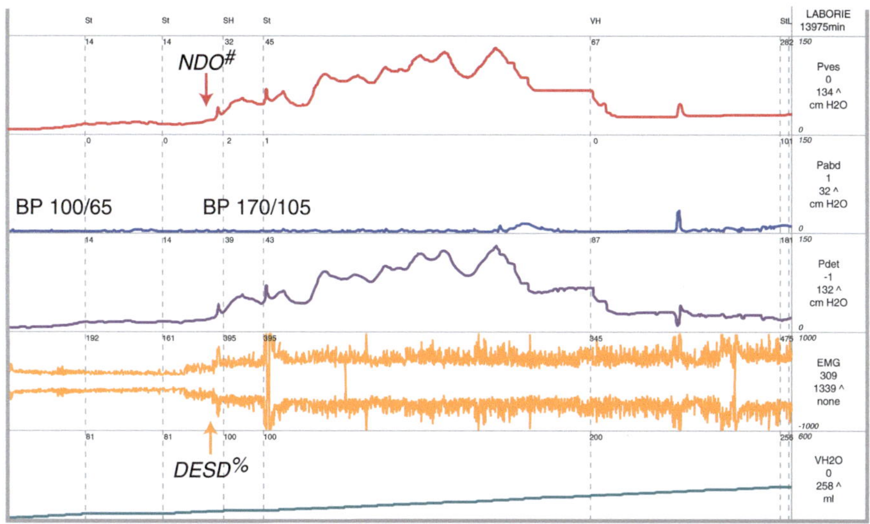

Fig. 9.1 Autonomic dysreflexia. Elevation in blood pressure associated with a detrusor contraction and detrusor-sphincter dyssynergia during UDS in a quadriplegic patient. #Neurogenic detrusor overactivity. %Detrusor external sphincter dyssynergia

patients presenting with these classic symptoms, some patients may be entirely asymptomatic. A study by Linsenmeyer et al. [15] demonstrated that 35 of 45 patients with SCI above T6 were asymptomatic with a significant elevation of BP. This stresses the importance of monitoring BP during procedures as AD may be missed in an asymptomatic patient with possible devastating outcomes including seizures, stroke, or even death. During a UDS study it is generally recommended to obtain a baseline BP and cycle the BP during regular intervals throughout the study (Fig. 9.1).

When AD is recognized, the first course of action should be removal of the stimulus. Usually this means ensuring that a patient's catheter is draining appropriately, checking for fecal impaction, or if performing a urologic procedure, immediate emptying of the bladder. It is also recommended to move the patient upright and remove any tight clothing or constrictive devices [16]. If this does not alleviate symptoms and/or decrease BP, one can move to pharmacologic agents. No particular pharmacologic agent is preferred for acute AD, and multiple drugs have been used: nifedipine, nitrates, captopril, terazosin, prazosin, phenoxybenzamine, and Prostagladin E2.

Nifedipine, a calcium channel blocker, has been the most popular pharmacologic agent for management of acute AD. The usual dose is 10 mg oral and the patient is asked to chew and swallow the medication for optimal absorption. The use of nifedipine is falling out of favor secondary to adverse events seen in management of hypertensive emergencies (not SCI), which include stroke, heart attack, severe hypotension, and death [17]. Nitrates have been used for acute AD, but should be used with caution, especially in patients who use PDE5 inhibitors because of drug interaction. Topical nitrates are easy to use and can be removed quickly if necessary. Typically they are placed on the shoulders or arms, above the level of injury. If patients have a history of AD, consideration of providing pharmacological prophylaxis 30 min prior to a urologic procedure including UDS would be appropriate.

Patients with recurrent AD can be managed prophylactically. Terazosin 5 mg nightly has been used without change in BP or erectile function [18]. Vaidyanathan et al. [19] titrated terazosin from 1 to 10 mg daily in 18 patients with resolution of AD in all patients. One patient did require discontinuation secondary to dizziness.

Although prophylaxis has been effective in prevention of AD, it is important to continue to monitor during any urologic procedure, including UDS. Other prophylactic medications include prazosin and phenoxybenzamine, and intravesical botulinum toxin and capsaicin have been demonstrated to decrease AD episodes, but further studies are required. If conservative measures still do not alleviate AD, sacral denervation has been described, but studies are conflicting on their effectiveness of eliminating AD.

Infection

UTI is a significant potential cause of morbidity as well as potential source for upper tract damage in patients with NGB. Patients with SCI are at a higher risk of infection simply due to how they manage their bladder, whether it is reflex voiding, intermittent catheterization, indwelling catheter, or urinary diversion. In a study of 112 patients with SCI, 75 % of patients had positive cultures as defined by $>10^3$ colony forming units (CFU) [20]. The patients managed by IC had lower rates of positive cultures, lower CFU, and lower number of species growing than those managed with indwelling SPT, urethral catheter, or reflex voiding. It is important to note, despite the use of IC, 70 % of these patients still had positive cultures. This is especially important when considering when to perform UDS.

Böthig et al. [21] looked at rates of UTI associated with UDS performed on hospitalized patients, excluding those who had already been treated or patients with indwelling catheters, finding that 30 % of patients had unsuspected bacteriuria defined as $\geq 10^5$ CFU. After patients underwent UDS, 88 % of the patients who were sterile prior to UDS remained sterile 3–5 days later, whereas 50 % of patients with bacteriuria prior to UDS had sterile cultures later. Patients who utilized reflex voiding were at highest risk to have UTI (defined as bacteriuria and ≥ 100 leukocytes/μL urine), though this group was only 19 patients.

In general it is not advised to give antibiotic prophylaxis to NGB patients undergoing UDS as there is no consistent evidence that prophylaxis provides significant benefit and may in fact promote antibiotic resistance, which is a common problem in NGB patients.

Use of Fluoroscopy or Video Urodynamics

Often patients with NGB have symptoms that are difficult to differentiate, especially when evaluating incontinence and incomplete bladder emptying. This is particularly challenging for aging male patients with concomitant benign prostatic enlargement (BPE) or female patients with concomitant prolapse. FUDS allows one to evaluate multiple aspects of both filling and voiding. AUA guidelines state, "When available, clinicians may perform fluoroscopy at the time of urodynamics (videourodynamics) in patients with relevant neurologic disease at risk for neurogenic bladder…" [22].

In the filling and voiding phases, upper tract dilation can be seen with elevated bladder pressures, and may be associated with vesicoureteral reflux (VUR) [9]. Upper tract dilation is seen much less commonly in females than males. FUDS allows one to assess bladder pressures and visualize the bladder and upper tracts to assess for VUR. Frequently patients with VUR and a poorly compliant bladder have a "Christmas tree" appearance with severe trabeculations and massively dilated upper tracts (Fig. 9.2). The clinical consequences of VUR include increased risk of pyelonephritis and permanent renal scarring.

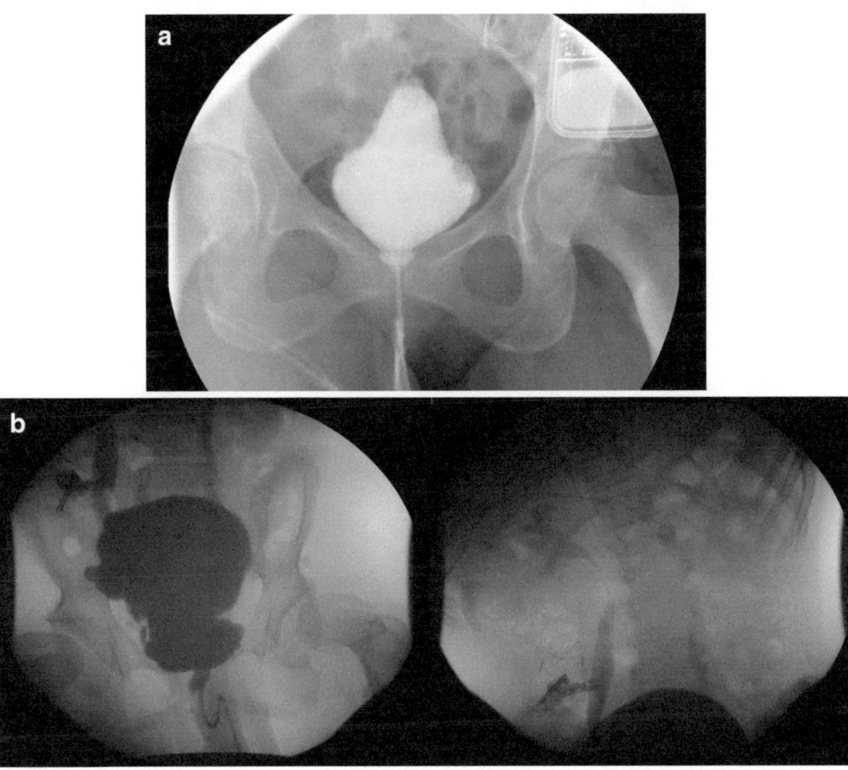

Fig. 9.2 Vesicoureteral Reflux. (**a**): Patient with a poorly compliant "Christmas Tree" appearance to her bladder without VUR. (**b**): Patient with a trabeculated bladder with bilateral VUR during voiding

During the voiding phase, the bladder outlet can be assessed for functional or anatomic obstruction. Patients with suprasacral SCI may have detrusor external sphincter dyssynergia (DESD) with or without bladder neck dyssynergy and in such patients the bladder neck will not open and funnel during voiding. In the case of BPE, incomplete bladder neck funneling may be present, but a prostate shadow may also be seen in the bladder. For assessment of patients with incontinence, FUDS provides visualization of the bladder neck during Valsalva maneuvers at which time leakage may be identified.

Fluoroscopy is also helpful in identifying other potential issues in patients with NGB including bladder stones, bladder diverticulae, and VUR.

Electromyelography

Also very useful in patients with NGB is the use of sphincter electromyelography (EMG). Sphincter EMG may be used to confirm denervation of the pelvic floor musculature or to identify discoordination of the urethral sphincter [10]. Sphincter EMG can be performed using surface electrodes, i.e., pads, or needle electrodes. Needle electrodes are usually reserved for SCI patients without sensation. In the past surface electrodes were mounted on sites on the urethral and anal catheters. However, currently sticky pads are used and placed around the anus.

EMG is very helpful to evaluate patients for DESD. Patients with DESD have increased sphincter activity during the voiding phase (Fig. 9.1), to the point where it might suppress a detrusor contraction and not allow satisfactory bladder emptying. This is often relevant when following patients after external sphincterotomy when assessing bladder emptying in such patients [23].

References

1. Wein AJ, Dmochowski RR. Neuromuscular dysfunction of the lower urinary tract. In: Wein AJ, Kavoussi LR, Novick AC, et al., editors. Campbell-Walsh urology. 10th ed. Philadelphia: WB Saunders; 2012. p. 1909–46.
2. McGuire EJ, Woodside JF, Borden TA, Weiss RM. Prognostic value of urodynamic testing in myelodysplastic patients. J Urol. 1981;126:205–9.
3. Schäfer W, Abrams P, Liao L, Mattiasson A, et al. Good urodynamic practices: uroflowmetry, filling cystometry, and pressure-flow studies. Neurourol Urodyn. 2002;21:261–74.
4. Bellucci CH, Wöllner J, Gregorini F, Birnböck D, et al. Neurogenic lower urinary tract dysfunction—do we need same session repeat urodynamic investigations? J Urol. 2012;187:1318–23.
5. Ockrim J, Laniado ME, Khoubehi B, Renzetti R, et al. Variability of detrusor overactivity on repeated filling cystometry in men with urge symptoms: comparison with spinal cord injury patients. BJU Int. 2005;95:587–90.
6. Virseda M, Salinas J, Esteban M, Méndez S. Reliability of ambulatory urodynamics in patients with spinal cord injuries. Neurourol Urodyn. 2013;32:387–92.
7. Nosseir M, Hinkel A, Pannek J. Clinical usefulness of urodynamic assessment for maintenance of bladder function in patients with spinal cord injury. Neurourol Urodyn. 2007;26:228–33.

8. Pannek J, Bartel P, Göcking K, Frotzler A. Clinical usefulness of ultrasound assessment of detrusor wall thickness in patients with neurogenic lower urinary tract dysfunction due to spinal cord injury: urodynamics made easy? World J Urol. 2013;31:659–64.

9. Thomas DG. Spinal cord injury. In: Mundy AR, Stephenson TP, Wein AJ, editors. Urodynamics: principles, practice and application. New York: Churchill Livingstone; 1984. p. 259–72.

10. Hald T, Bradley WE. Cystometry. In: Hald T, Bradley WE, editors. The urinary bladder: neurology and dynamics. Baltimore: Williams and Wilkins; 1982. p. 110–7.

11. Hilton J. Pain and therapeutic influence of mechanical physiological rest in accident and surgical disease. Lancet. 1860;2:401.

12. Head H, Riddoch G. The autonomic bladder, excessive sweating, and some other reflex conditions in gross injuries of the spinal cord. Brain. 1917;40:188.

13. Talaat M. Afferent impulses in nerves supplying the bladder. J Physiol. 1938;32:121.

14. Guttman L, Whitteridge D. Effects of bladder distension on autonomic mechanisms after spinal cord injuries. Brain. 1947;70:361.

15. Lisenmeyer TA, Campagnolo DI, Chou IH. Silent autonomic dysreflexia during voiding in men with spinal cord injuries. J Urol. 1996;155:519–22.

16. Consortium for Spinal Cord Medicine. Paralyzed Veterans of America. Bladder management for adults with spinal cord injury: a clinical practice guideline for health-care providers. J Spinal Cord Med. 2006;29(5):527–73.

17. Grossman E, Messerli FH, Grodzicki T, Kowey P. Should a moratorium be placed on sublingual nifedipine capsules given for hypertensive emergencies and pseudoemergencies? JAMA. 1996;276:1328–31.

18. Chancellor MB, Erhard MJ, Hirsch IH, Stass Jr WE. Prospective evaluation of terazosin for the treatment of autonomic dysreflexia. J Urol. 1994;151:111–3.

19. Vaidyanathan S, Soni BM, Sett P, Watt JW, et al. Pathophysiology of autonomic dysreflexia: long-term treatment with terazosin in adult and pediatric spinal cord injury patients manifesting recurrent dysreflexic episodes. Spinal Cord. 1998;36:761–70.

20. Ryu KH, Kim YB, Yang SO, Lee JK, et al. Results of urine culture and antimicrobial sensitivity tests according to the voiding method over 10 years in patients with spinal cord injury. Korean J Urol. 2011;52:345–9.

21. Böthig R, Fiebag K, Thietje R, Faschingbauer M, et al. Morbidity of urinary tract infection after urodynamic examination of hospitalized SCI patients: the impact of bladder management. Spinal Cord. 2013;51:70–3.

22. Winters JC, Dmochowski RR, Goldman HB, Herndon CD, et al. Urodynamic studies in adults: AUA/SUFU guideline. J Urol. 2012;188(supp 6):2464–72.

23. Kim YH, Kattan MW, Boone TB. Bladder leak point pressure: the measure for sphincterotomy success in spinal cord injured patients with external detrusor-sphincter dyssynergia. J Urol. 1998;159:493–6.

Part II
Interpretation of Tracings

Chapter 10
The Normal Study

Michelle E. Koski and Eric S. Rovner

Introduction

In practice, particularly in a specialized practice, it may be rare that one encounters a normal urodynamic study. Generally, patients may be referred for refractory or complex issues. Patients with less complicated issues may show treatable etiologies based on symptoms, physical exam, or other non-invasive studies such as voiding diaries and post-void residual determination. Other patients may improve with symptom directed therapies, precluding the need for urodynamics. In order to define and assess a normal study, one must be aware of the normal values in each measurable parameter, as well as the appearance, pattern, and configuration of the graphic display, and the variability that is noted in these parameters, even in normal, asymptomatic patients [1, 2]. Additionally, it is important to take into account possible issues with symptom reproducibility that would require a need to optimize the study to better capture urodynamic findings associated with symptoms (as discussed in Chaps. 5 and 7) or whether catheter dampening or other artifact may be masking actual existing findings (discussed in Chap. 6).

M.E. Koski, MD (✉)
Department of Urology, Medical University of South Carolina,
96 Jonathan Lucas St., CSB 644, Charleston, SC 29425, USA

Department of Urology, Kaiser Permanente Southern California,
400 Craven Road, San Marcos, CA 92078, USA
e-mail: mkoski82@hotmail.com

E.S. Rovner, MD
Department of Urology, Medical University of South Carolina,
96 Jonathan Lucas St., CSB 644, Charleston, SC 29425, USA
e-mail: rovnere@musc.edu

© Springer Science+Business Media New York 2015
E.S. Rovner, M.E. Koski (eds.), *Rapid and Practical Interpretation of Urodynamics*, DOI 10.1007/978-1-4939-1764-8_10

Normal Filling Cystometry

Normal urine storage is facilitated by sympathetic reflexes as well as somatic input. Sympathetic inflow inhibits bladder activity during bladder filling while promoting closure of the bladder outlet. Somatic reflexes mediated through the pudendal nerve augment bladder outlet closure forces and may also suppress activity of the detrusor. Viscoelastic properties of the bladder wall allow filling without an appreciable rise in bladder pressure. On fluoroscopy during filling cystometry with a radiopaque contrast agent, the bladder will be visualized as a smooth walled, distensible viscus, without visualization of the ureters (absence of vesicoureteral reflux), or urethra (absence of incontinence), with the bladder outlet closed at rest. The location of the vesicourethral junction or bladder neck can be identified by the location of the filling urethral (vesical) catheter as it is filled with the radiopaque contrast agent.

Coarse Sensation and Capacity

It has been noted that there is significant variability in sensation parameters in cystometry in normal patients. This is even in nominally similar patients accounting for variations associated with differences in filling rate, infusate temperature, or patient temperature [1]. The ICS defines normal bladder sensation by three defined points during filling cystometry, as listed in Table 10.1 [3]. Maximum cystometric capacity is the bladder volume at which the patient cannot delay micturition and is the sum of the volume voided and residual volume. In eight different studies, mean first sensation of filling (FSF) varied from 100 to 350 cc, mean first desire to void (FDV) ranged from 170 to 325 cc, and mean strong desire to void (SDV) 260–450 cc [1]. The 4th International Consultation on Incontinence [1] attributes this to a possible lack of standardization of definition between studies.

The ICI cites a general guideline for normal sensation parameters during filling cystometry in healthy adult subjects as follows: FSF at 170–200 ml, FDV at 250 ml, and SDV at about 400 ml, with maximum cystometric capacity at around 480 ml [1]. However this is only a guideline and actual values in the "normal" population may

Table 10.1 ICI guideline for normal sensation parameters

Bladder sensation during filling cystometry	Definition	Suggested normal range (ml)
First sensation of bladder filling	Sensation when the patient first becomes aware of the bladder filling	170–200
First desire to void	Feeling that would lead the patient to pass urine at the next convenient moment, but voiding can be delayed if necessary	~250
Strong desire to void	A persistent desire to void without the fear of leakage	~400

vary considerably. In a group of 50 normal volunteers, Wyndaele and De Wachter [4] found that cystometric sensation points were significantly lower in females than males, but also found that there was a significant difference in weight in the two groups which could influence bladder capacity. In children, the expected bladder volume (EBV) may be calculated from the Koff formula ([age in years+2]×30=EBV ml) in older children, and by the formula (38+[2.5×age in months]=EBV in ml) in infants [5]. Ultimately, bladder sensation is dependent on a subjective report from a patient who is in extraordinarily unnatural circumstances. Such factors as indwelling urethral and rectal catheters, pain from urethral catheterization, abnormal positioning on a chair (not a toilet), while being publicly observed by the study technician during a very private act can significantly alter a patients perspective and thus likely accounts for some variability and even artifact. Techniques to improve patient comfort and understanding of filling sensation points are outlined in Chap. 7. However, ultimately there are studies that show correlation of patient report with objective data. In healthy volunteers it has been found that the cystometric bladder filling sensations correspond to the filling sensations reported on frequency volume charts [6].

Compliance

Bladder compliance is the relationship between change in bladder volume and change in detrusor pressure and is measured in ml/cm H_2O. Per ICS recommendation, compliance is usually calculated over the change in volume from an empty bladder to that at MCC or immediately before the start of any detrusor contraction that causes significant leakage. Both detrusor pressure measurements (at the start of filling and at MCC respectively) in the calculation of compliance are measured excluding any detrusor contraction [1, 3].

The rise in bladder pressure in a normal individual is barely perceptible in the absence of an involuntary bladder contraction. This unique property of bladder smooth muscle is likely due to a combination of active and passive phenomena. Studies of filling cystometry with physiologic filling rates in healthy subjects reveal mean compliance values from 46 to 124 ml/cm H_2O. The overall range in these studies of normal, asymptomatic subjects is broad, 11–150 ml/cm H_2O in one study of 17 subjects and 31–800 ml/cm H_2O in another [1]. Additionally, the actual performance of filling cystometry may provoke higher pressure increases than what is seen with physiological filling of the bladder, as has been seen in studies comparing filling cystometry to ambulatory urodynamics [7]. In a study of adult patients, Weld et al. [8] proposed a critical compliance value of 12.5 ml/cm H_2O, based on studies of adults with neurogenic bladder.

In defining normative values and placing such numbers in a clinical context, it is important to understand that compliance is a mathematical calculation: intravesical pressure divided by the bladder volume at bladder capacity. From prior studies of intravesical pressure, 40 cm H_2O bladder storage pressure is the value at which the antegrade transport of urine from the upper tract function is compromised and such a pressure puts the kidneys at jeopardy [9]. In patients with diminished compliance and sustained high intravesical storage pressure during filling, it is clinically advantageous to maintain low bladder volumes such that intravesical pressure is consistently kept below this critical level. This is most often done by continuous bladder drainage (catheterization) or frequent voiding or catheterization intervals such that intravesical volume and thus pressure is maintained in a safe range. It should be noted that this often quoted study regarding the risk of elevated intravesical pressure is related to children with myelodysplasia and may not be relevant for non-pediatric age groups and furthermore, the risk of upper tract deterioration may occur at pressures less than 40 mm H_2O.

It has been suggested that bladder compliance is a more complicated entity in pediatric practice because it is related to bladder volume which increases with age. Small pediatric bladders may be more affected by filling rates during urodynamics, and as such, slow filling rates are preferable. The Committee of the International Childrens' Continence Society cites a rule of thumb that 10 cm H_2O or less as an absolute value at expected bladder capacity is acceptable. Additionally, they recommend that as there are no reliable reference ranges for compliance in infancy and childhood, attention be directed more toward the shape of the curve than numbers, looking to see if it is linear or nonlinear, and if nonlinear, in what way it deviates from linearity [5].

Contractions

The occurrence of involuntary detrusor contractions or detrusor overactivity (DO) may be observed in normal, asymptomatic patients during urodynamics. A variety of studies have shown DO in up to 17 % of normal patients, with a mean occurrence of roughly 8 % [1]. The significance of this is unknown. It may be situational, due to sensitivity or trauma of the urethral catheter or to infusate temperature or rate. Although it can occur in normal patients, in the majority of studies, DO comprises a significant urodynamic finding that may explain a number of storage symptoms especially in those cases where it reproduces the patient's presenting complaints.

Continence

For continent individuals there should not be a demonstrable Valsalva or abdominal leak point pressure. Patients with adequate sphincter function and without symptoms of stress incontinence will not leak under any increased physiologic abdominal pressure [10]. There is no "normal" abdominal leak point pressure. Thus, when doing an urodynamic study, the demonstration of urinary leakage during stress maneuvers such as cough or Valsalva in an individual without complaints of urinary incontinence is potentially artifactual due to the circumstances of the study. Of course, the patient who demonstrates a Valsalva leak point pressure on urodynamics but does not have the complaint of SUI should be carefully requestioned to be sure that this does not reproduce any of their symptoms. It is important to note that a lack of leakage in a symptomatic patient with complaints of urinary incontinence should be further investigated. In such individuals, particular provocative maneuvers such as shifting position, or running water during the UDS exam will potentially unmask and demonstrate incontinence. Furthermore, 15 % of women with SUI and 35 % of men with postprostatectomy SUI who are stress continent during the UDS exam will demonstrate an ALPP with the urethral catheter removed [10]. If prolapse is present, stress incontinence should be tested for with the prolapse reduced in order to exclude occult stress incontinence.

Normal Emptying

The normal voiding sequence is a coordinated neuromuscular event initiated with the activation of the micturition reflex. The first recordable event in both voluntary and involuntary voiding is the relaxation of the urethral sphincteric complex, which can be visualized on EMG as a decreased signal. This relaxation results in a decrease in urethral pressure followed closely by a rise in detrusor pressure with opening of the bladder neck and urethra and initiation of urine flow [11]. Flouroscopy during voiding in a normal patient will demonstrate bladder neck funneling and an open urethra with no narrowing or abnormal dilation.

Contractility, Clinical Obstruction, and Complete Emptying

The ICS defines normal voiding as a voluntary continuous contraction that leads to complete emptying in a normal time span in the absence of obstruction [3]. In the normal bladder, as volume increases and the detrusor muscle fibers become more progressively stretched, there is an increase in the potential bladder power and work associated with a contraction. This is most pronounced in the range from empty up to 150–250 ml bladder filling volume. At volumes higher than 400–500 ml, the detrusor may become overstretched and contractility may decrease again [12]—however, this number may be higher in patients who have exceptionally large bladder volumes [11]. Normal detrusor function is incompletely defined solely by absolute values of detrusor pressure because emptying is also related to outlet resistance. For this reason, emptying is best defined through comparison of contractile pressures to their resulting flow rates. Multiple nomograms have been developed to classify this relationship, which will be discussed in Chap. 19. The majority of these nomograms were developed in male patients. The bladder outlet obstructive index (BOOI) (Fig. 10.1), which was derived from the Abrams Griffiths and Schafer nomograms

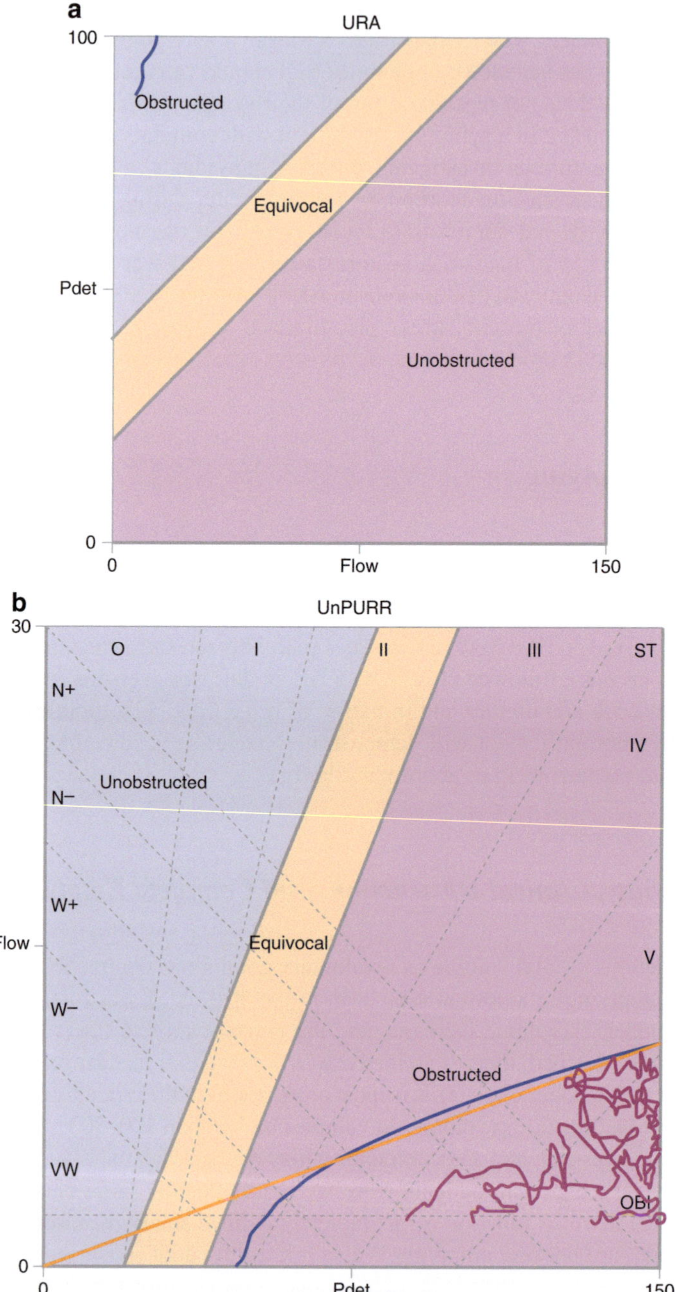

Fig. 10.1 (**a**) Nomograms and formulas defining obstruction and contractility. $BOOI = P_{det}Q_{max} - (2 \times Q_{max})$, $BCI = P_{det}Q_{max} + 5(Q_{max})$, ICS nomogram. (**b**) Composite nomogram

and is the basis for the ICS provisional nomogram, plots Q_{max} against $P_{det}@Q_{max}$ to categorize (male) patients as obstructed, unobstructed, or equivocal. Men are considered obstructed if BOOI is greater than 40, unobstructed if BOOI is less than 20, and equivocal if 20–40. The bladder contractility index (BCI) is derived from Schafer's nomogram (formula in Fig. 10.1). Strong contractility is a BCI greater than 150, normal contractility a BCI of 100–150, and weak contractility a BCI of less than 100 [10]. A composite nomogram incorporates the BOOI and BCI to categorize patients into one of nine groups characterizing the spectrum of obstruction and contractility (Fig. 10.1) [10].

Female patients generally show lower $P_{det}@Q_{max}$ values than men. Empirically, in women, although somewhat controversial, urethral obstruction has been defined by some authors as $P_{det}@Q_{max} > 20$ cm H_2O and $Q_{max} < 12$ ml/s and impaired detrusor contractility as $P_{det}@Q_{max} < 20$ cm H_2O and $Q_{max} < 12$ ml/s (as compared to an empiric cutoff of 40 cm H_2O for $P_{det}@Q_{max}$ in male patients) [11].

Impaired detrusor contractility is characterized by a weak detrusor contraction and a low uroflow. It should be noted that in some patients with low urethral resistance, complete voiding may be accomplished by pelvic relaxation without a significant rise in detrusor pressure. This is considered a normal variant by some authors, explained by the fact that when the detrusor reflex is activated there is no counteractive urethral resistance and the energy is converted to flow. In these patients there may be a very low or no visible rise in detrusor pressure [11].

In all considerations of the pressure flow study it should be kept in mind that the maximum flow rate recorded during pressure flow studies is lower than during free flow. The explanation is not as basic as simple obstruction from the catheter, as this phenomenon has been observed in suprapubic pressure flow studies as well. Possible complex causes might include psychogenic or physiologic causes related to artificial bladder filling [12]. It is recommended that a free uroflow and post-void residual be compared to the pressure flow voiding findings [1]. A normal uroflow curve should be roughly bell shaped, continuous, and not fluctuating. Uroflow is dependent on the voided volume, and nomograms such as the Siroky et al. [13] (developed for male patients) and Liverpool [14] (developed for male and female patients) nomograms which standardize maximum and average flow rates for voided volumes. Normal maximum flow rate ranges are about 20–25 ml/s in men and 25–30 ml/s in women.

Post-void residual (PVR) volumes vary, and one given measurement of PVR may not be accurately representative of typical voiding patterns [1]. PVR, as a measurement in general, increases in reliability when measured on multiple occasions. The ICI has concluded that in review of the literature, there is not an evidence based specific maximum PVR that is considered normal [1]. The Agency for Health Care Policy and Research cite a general rule of PVR less than 50 ml to be adequate emptying and over 200 ml to be inadequate bladder emptying [15]. Lastly, and importantly, in the setting of urodynamics, it should always be taken into account whether the patient felt that the study represented a typical voiding pattern.

Coordination of Sphincters

Normal urine storage is facilitated by a number of physiologic mechanisms that may be seen on the EMG tracing [11]. As the bladder fills, there should be a gradual increase in sphincter EMG activity. Oftentimes, such a subtle increase is not seen on the urodynamic tracing due to the artifact resulting from the use of patch as opposed to needle EMG electrodes. During cough or strain, a reflex increase in sphincter activity should register on the EMG in a normal patient. Suppression of involuntary detrusor contractions by pelvic floor contraction may also be seen (example in Fig. 10.2). Assessment of EMG tracings is complicated by the fact that it may be technically difficult to obtain good quality EMG signals of the desired muscle groups with patch electrodes which are the type most commonly utilized in clinical practice. Needle electrodes, while more accurate in recording pelvic floor activity, are technically difficult to place, painful for the sensate patient, invasive, and expensive. Remarkably, there have been no publications in the last 20 years investigating the benefits of combining EMG with cystometry [1].

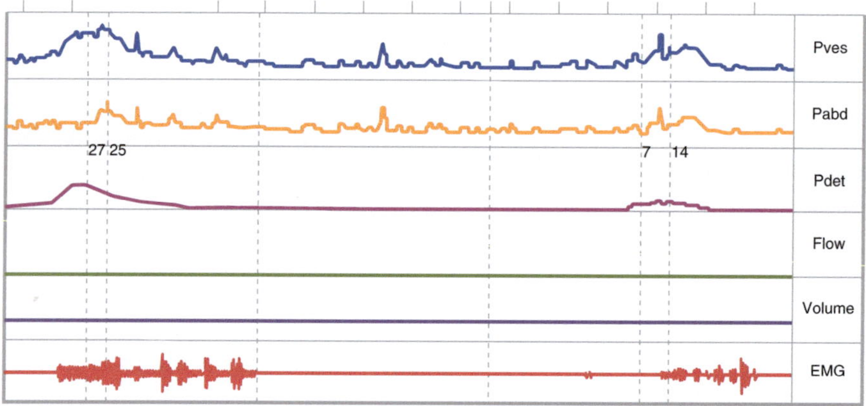

Fig. 10.2 Filling cystometry: patient suppresses detrusor contraction with directed pelvic floor contraction

Example 1

Clinical History: 65-year-old female presenting with urge predominant mixed urinary incontinence, using 2–3 light pads per day ("silver-dollar-sized leakage"). Stress incontinence is rare and is precipitated by cough or sneeze. She has had unsatisfactory response to anticholinergics and significant dry mouth. She has no prolapse or demonstrable stress incontinence on exam (Fig. 10.3).

Commentary on Example 1

This tracing demonstrates no increase in P_{det} over the course of filling. There is normal compliance and no detrusor overactivity. There was no stress incontinence

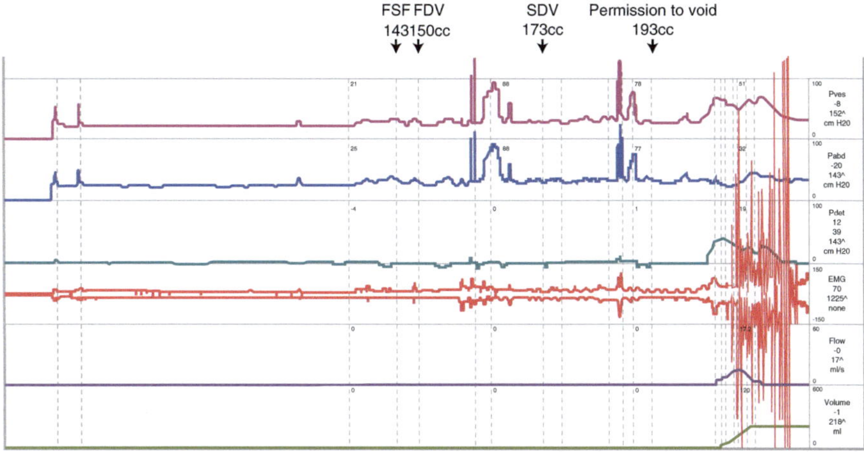

Fig. 10.3 Example 1

with cough or graduated Valsalva at 150 cc and 193 cc. Initial sensation was appropriate, with first sensation of filling at 143 cc, but first desire to void (150 cc) and strong desire to void (173 cc) followed shortly thereafter and bladder capacity was low, at 218 cc. She voids with an appropriate and adequate detrusor contraction, with complete emptying. The flow curve is continuous, but slightly blunted. Q_{max} is 17.2 ml/s. The EMG tracing was quiet throughout filling, with appropriate flaring with cough and Valsalva. There is artifact present in the voiding tracing in the EMG portion, when the transducer became wet.

The quality of the tracing is good. The catheters transmit appropriately, and the only artifact present is in the EMG.

This is a normal study, with the exception of perhaps an increased bladder sensation and reduced capacity. It should be noted, though, that provocative maneuvers on a subsequent fill provoked findings to further support the patient's symptoms.

Example 2
Clinical History: 70-year-old female presenting with urinary frequency and urge incontinence, initially improved with anticholinergics with declining effect. Past medical history is significant for craniotomy for an anterior fossa tumor 6 years prior and hysterectomy 30 years prior for metromenorrhagia. This study is presented in two pages due to the length of the study (Fig. 10.4a–c).

Clinical Commentary for Example 2
This tracing demonstrates essentially normal filling. Initial sensation of bladder filling was appropriate with FSF at 175 cc, although capacity is low, at 284 cc. There was no detrusor overactivity, despite provocative maneuvers of change in fill rate and positional change. There was no stress incontinence with cough and

Valsalva at 150 cc or 225 cc, or with vesical catheter removed. The P_{det} line shows rhythmic decreases secondary to rectal contractions causing isolated increases in the P_{abd} line. Bladder compliance was normal. She was unable to void with the vesical catheter in. Once the vesical catheter was removed, visualized in the second frame with the precipitous drop in P_{ves} and P_{det}, she was able to void. Since the P_{ves} catheter was removed, detrusor contractility cannot be assessed. However, we can see that she did not mount any increase in abdominal pressure during her void suggesting that she did not void by Valsalva. The EMG is appropriately quiet, the uroflow curve is continuous and bell shaped, and on fluoroscopy she has normal bladder neck funneling and an open and nondilated urethra. Her Q_{max} is 25 ml/s. She empties completely. This would indicate a normal void.

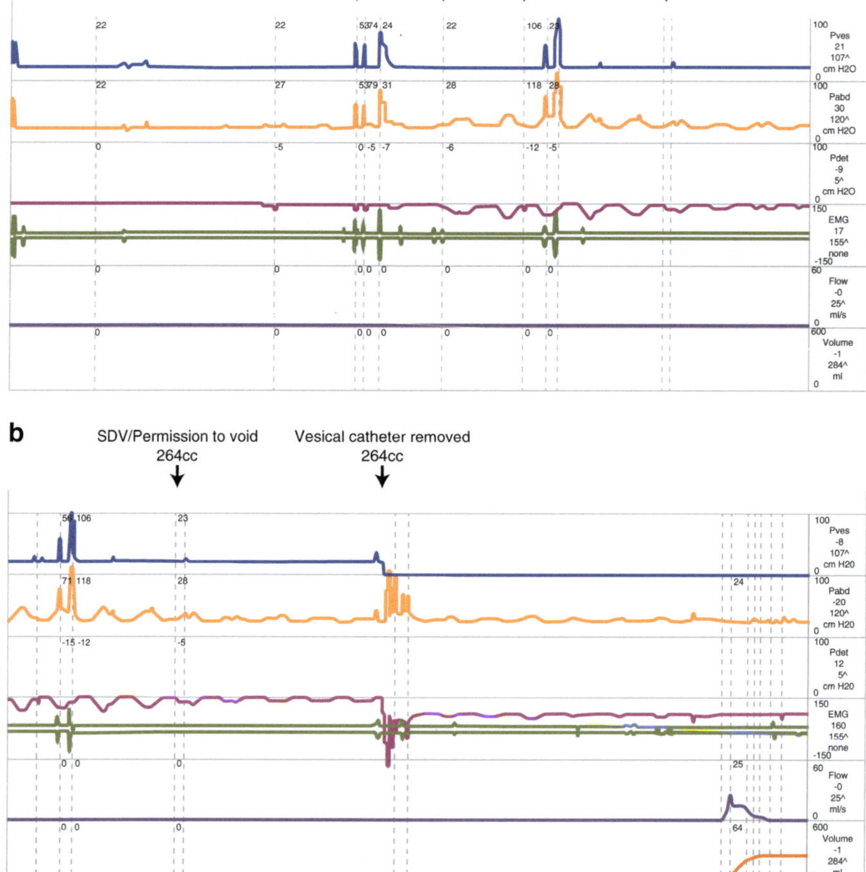

Fig. 10.4 (**a–c**) Example 2

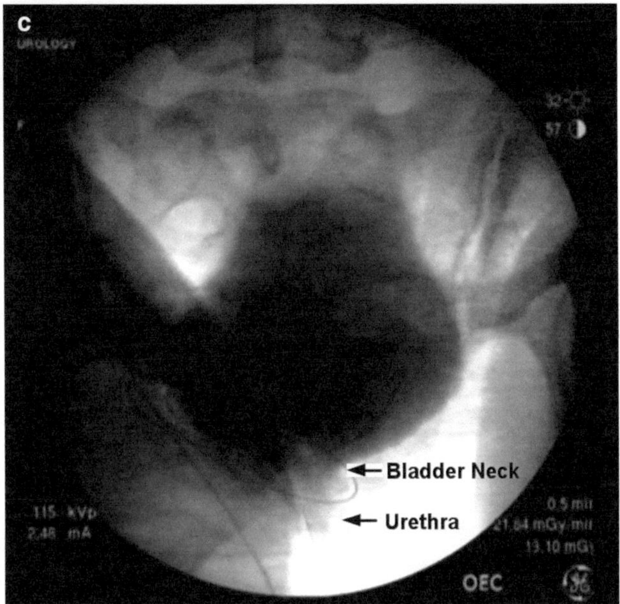

Fig. 10.4 (continued)

The quality of the tracing is good. There is appropriate catheter calibration and transmission and no artifact. The fact that she could only void with the catheter out is a shortcoming, but not uncommon, and there is adequate supplemental information that can be derived from the study to support her voiding pattern. However, her urgency and urge incontinence were not able to be replicated.

Example 3
A 57-year-old male who sustained a fall at work that led to an L3–L4 laminectomy. Two years later he informed his workers compensation insurance company that he was having urinary urgency, frequency, and urge incontinence and erectile dysfunction, reportedly since the time of the initial injury, and he was sent for urodynamic study. Pad test yielded 36 g (Figs. 10.5 a and b).

Clinical Commentary for Example 3
This tracing demonstrates a slight decrease in P_{abd} without a concomitant rise in P_{ves} (annotated by arrow on P_{det} line) which causes a transient increase in P_{det}. However, compliance is normal. There was no detrusor overactivity. Sensation of filling was normal (first desire to void at 225 cc and strong desire at 469 cc), as was capacity at 525 cc. The EMG tracing was quiet throughout with appropriate flaring with coughing and laughing, and also with a slight flare midway through his void, consistent

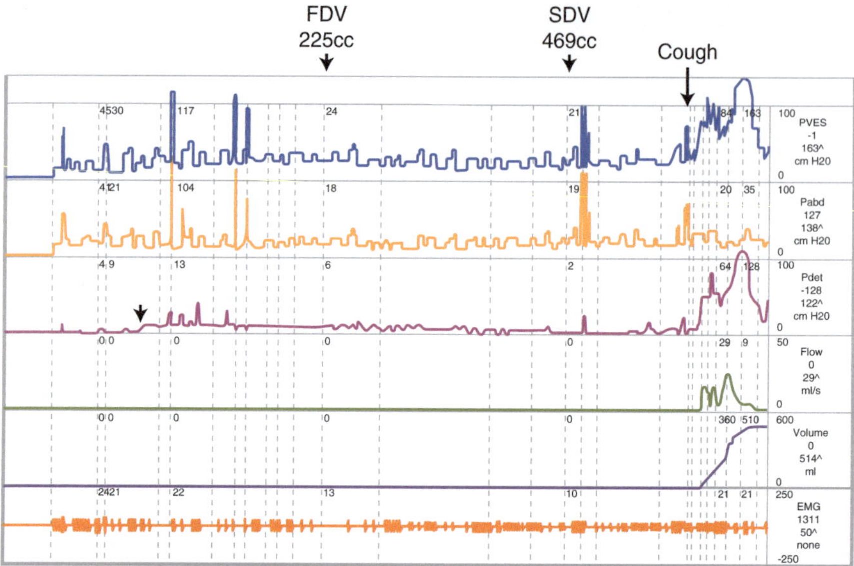

Fig. 10.5 a Example 3

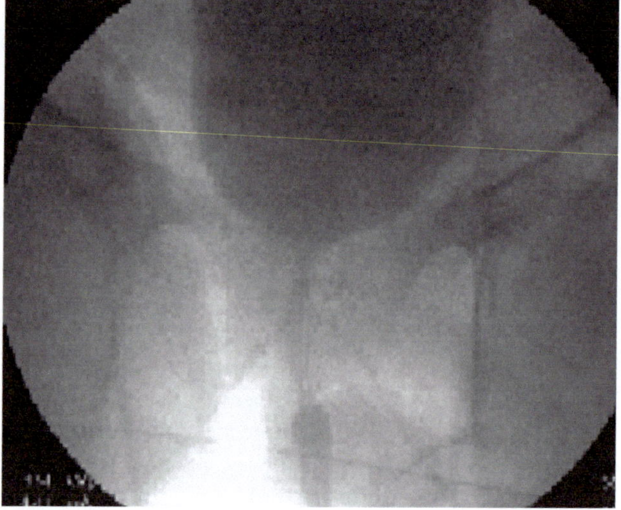

Fig. 10.5 b Voiding image

with guarding. There is a decrease in P_{det} concomitant with the EMG flare. He felt that this void was not indicative of his home voiding pattern. Bladder emptying was accomplished by an adequate detrusor contraction and was complete. The flow curve is somewhat irregular in the first third, but then becomes parabolic in shape.

He does show a suggestion of an aftercontraction, which would be consistent with his clinical history of urgency, as this is sometimes related to overactivity, although no DO was demonstrated on the study. P_{det} at Q_{max} was 64 with Q_{max} of 29, yielding a BOOI of 6. There was no evidence of obstruction. An uninstrumented uroflow showed a normal flow curve. Flouroscopy imaging demonstrates closed bladder neck and a smooth walled bladder at rest (not shown), and normal bladder neck funneling and delineation of the urethra with voiding. There is an artifactual appearance of widening in the distal urethra secondary to a turn in the urethra.

The clinical significance of the finding on this tracing is inconclusive, in terms of looking for neurogenic characteristics related to his back injury. It is a normal study, with the exception of the aftercontraction and the initially abnormal appearance of the uroflow. It is important to recognize that DO may not be reproduced on an urodynamic tracing, again emphasizing the importance of reproducing the patients symptoms during the study. Repeating the study with provocative maneuvers may result in DO.

References

 1. Hosker G, Rosier P, Gajewski J, et al. Dynamic testing. In: Abrams/Cardozo/Khoury/Wein 4th International Consultation on Incontinence. Paris: Health Publication Ltd.; 2009. p. 417–34.
 2. Mahfouz W, Al Afraa T, Campeau L, et al. Normal urodynamic parameters in women. Part II – invasive urodynamics. Int Urogynecol J. 2012;23:269–77.
 3. Abrams P, Cardozo L, Fall M, et al. The standardization of terminology in lower urinary tract function: report from the standardization sub-committee of the International Continence Society. Urology. 2003;61:37–49.
 4. Wyndaele JJ, De Wachter S. Cystometrical sensory data from a normal population: comparison of two groups of young healthy volunteers examined with 5 years interval. Eur Urol. 2002;42(1): 34–8.
 5. Neveus T, von Gontard A, Hoebeke P, et al. The standardization of terminology of lower urinary tract function in children and adolescents: report from the Standardisation Committee of the International Children's Continence Society. J Urol. 2006;176(1):314–24.
 6. De Wachter S, Wyndaele JJ. Frequency–volume charts: a tool to evaluate bladder sensation. Neurourol Urodyn. 2003;22:638–42.
 7. Heslington K, Hilton P. Ambulatory monitoring and conventional cystometry in asymptomatic female volunteers. B J Obstet Gynaecol. 1996;103(5):434–41.
 8. Weld KJ, Graney MJ, Dmochowski RR. Differences in bladder compliance with time and associations of bladder management with compliance in spinal cord injured patients. J Urol. 2000;163:1228–33.
 9. Kaufman AM, Ritchey MI, Roberts AC, et al. Decreased bladder compliance in patients with myelomeningocele treated with radiological observation. J Urol. 1996;156:2031–3.
10. Nitti V. Urodynamic and videourodynamic evaluation of the lower urinary tract. In: Wein AJ, Kavoussi LR, NOvick AC, Partin AW, Peters CA, editors. Campbell-Walsh urology. 10th ed. Philadelphia: Elsevier; 2012.
11. Blaivas JG, Chancellor M, Weiss J, Verhaaren M, editors. Atlas of urodynamics. Milton: Blackwell; 2007.
12. Schafer W, Abrams P, Liao L, et al. Good urodynamic practices: uroflowmetry, filling cystometry, and pressure-flow studies. Neurourol Urodyn. 2002;21(3):261–74.

13. Siroky MB, Olsson CA, Krane RJ. The flow rate nomogram. I. Development. J Urol. 1979;122:665–8.
14. Halen BT, Ashby D, Stherest JR, et al. Maximum and average urine flow rate in normal male and female populations – the liverpool nomogram. Br J Urol. 1989;64:30–8.
15. Agency for Health Care Policy and Research. Clinical practice guideline: urinary incontinence in adults. AHPCR Pub No. 96-0682. Rockville: Dept of Health and Human Services (US), Agency for Health Care Policy and Research; 1996.

Chapter 11
Bladder Filling and Storage: "Capacity"

Ariana L. Smith, Mary Y. Wang, and Alan J. Wein

Introduction

Bladder capacity is a measure used to estimate the volume of urine a patient can comfortably hold. It can be determined in many ways and often changes from void to void making it a rather imprecise measure of the true amount of urine the bladder is able to hold. The ability of bladder capacity measures to accurately predict the cause of bladder symptoms such as frequency or urgency of urination is limited but provides the clinician with a general idea of bladder dynamics, toileting patterns, and impact on patient quality of life. Patients often report decreased bladder capacity, or the subjective symptom that their bladder does not hold as much as it used to, based on a more frequent desire to go to the toilet. Complaints such as "I have a small bladder" or "my bladder shrunk" are common reports as are "I must rush" and "sometimes I don't make it." A frequency–volume chart or voiding diary may provide slightly more objective measures of bladder capacity but does not insure the bladder was actually *full* at the time of voiding since the decision to void is often made out of convenience, opportunity, or fear of needing a toilet when one may not be available. Frequency–volume chart measures reflect a large range of volumes at which the patient chose to go to the toilet (Table 11.1) and rarely are these annotated with the reason why the patient chose to void.

From the frequency–volume chart maximum and average-voided volumes can be determined as can the median functional bladder capacity which is defined as the median maximum voided volume during every day activities [1]. A 3-day chart is preferred and will likely demonstrate a greater range of voided volumes and a larger maximum voided volume than a 1-day diary [2].

A.L. Smith, MD (✉) • M.Y. Wang, MSN, CRNP • A.J. Wein, MD, PhD(hon), FACS
Penn Medicine Division of Urology, University of Pennsylvania Health System,
Perelman Center for Advanced Medicine, West Pavilion, 3rd Floor 3400
Civic Center Boulevard, Philadelphia, PA 19104, USA
e-mail: ariana.smith@uphs.upenn.edu

© Springer Science+Business Media New York 2015
E.S. Rovner, M.E. Koski (eds.), *Rapid and Practical Interpretation
of Urodynamics*, DOI 10.1007/978-1-4939-1764-8_11

Table 11.1 Bladder diary

Time Interval	Urinated in Toilet	Incontinent Episode Amount L/S	Reason for Urine Leakage	Type/Amount of Liquid Intake
6 am				
7 am	450			
8 am				Coffee
9 am	200			
10 am				Coffee
11 am				
Noon	200			Iced Tea
1 pm				
2 pm	300			
3 pm				
4 pm				
5 pm	200			
6 pm				wine/water
7 pm				
8 pm	300			
9 pm				
10 pm-Midnight	200			
Midnight-2 am				
2-4 am				
4-6 am				

Type of Pad______None__________________   # Pads Used________0________

Normal bladder capacity should be considered as a wide range of acceptable values and likely varies with age and 24-h urine volume [2]. In children, normative values for bladder capacity were initially estimated using linear functions versus age; [3] however, this method was found to substantially underestimate bladder capacity and not account for the upper and lower limits of normal [4]. Despite its shortcomings linear equation estimates are often referenced as a measure of normative values [5]. Further studies have suggested that bladder capacity correlates logarithmically with age in children to account for a growing bladder and should be interpreted as normal within two standard deviations of the mean (between the 5th and 95th percentiles) [6].

Cystometry is a component of urodynamic testing that measures the pressure–volume relationship of the bladder. It is also used to assess bladder capacity, compliance, sensation, and uninhibited bladder contractions. The cystometrogram is a graphic representation of the pressure volume relationship annotated with patient reported sensations and other important findings. Sensations are purely subjective and therefore depend on a cooperative and informed patient for reliability. The artificial environment in which cystometry is performed including the non-physiologic retrograde filling of the bladder can produce artifacts in the results. A nervous or fearful patient, or one who is experiencing discomfort from the urodynamic catheter,

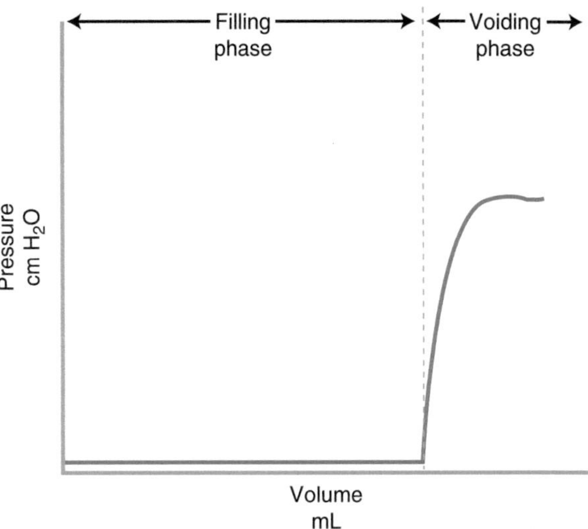

Fig. 11.1 Idealized pressure–volume relationship demonstrating low pressure storage during the filling phase and a rise in pressure during the voiding phase. Adapted from Campbell-Walsh urology, 10th ed., Elsevier; 2012

may report sensations and symptoms that are not reflective of their presenting bladder complaint. Conversely, a sedated or stoic patient may not report sensations reflective of their complaint.

Cystometric capacity is the bladder volume at the end of filling cystometry when the patient reports a normal desire to void. It is generally the point where permission to void is given; however, in some situations further volume may be infused. Maximum cystometric capacity is the volume at which a patient reports that they cannot hold any more in their bladder and can no longer delay voiding [1]. The end point for bladder filling should be well annotated on an urodynamics tracing such that the clinician interpreting the information can properly categorize the final infused volume as either cystometric capacity or maximum cystometric capacity. Capacity measures reflect not only voided volume, but also post-void residual urine. An idealized pressure–volume relationship demonstrates a detrusor pressure near zero during the filling phase until cystometric capacity is reached, and generation of detrusor pressure corresponding to the initiation of voluntary voiding (Fig. 11.1).

Measuring Cystometric Capacity

Good Urodynamics Practices are outlined in Part 1 of this book but are briefly reviewed here in relation to cystometric capacity measurement. Initial bladder volume and detrusor pressure should be zero at the start of an urodynamic study. This is achieved by emptying the bladder to completion with a catheter prior to placing the sensor tipped urodynamic catheter. In addition, vesical pressure and abdominal pressure should be equalized to establish a subtracted detrusor pressure of zero.

Bladder filling begins at a rate determined by the urodynamicist, usually between 10 and 100 ml s/min. This rate may be held constant throughout the study or may be altered in response to patient parameters. The patient will also make urine at a rate determined by their hydration status and underlying renal function contributing to the volume in the bladder during the study. Given the short duration of time over which an urodynamic study is typically performed this latter contribution is often ignored. There is data to suggest however that natural filling during cystometry should be accounted for since it may occur at a rate of 6.1 ml/min, increasing bladder capacity 14 % [7]. Other studies have suggested a rate of 1.4 ml/min increasing capacity 12.1 % [8]. Instructions given to patients regarding hydration and the "need to come with a full bladder" may influence the rate of urine production during the urodynamics test. Specifically, when patients are informed that they must give a urine sample or perform a non-invasive uroflow on arrival they may drink excessively before testing [7]. In addition, prolonged set up and testing time can further increase the contribution of natural filling to infused volume, impacting the accuracy of capacity measures [8].

Sensation during filling cystometry is reported by the patient and documented on the urodynamics tracing. Once a normal desire to void is reported by the patient, cystometric capacity is documented. Next, the patient may be instructed to report when he or she can no longer delay micturition and this volume is recorded as maximum cystometric capacity. The capacity measures obtained should be compared to the voided volumes noted on the frequency–volume chart to ensure consistency and reliability of the urodynamic test measures. Artifact secondary to the non-physiologic fill rate and abnormal situation of being observed during a normal private process can impact measurements obtained. Repeat fill cycles of the bladder may be needed and are encouraged to accurately interpret bladder capacity. Abrams has correlated patient reported sensation during urodynamic testing with maximum cystometric capacity. He found that first sensation of bladder filling correlated with roughly 50 % of maximum capacity while normal desire to void and strong desire to void correlated with 75 and 90 %, respectively [9].

In situations where abnormal bladder function exists, cystometric capacity may be reached before the patient can report a desire to void. For example, in patients with impaired sensation, cystometric capacity is the volume at which bladder filling was stopped. There can be several reasons for stopping and this should be well annotated on the urodynamics tracing. With impaired compliance, high detrusor pressures may prompt the urodynamicist to stop filling; in other situations, pain, involuntary voiding, or a maximum predetermine filling volume may prompt discontinuation. Detrusor overactivity or impaired compliance may lead to leakage of urine before the patient reports sensation of fullness; in these situations, cystometric capacity is measured as the volume at which leakage began. In the setting of sphincteric incompetence, capacity measures may be artificially low due to passive leakage across the sphincter. Occluding the urethral outlet with a catheter balloon can increase capacity measures. Maximum cystometric capacity is only defined for patients with normal bladder sensation and therefore generally only cystometric capacity is reported in this population.

Definitions of Normal and Abnormal

Normal cystometric capacity should be interpreted as a wide range of acceptable values. Reference ranges for normal cystometric capacity in adults have not been universally agreed upon primarily because the question still remains on how well this reflects pragmatic functional bladder capacity. Normal cystometric capacity is generally defined as 300–550 ml with larger values obtained in men compared to women [10]. These reference values represent mean values obtained on a sample of only 28 men and 10 women with no history of urologic disease. Mean age was only 24 years, which is hardly comparable to the population of patients generally undergoing urodynamic testing. In another study of 32 highly selected, middle aged volunteers without urologic disease, mean cystometric capacity was 586 ± 193 ml; this is much higher than several previous reports [11].

Abnormal cystometric capacity can be either too small or too large. Small capacity may result from involuntary bladder contractions, bladder pain, impaired compliance, or bladder oversensitivity. Yoon and Swift [12] defined abnormally small maximum cystometric capacity as less than 300 ml but advised using caution in interpreting low cystometric capacity as abnormal in the setting of a normal functional bladder capacity on frequency–volume charts. Large capacity may result from poor or absent bladder sensation during filling or neurologic bladder dysfunction. Large bladder capacity, outside of the range of normal, is generally not interpreted to be pathologic in the absence of neurologic disease. Artifact, as noted above, from catheter placement, filling rate, media temperature, media type, patient positioning, provocative measures such as coughing, patient discomfort or patient anxiety may impact reliability of this measure [13, 14]. For example, during cystometry a patient is generally positioned in either the seated or the standing position for the duration of the test. When completing a 24-h frequency–volume chart a patient generally changes body positions throughout the day and night with the largest voided volumes generally recorded after sleeping in the recumbent position. The impact of patient position on the variability in daytime voided volumes has not been reported. Faster filling rates during cystometry have been shown to produce lower maximum cystometric capacity measures [13]. Room temperature filling media which is much cooler than body temperature urine has been shown to result in lower maximum cystometric capacity measures as well [14]. The non-physiologic fill rate used during urodynamic testing may impact bladder sensations as well as bladder compliance. Prior studies have shown that supraphysiologic fill rates used during urodynamic testing produce an increase in bladder wall pressure and a decrease in bladder compliance [15]. It is unclear if bladder wall pressure influences bladder sensation and ultimately diminishes maximum cystometric capacity.

Relation to Functional Capacity

Frequency–volume charts and bladder diaries are felt to be more accurate representations of true bladder capacity since these measures document the patients voiding patterns in a more natural environment than cystometry during urodynamic testing. However, the act of keeping the journal may influence voiding patterns making the patient more in tune with their bladder sensations. Diokno et al. [16] reported that moderate correlation exists between functional bladder capacity and cystometric capacity thus establishing validity of the cystometric bladder capacity measure ($r=0.493$, $p<0.01$). Further studies on women with incontinence confirmed correlation between the two measures but showed a statistically significant difference in volumes obtained, with a smaller volume recorded at the time of cystometry. Thus they interpreted the data as displaying a weak clinical relationship between the two measures [12]. Yoon and Swift report poor positive predictive value (51.4 %) of cystometry in detecting abnormalities in bladder capacity but good negative predictive value (84.0 %). Thus, *normal* bladder capacity during cystometry correlates strongly with *normal* functional bladder capacity.

Videourodynamic Assessment

Radiologic imaging of the bladder and urethra during urodynamic testing can be performed with synchronous fluoroscopy termed videocystourethrography. This is generally reserved for patients with more complex clinical presentations or those with neurologic dysfunction. Concomitant imaging of the bladder and urethra allows direct observation of the effects of bladder events. During bladder filling and at capacity, an assessment of bladder shape, position with respect to the pubic symphysis, conformation of the bladder neck, diverticuli and vesicoureteral reflux (VUR) is undertaken (Fig. 11.2a, b). Leakage of urine can be detected at earlier time points and at smaller volumes using fluoroscopy than the standard uroflow sensor.

Urodynamic Examples of Conditions of Altered Capacity

Bladder oversensitivity is defined as an increase in bladder sensation or urgency that may occur during filling cystometry in the absence of a rise in detrusor pressure [1]. This term is reserved for situations where sensations are reported at volumes felt to be lower than normal. Generally an early first sensation, an early first desire to void, an early strong desire to void, and low maximum cystometric capacity are noted (Fig. 11.3).

Several conditions such as overactive bladder, bladder pain syndrome (BPS), and urinary tract infection (UTI) are associated with bladder oversensitivity. Urodynamic tracings similar to Fig. 11.3 are commonly seen with each of these conditions. The

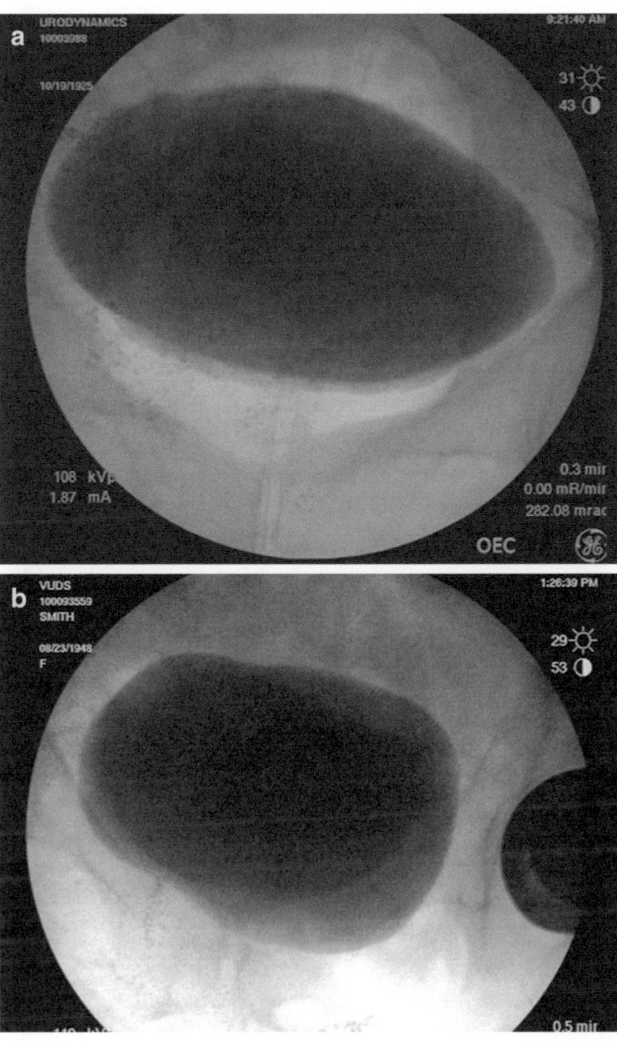

Fig. 11.2 (**a** and **b**) Videofluoroscopic images corresponding to maximum cystometric capacity showing a smooth contoured bladder without evidence of diverticuli, vesicoureteral reflux, bladder neck funneling, or bladder prolapse

hallmark signs on urodynamics are early reported sensations and low cystometric capacity and maximum cystometric capacity.

Overactive bladder syndrome (OAB) is a clinical condition consisting of bothersome urinary symptoms. The International Continence Society has defined OAB as urgency of urination, with or without urgency urinary incontinence (UUI), usually accompanied by frequency and nocturia [17]. OAB may produce urgency during urodynamic testing, which can be purely sensory in nature or have a

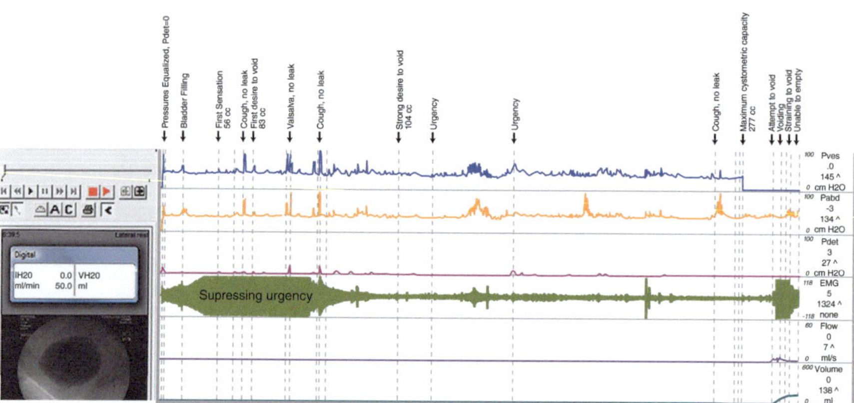

Fig. 11.3 Cystometrogram showing small cystometric capacity. Vesical pressure and abdominal pressure were equalized at the start of the study with a corresponding detrusor pressure of zero. Valsalva followed by cough were performed during the filling phase of the study without associated leakage of urine. With increasing fill volume the patient reports early first sensation (56 cc), early first desire to void (83 cc), and early strong desire to void (104 cc). Increased EMG activity is noted as the patient is suppressing urgency. The patient could no longer delay micturition and reached maximum cystometric capacity at 277 cc. This cystometrogram represents bladder oversensitivity

corresponding rise in detrusor pressure (see detrusor overactivity below). OAB impacts cystometric and maximum cystometric capacity and effective treatment can improve urodynamic parameters as well as patient complaints [18].

BPS is the preferred term for the clinical condition previously referred to as interstitial cystitis. It is defined as the complaint of suprapubic pain related to bladder filling, accompanied by other symptoms such as increased daytime and nighttime frequency, in the absence of proven urinary infection or other obvious pathology [17]. BPS often produces bladder discomfort at low cystometric capacity in the absence of a rise in detrusor pressure during urodynamic testing. Effective treatment can improve cystometric and maximum cystometric capacity as well as patient symptoms [19].

UTI can be defined clinically as the presence of dysuria or bladder pain associated with voiding, and pathologically as the presence of bacteria in a properly obtained urine culture associated with a pyuria, or by several other heterogeneous parameters [20]. Generally, UTI causes increased bladder sensitivity and bladder discomfort at low cystometric capacity. Urodynamic testing should be avoided in the setting of acute UTI. If performed, urgency and/or discomfort in the presence or absence of a rise in detrusor pressure will likely be noted.

Detrusor overactivity (DO) is an involuntary bladder muscle contraction that occurs during filling cystometry often producing a sensation of urgency corresponding to a rise in detrusor pressure (Fig. 11.4a, b). DO can be phasic, which can occur once or several times throughout an urodynamic study and may or may not lead to

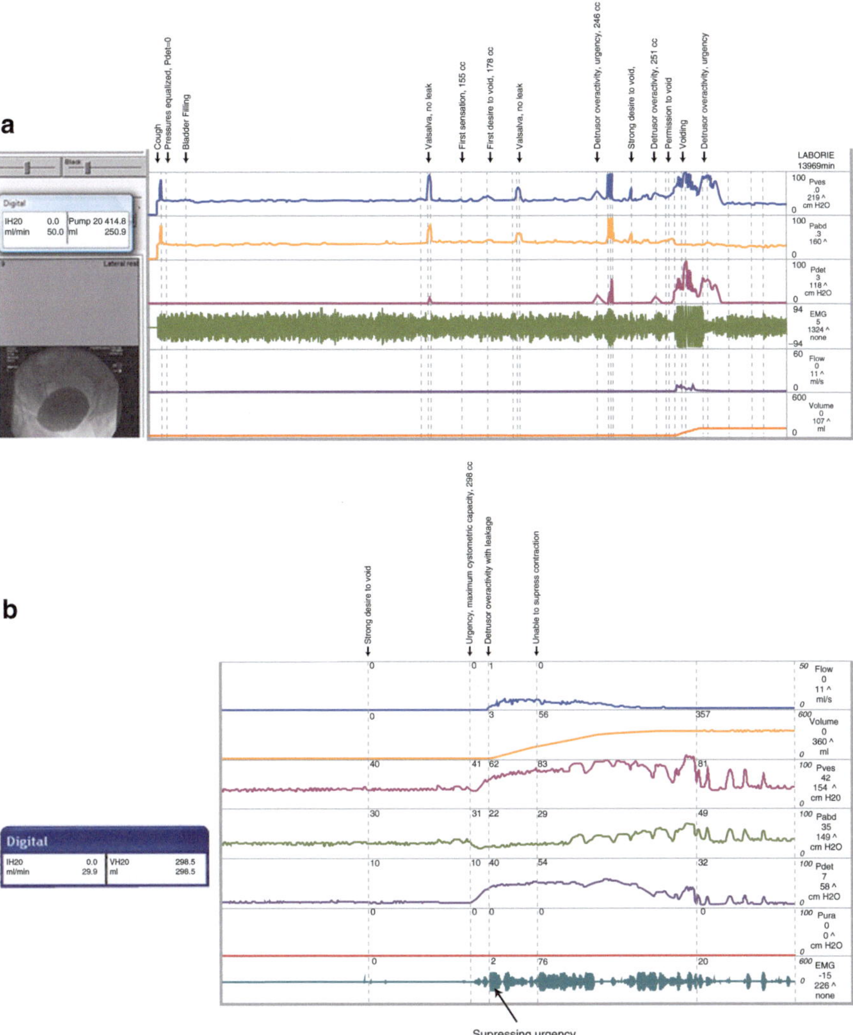

Fig. 11.4 (**a**) Cystometrogram showing detrusor overactivity associated with patient reported urgency. Videofluoroscopic image at cystometric capacity demonstrates a smooth bladder without evidence of trabeculation, diverticuli, vesicoureteral reflux, or bladder neck funneling. Vesical pressure and abdominal pressure were equalized at the start of the study with a corresponding detrusor pressure of zero. With increasing fill volume the patient reports first sensation at 155 cc, desire to void at 178 cc, and strong desire to void at 251 cc. Phasic detrusor overactivity is seen at 246 and 251 cc. After the involuntary contraction subsided, permission to void was granted and the patient volitionally voided. Following voiding another detrusor contraction with associated urgency was noted. (**b**) Cystometrogram demonstrating terminal detrusor overactivity associated with patient reported urgency and leakage of urine. Vesical pressure and abdominal pressure were equalized at the start of the study with a corresponding detrusor pressure of zero. At a maximum cystometric capacity of 298 cc the patient reported urgency and a strong desire to void. Detrusor overactivity and associated leakage followed. Increased EMG activity was noted as the patient attempted to suppress the involuntary bladder contraction

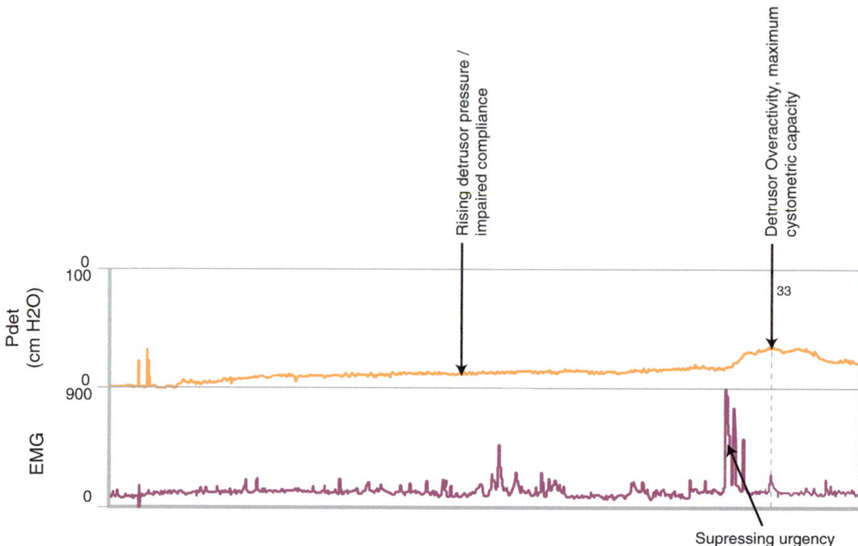

Fig. 11.5 Cystometrogram with impaired bladder compliance. Vesical pressure and abdominal pressure were equalized at the start of the study with a corresponding detrusor pressure of zero. With increasing fill volume the detrusor pressure steadily rises to a peak of 33 cm H_2O. Increased EMG activity is noted as the patient is suppressing urgency associated with increasing detrusor pressure. Maximum cystometric capacity corresponds to the volume at which the patient could no longer delay micturition

urinary incontinence; or terminal, which is a single involuntary contraction that leads to complete bladder emptying [21]. DO can elicit urinary leakage ranging from drops of urine to complete bladder loss; regardless of amount, this is termed detrusor overactivity leakage. DO may be the result of neurogenic bladder dysfunction, or idiopathic OAB. DO generally decreases cystometric capacity.

Impaired bladder compliance produces an abnormal rise in detrusor pressure during filling cystometry (Fig. 11.5). This rise in pressure is generally felt to be due to impaired visco-elastic properties of the detrusor muscle. The patient may or may not report urgency as the pressure rises and leakage of urine may occur if the detrusor leak point pressure is reached. VUR or impaired drainage from the upper urinary tract may occur secondary to high pressure in the bladder. Impaired compliance generally decreases cystometric bladder capacity.

Neurogenic bladder dysfunction can produce a variety of clinical and urodynamic effects depending on the exact location of the neurologic lesion. When lesions are located above the level of the brainstem detrusor overactivity may be seen leading to decreased bladder capacity and symptoms of OAB (Fig. 11.6).

When lesions are located between the brainstem and the sacral spinal cord, detrusor sphincter dyssynergia (DSD) as well as detrusor overactivity may be seen, generally leading to a decrease in bladder capacity with or without impaired compliance and symptoms of both OAB and difficulty emptying/urinary retention. DSD

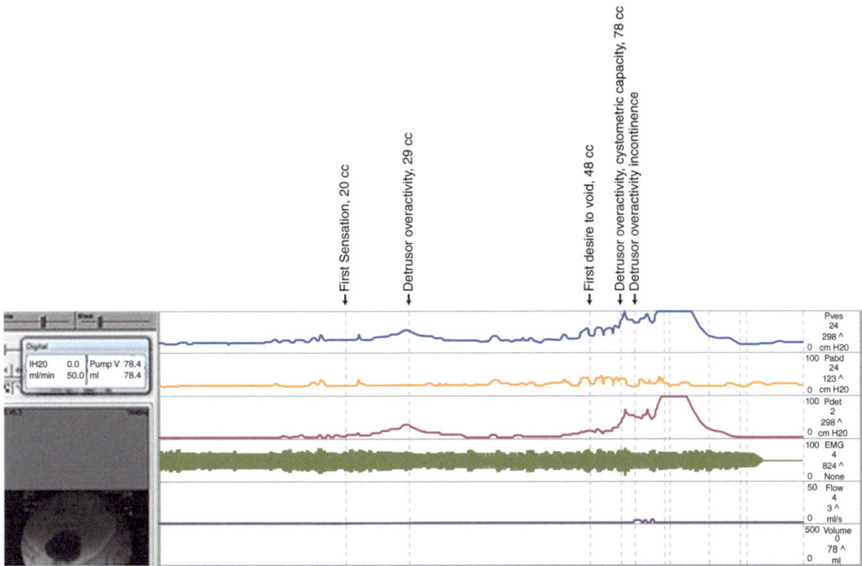

Fig. 11.6 Cystometrogram in a patient with neurogenic bladder dysfunction and severely diminished cystometric capacity. Vesical pressure and abdominal pressure were equalized at the start of the study with a corresponding detrusor pressure of zero. First sensation was reported at 20 cc, detrusor overactivity was seen at 29 cc, and first desire to void reported at 48 cc. A second involuntary contraction was seen at 78 cc with corresponding leakage of urine

can produce drastic changes in bladder function and anatomy as a result of obstruction at the level of the urethral sphincter (Fig. 11.7a, b).

When lesions are located at or below the sacral spinal cord an atonic bladder or a poorly contractile bladder with or without impaired compliance may be seen associated with symptoms of difficulty emptying, complete urinary retention, and incontinence without sensation. Diabetic cystopathy is a peripheral neuropathy producing a hypotonic or atonic bladder. Large capacity is generally noted and can be associated with detrusor overactivity (Fig. 11.8).

Anatomic Considerations of Bladder Capacity

Bladder diverticula can be the result of obstructed voiding, surgical intervention or can be congenital (Fig. 11.9). Bladder capacity is the sum of the volume held in the bladder and the diverticulum. This measured bladder capacity during urodynamic testing is likely an overestimate of functional bladder capacity. Most diverticuli have fairly small ostia and as a result empty poorly during voiding. The diverticulum remains distended with stagnant urine and can be a nidus of infection and stone formation. When the bladder is emptied to completion using a catheter

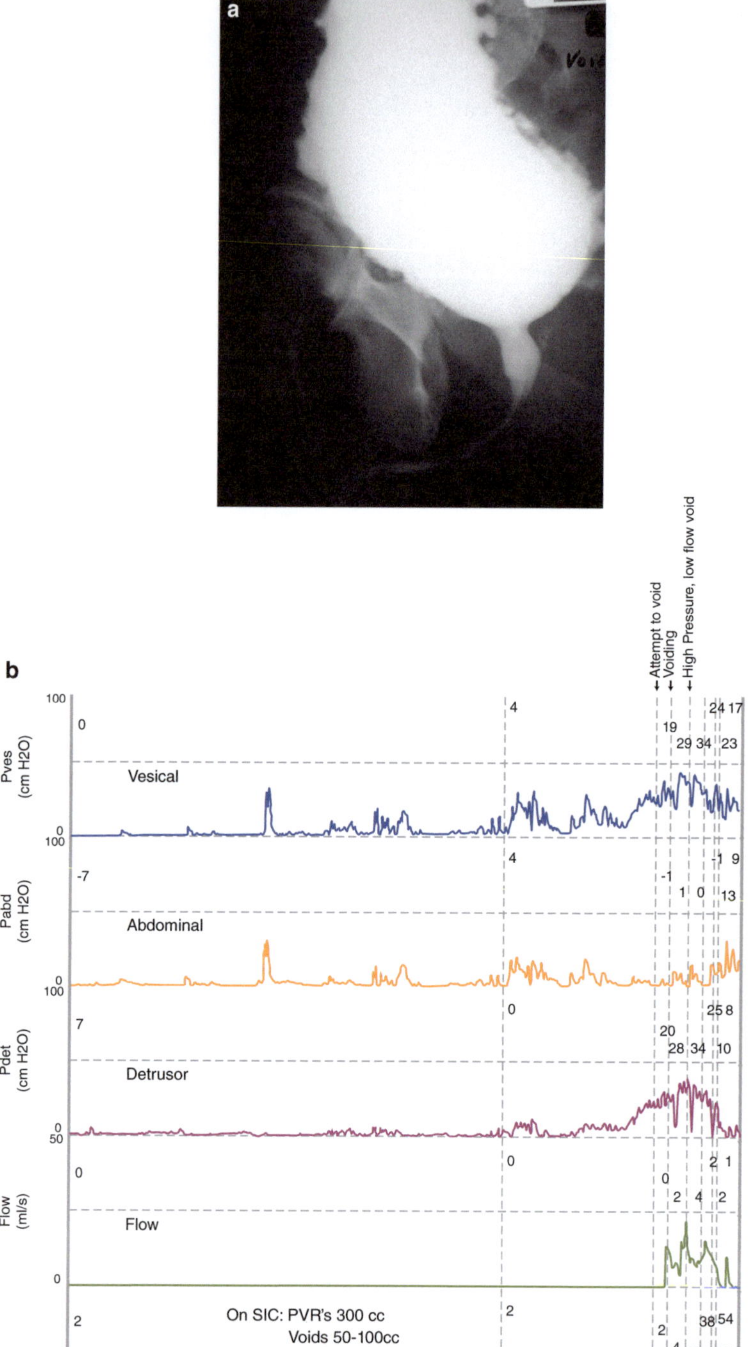

Fig. 11.7 (**a** and **b**) Videofluoroscopic image and accompanying cystometrogram in a patient with DSD producing and obstructed voiding pattern and anatomic distortion of the bladder and urethra. Failure of the urinary sphincter to relax during voiding produces a high-pressure detrusor contraction, low flow across the urethra, and incomplete bladder emptying. With time bladder trabeculation, diverticuli and proximal urethral dilation result

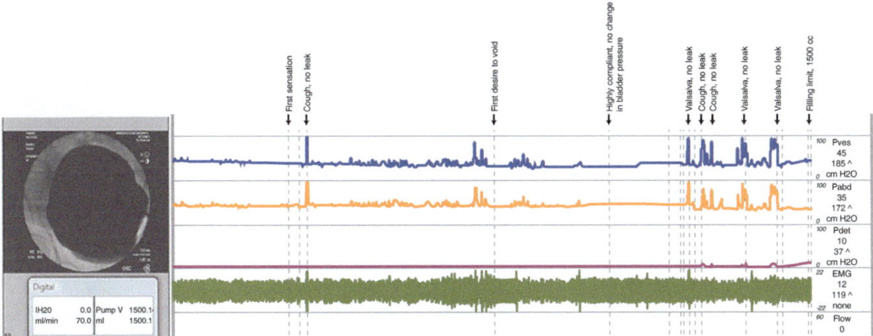

Fig. 11.8 Cystometrogram of a patient with diabetic cystopathy showing a hypocontractile large capacity bladder, maximum cystometric capacity was never reached. Vesical pressure and abdominal pressure were equalized at the start of the study with a corresponding detrusor pressure of zero. Filling was discontinued at a volume of 1,500 cc. This bladder is highly compliant without evidence of detrusor overactivity

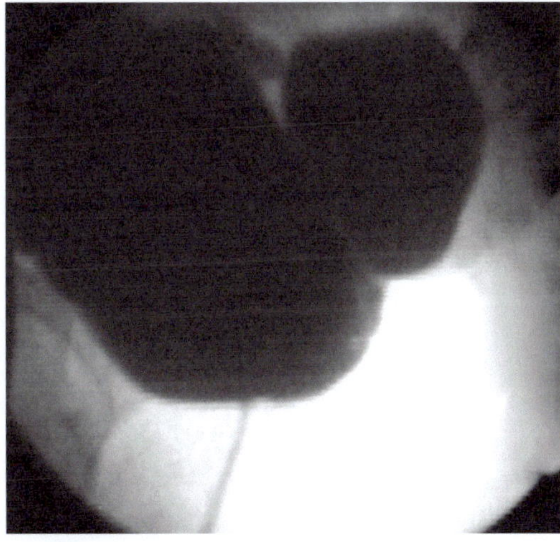

Fig. 11.9 Videofluoroscopic image of a large bladder diverticulum. Cystometric capacity reflects the sum of the bladder and diverticular volume

at the start of urodynamic testing the diverticulum may empty thereby allowing it to fill during the filling phase of the study. The capacity measures obtained will therefore reflect the cumulative volume of the bladder and the diverticulum. This overestimation of functional capacity may be significant when the diverticulum is large in size.

Pelvic organ prolapse can produce urinary tract obstruction. Cystoceles can be visualized during fluoroscopy as the bladder fills to capacity (Fig. 11.10). Capacity includes the volume of urine held in the normally positioned bladder as well as the prolapsing portion. Much like a diverticulum, the prolapsing portion of the bladder may fail to empty during voiding thereby diminishing the functional bladder capacity. When a catheter is placed to drain the bladder at the start of urodynamic testing,

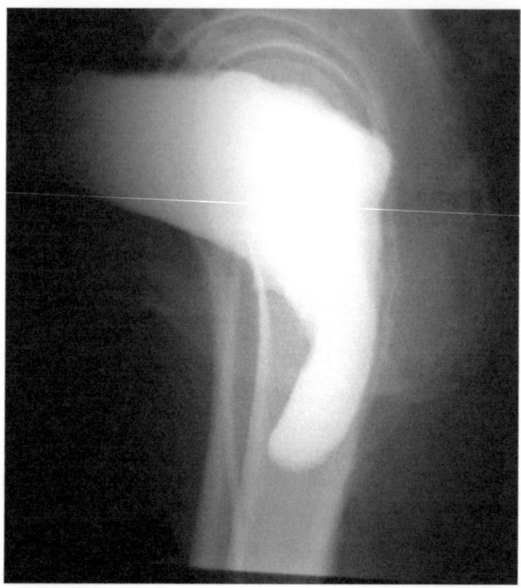

Fig. 11.10 Videofluoroscopic image of significant cystocele. Cystometric capacity reflects the sum of the orthotopic and prolapsing bladder volume

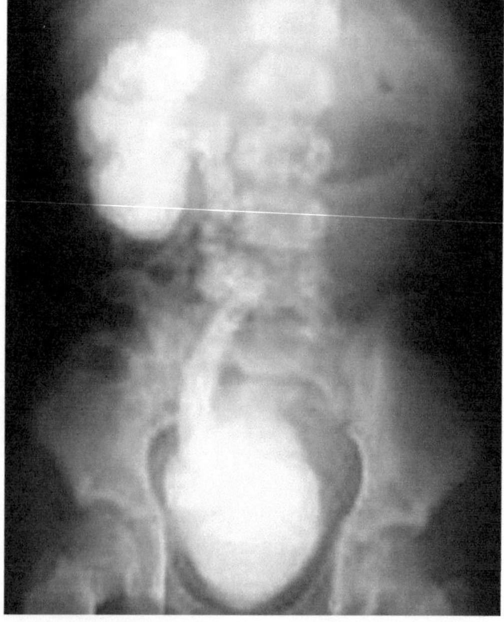

Fig. 11.11 Videofluoroscopic image of severe right-sided vesicoureteral reflux. Cystometric capacity reflects the sum of the bladder volume and the collecting system volume

the prolapsing portion may have the opportunity to drain to completion thereby elevating the capacity measured obtained during the test. The overestimation of functional bladder capacity may be significant especially when the prolapsing portion of the bladder is large and kinked during voiding.

VUR may be seen on fluoroscopy as the bladder fills to capacity or during the voiding phase (Fig. 11.11). Bladder capacity is the sum of the volume held in the bladder as well as the collecting system (kidney and ureter) of the refluxing unit. The collecting system may fail to empty during voiding thereby diminishing the functional bladder capacity. When a catheter is placed to drain the bladder at the start of urodynamic testing, the refluxing unit may have the opportunity to drain to completion thereby elevating the capacity measure obtained during the test. The overestimation of functional bladder capacity may be significant especially when the reflux is high grade into a dilated upper urinary tract.

References

 1. Haylen BT, de Ridder D, Freeman RM, Swift SE, Berghmans B, Lee J, Monga A, Petri E, Rizk DE, Sand PK, Schaer GN. An International Urogynecological Association (IUGA)/ International Continence Society (ICS) joint report on the terminology for female pelvic floor dysfunction. Int Urogynecol J. 2009;21(1):5–26.
 2. Amundsen CL, Parsons M, Tissot B, Cardozo L, Diokno A, Coats AC. Bladder diary measurements in asymptomatic females: functional bladder capacity, frequency, and 24-hr volume. Neurourol Urodyn. 2007;26(3):341–9.
 3. Berger RM, Maizels M, Moran GC, Conway JJ, Firlit CF. Bladder capacity (ounces) equals age (years) plus 2 predicts normal bladder capacity and aids in diagnosis of abnormal voiding patterns. J Urol. 1983;129(2):347–9.
 4. Zerin JM, Chen E, Ritchey ML, Bloom DA. Bladder capacity as measured at voiding cystourethrography in children—relationship to toilet training and frequency of micturition. Radiology. 1993;187:803.
 5. Hamano S, Yamanishi T, Igarashi T, Ito H, Murakami S. Functional bladder capacity as predictor of response to desmopressin and retention control training in monosymptomatic nocturnal enuresis. Eur Urol. 2000;37(6):718–22.
 6. Bael AM, Lax H, Hirche H, Hjälmš K, Tamminen-Möbius T, Van Hoeck KM, van Gool JD. Reference ranges for cystographic bladder capacity in children—with special attention to vesicoureteral reflux. J Urol. 2006;176(4 Pt 1):1596–600. On behalf of the International Reflux Study in Children.
 7. Heesakkers JP, Vandoninck V, van Balken MR, Bemelmans BL. Bladder filing by autologous urine production during cystometry: a urodynamic pitfall! Neurourol Urodyn. 2003;22(3):243–5.
 8. Lee SW, Kim JH. The significance of natural bladder filling by the production of urine during cystometry. Neurourol Urodyn. 2008;27(8):772–4.
 9. Abrams P. Urodynamic technique. In: Abrams P, editor. Urodynamics. 3rd ed. London: Springer; 2006. p. 17–116.
10. Wyndaele JJ. Normality in urodynamics studied in healthy adults. J Urol. 1999;161:899–902.
11. Pauwels E, De Wachter S, Wyndaele JJ. Normality of bladder filling studied in symptom-free middle-aged women. J Urol. 2004;171(4):1567–70.
12. Yoon E, Swift S. A comparison of maximum cystometric bladder capacity with maximum environmental voided volumes. Int Urogynecol J. 1998;9(2):78–82.
13. Cass AS, Ward BD, Markland C. Comparison of slow and rapid fill cystometry using liquid and air. J Urol. 1970;104:104–8.
14. Jensen JK. Urodynamic evaluation. In: Ostergard DR, Bent AE, editors. Urogynecology and urodynamics. 4th ed. Baltimore: Williams and Wilkins; 1991. p. 116–21.
15. Klevmark B. Volume threshold for micturition. Influence of filling rate on sensory and motor bladder function. Scand J Urol Nephrol Suppl. 2002;210:6–10.
16. Diokno AC, Wells TJ, Brink CA. Comparison of self-reported voided volume with cystometric bladder capacity. J Urol. 1987;137(4):698–700.

17. Abrams PH, Cardozo L, Fall M, Griffiths D, Rosier P, Ulmsten U, Van Kerrebroeck PEV, Wein AJ. The standardisation of terminology of lower urinary tract function: report from the Standardisation Sub-committee of the International Continence Society. Neurourol Urodyn. 2002;21:167–78.
18. Herbison P, Hay-Smith J, Ellis G, Moore K. Effectiveness of anticholinergic drugs compared with placebo in the treatment of overactive bladder: systematic review. BMJ. 2003;326(7394): 841–4.
19. Smith CP, Radziszewski P, Borkowski A, Somogyi GT, Boone TB, Chancellor MB. Botulinum toxin a has antinociceptive effects in treating interstitial cystitis. Urology. 2004;64(5):871–5.
20. Johansen TE, Botto H, Cek M, Grabe M, Tenke P, Wagenlehner FM, Naber KG. Critical review of current definitions of urinary tract infections and proposal of an EAU/ESIU classification system. Int J Antimicrob Agents. 2011;38(Supple):64–70.
21. Abrams P. Describing bladder storage function: overactive bladder syndrome and detrusor overactivity. Urology. 2003;62(5 Suppl 2):28–37.

Chapter 12
Bladder Filling and Storage: "Compliance"

Elizabeth Timbrook Brown, Kristi L. Hebert, and J. Christian Winters

Introduction

During normal bladder filling, the bladder accommodates increasing volumes of urine while maintaining low storage pressure. This accommodation is unique due to the viscoelastic properties of the bladder. Compliance is an urodynamic measurement which assesses bladder filling, and describes the relationship between change in bladder volume and change in detrusor pressure (Pdet) [1]. Compliance is measured during multichannel filling cystometry. As shown in Fig. 12.1a, b compliance is calculated by dividing the change in detrusor pressure (ΔPdet) during the associated change in bladder volume (ΔV) [1]. Compliance is generally thought to be one of the most reproducible and reliable urodynamic measurements. It is a passive measurement which records detrusor pressure over a defined volume. It is not dependent on provocative maneuvers or on patient cooperation. It is easily measured with properly functioning and calibrated urodynamic equipment.

When analyzing compliance on an urodynamic tracing, the International Continence Society (ICS) recommends choosing two standard points for comparison: "the detrusor pressure at the start of bladder filling and the corresponding bladder volume (usually zero), and the detrusor pressure (and corresponding bladder volume) at cystometric capacity or immediately before the start of any detrusor contraction that causes significant leakage (and therefore causes the bladder volume to decrease, affecting compliance calculation). Both points are measured excluding any detrusor contraction" [1].

E.T. Brown, MD, MPH (✉) • K.L. Hebert, MD • J.C. Winters, MD
Department of Urology, Louisiana State University School of Medicine,
1542 Tulane Ave, Suite 547, New Orleans, LA 70112, USA
e-mail: brookbrownmd@gmail.com

© Springer Science+Business Media New York 2015

E.S. Rovner, M.E. Koski (eds.), *Rapid and Practical Interpretation of Urodynamics*, DOI 10.1007/978-1-4939-1764-8_12

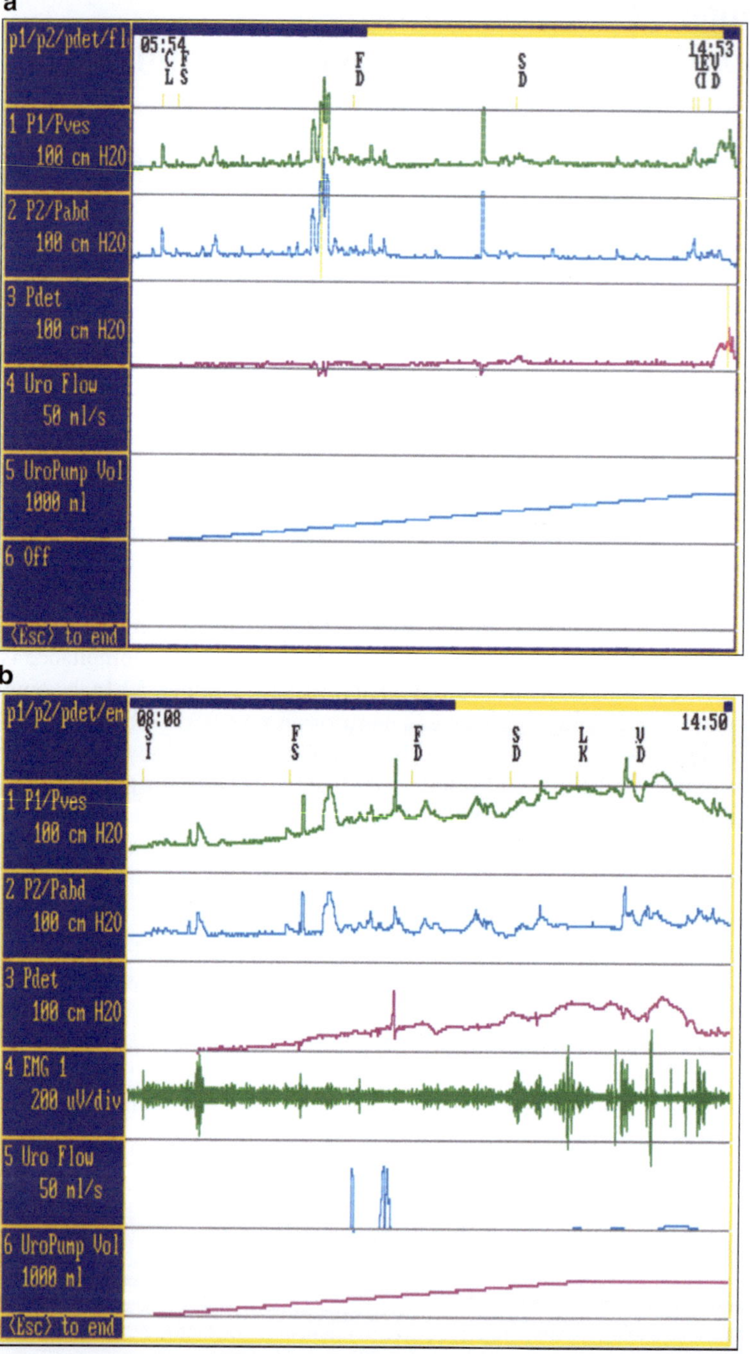

Fig. 12.1 (**a**) Calculating compliance. $A = 495$ ml/3 cm H_2O $A = 165$ ml/cm H_2O (**b**) Calculating Compliance. $B = 400$ ml/62 cm H_2O $B = 6.5$ ml/cm H_2O

Low bladder compliance is consistent with an abnormal increase in detrusor pressure between these two given points. Over the past few decades there have been several studies attempting to define "normal compliance." Unfortunately, however, there has never been an agreed upon absolute value for bladder compliance. Topercer and Tetreault [2] attempted to define abnormal compliance in their 1979 study comparing asymptomatic women to women with stress urinary incontinence, but could not establish a definitive value due to the lack of a data pattern among study participants. Weld et al. [3] found that there was a significant change in the risk of upper tract damage between compliance values of 12.5 and 15 cc/cm H_2O, and thus recommended using a cut-off value of 12.5 cc/cm H_2O to define abnormal compliance. However, Churchill et al. [4, 5] define abnormal compliance as greater than 10 cc/cm H_2O.

While there are various measurements used to define abnormal compliance, it is widely agreed upon that a sustained bladder pressure of greater than 40 cm H_2O can cause significant risk to the upper tracts [6]. It is also thought that the amount of time that the bladder experiences high pressures is directly proportional to the risk of upper tract deterioration [4]. Thus, a patient whose urodynamic tracing demonstrates a sustained tonic elevation in detrusor storage pressure appears to be more at risk for upper tract complications (see case #1) than a patient who has intermittent, phasic rises in detrusor pressure that return to baseline (see case #7).

Sustained pathologic increases of detrusor pressure which can cause upper tract complications can be measured in two ways. First, consistently high abnormal storage pressures should be approached with caution and may signify upper tract risk [7]. The absolute value of sustained pressure elevation during filling is not standardized, but clinicians should be wary of sustained filling pressures exceeding 25 cm H_2O. Second, a widely agreed upon measurement assessing upper tract risk is the detrusor leak point pressure (DLPP). It is defined as the lowest detrusor pressure at which urine leakage occurs in the absence of either a detrusor contraction or increased abdominal pressure [1]. Studies have shown that a sustained Pdet greater than 40 cm H_2O is consistent with upper tract deterioration [6].

Many pathologic conditions can result in abnormal compliance. For example, decreased bladder compliance can result from neurogenic causes like multi-system atrophy (MSA), spina bifida, spinal cord injury (SCI), or iatrogenic causes such as resultant nerve damage from pelvic surgery, such as radical hysterectomy or abdominoperineal resection (APR). Other non-neurogenic causes can include bladder outlet obstruction (BOO), chronic cystitis, or a defunctionalized bladder [8, 9].

The measurement of compliance may be misleading in the presence of anatomic variations which may result in a buffering of intraluminal detrusor pressure. In cases such as vesicoureteral reflux or bladder diverticuli in the setting of a poorly compliant bladder, the detrusor pressure may appear falsely low due to a "pressure sink" effect. In these cases, the urine storage pressure is actually being dissipated into the expanding bladder diverticulum or refluxing upper tracts. These are clinical scenarios in which videourodynamics can provide invaluable information [7]. In addition, in severe intrinsic sphincter deficiency, the bladder storage pressures may appear low as a result of urethral loss or urethral leakage. In these cases urethral occlusion is necessary to determine the filling properties of the bladder.

Detrusor overactivity (DO) is an urodynamic observation characterized by involuntary detrusor contractions (IDC) during the filling phase which may be spontaneous or provoked. Phasic DO is defined by a characteristic waveform and may or may not lead to urinary incontinence [1]. Phasic IDC generally have shorter periods of pressure elevations with a return to baseline. Sustained involuntary detrusor pressure elevation caused by continuous bladder tension reflects a tonic increase in bladder pressure. This is indicative of low compliance. Phasic detrusor overactivity can sometimes be misleading and confused for abnormal compliance as well. This can especially occur if it is prolonged and of low amplitude. To differentiate between an IDC and abnormal compliance during filling, simply stop the infusion. If the Pdet returns to baseline, then the rise in Pdet is due to an IDC; if the Pdet remains elevated, then the rise in Pdet is due to a compliance abnormality [8].

This chapter will present urodynamic tracings and discuss the differential diagnosis, clinical interpretation, and treatment options for each given condition with regards to abnormal compliance (Fig. 12.1a, b).

Case Scenarios

Case #1

A 47-year-old male with a 10-year history of transverse myelitis presents with a chief complaint of persistent urinary leakage despite performing clean intermittent catheterization (CIC). He has been catheterizing three times a day for the last 10 years and has been managed with a daily extended release anticholinergic. His urodynamic tracing, shown below in Fig. 12.2, demonstrates an abnormal constant increase in detrusor pressure during the filling phase. This persistent elevation in Pdet can be characterized as a tonic abnormality of filling, representing abnormal compliance. During the filling phase, the patient also demonstrates an early sensation abnormality, followed by superimposed IDC with leakage. The DLPP is 36 cm H_2O. While 36 cm H_2O is borderline, one can infer that this patient is at higher risk for long-term upper tract deterioration based on the sustained, tonic compliance abnormality as well as further sustained rise in detrusor storage pressure. With the patient's clinical history and urodynamic tracing, a renal ultrasound would certainly be warranted to establish a baseline and evaluate for hydronephrosis. Initially, treatment options for this patient could include increasing the frequency of CIC as well as increasing anticholinergic therapy as tolerated. The rate-limiting dosage for anticholinergic therapy would be determined by tolerable side effects including dry mouth, constipation, and heat intolerance, most commonly. After a trial of a more aggressive CIC and anticholinergic regimen, further treatment options would include onabotulinum-toxinA injection or even possibly augmentation cystoplasty (Fig. 12.2).

Case #2

A 57-year-old male underwent a laparoscopic proctosigmoidectomy for colon cancer, and, subsequently, developed a neurogenic bladder. His urodynamic tracing in Fig. 12.3 demonstrates a tonic increase in detrusor pressure throughout the filling/

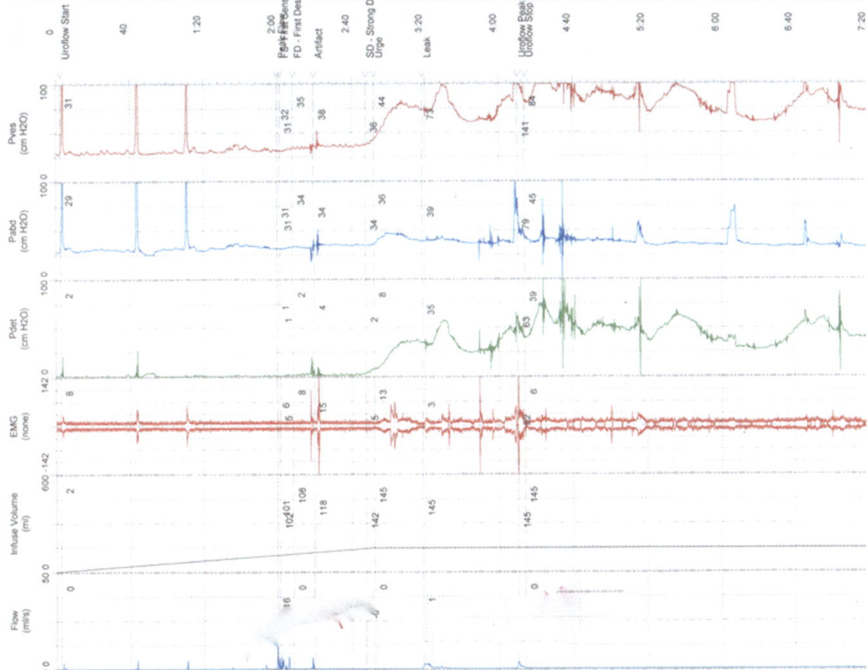

Fig. 12.2 Transverse myelitis. Filling phase

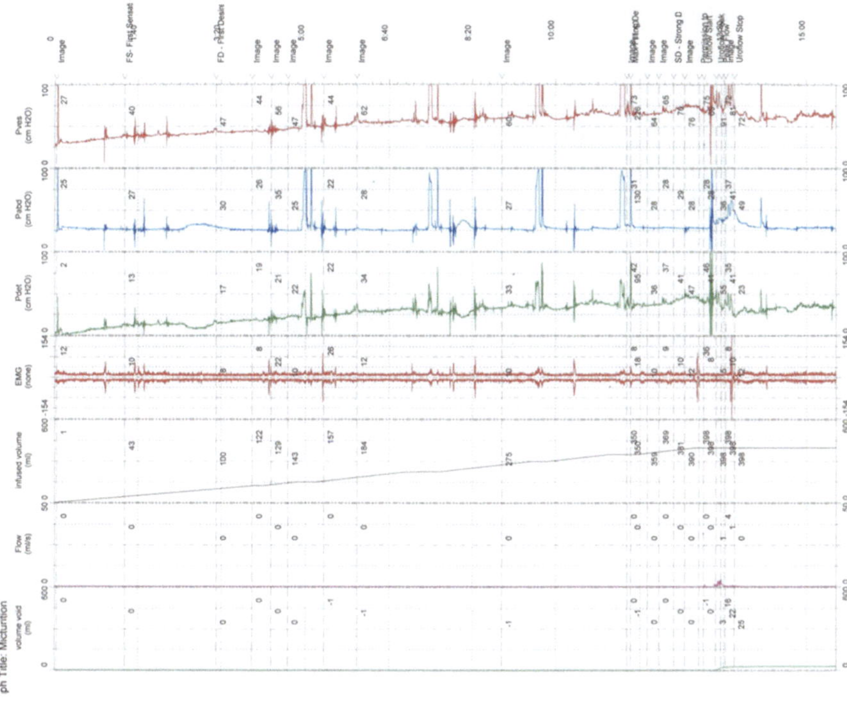

Fig. 12.3 Neurogenic bladder after a laparoscopic proctosigmoidectomy

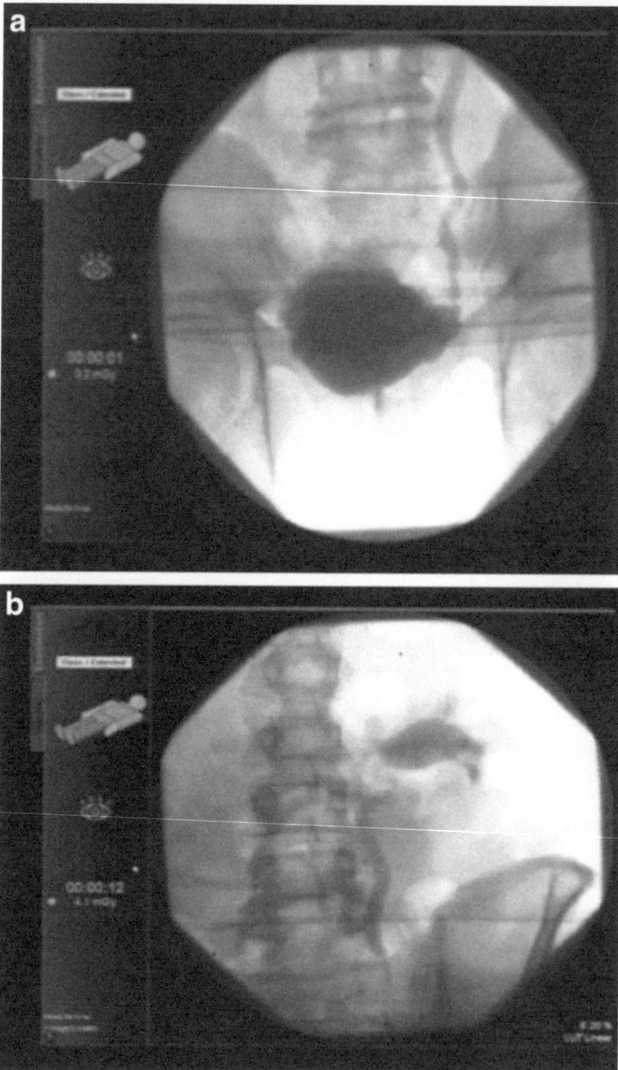

Fig. 12.4 Left grade IV vesicoureteral reflux with bladder diverticuli. (**a**) Left vesicoureteral reflux with bladder diverticuli (**b**) Left grade IV vesicoureteral reflux to upper tract

storage phase, as with case #1. Neurogenic bladder can develop as a result of a denervation injury during many colorectal, urologic, and gynecologic procedures. Most commonly, neurogenic bladders are seen as a result of APR.

The fluoroscopic images above in Fig. 12.4 demonstrate the utility of videourodynamic studies. Without imaging, this patient's Pdet falsely appears much lower than it actually is. When a patient develops poor bladder compliance, due to a decrease in the native viscoelastic properties of the bladder, the intrinsic detrusor pressure can be transmitted to the upper tracts as a "pop-off" type mechanism. This is best demonstrated by videourodynamics to delineate vesicoureteral reflux or bladder diverticuli. This patient's imaging combined with cystoscopy demonstrates a posterior bladder diverticulum as well as a left hutch diverticulum with grade IV vesicoureteral reflux. The voiding phase of the study is consistent with detrusor areflexia. In this setting of iatrogenic neurogenic bladder, treatment options again include an increase in CIC frequency and anticholinergic therapy, onabotulinumtoxinA injection or an augmentation cystoplasty.

Another important point in the diagnostic work-up can include a voiding diary. Determining the typical volume of urine during each catheterization can give invaluable information as well as help guide the urodynamic study itself. It can also be a useful tool during treatment with the goal to increase catheterization frequency and decrease storage volumes. This patient underwent an aggressive CIC and anticholinergic regimen with a marked improvement in his catheterized volumes at follow-up. Figure 12.5 shows the repeat urodynamics after a 3-month intervention, showing a marked improvement in bladder compliance with conservative therapy alone (Figs. 12.3, 12.4, and 12.5).

Case #3

A 37-year-old female presents with a history of a C6 SCI. She previously underwent an augmentation cystoplasty with a catheterizable, continent stoma using the modified Indiana technique. She is now referred for a persistent compliance abnormality on urodynamics and concern for upper tract deterioration.

On cursory review of her urodynamics, shown in Fig. 12.6, there appears to be early sensation, reduced cystometric capacity, and terminal detrusor overactivity which she does not suppress. This consists of a phasic involuntary rise with a return to baseline. Thus, this is not considered a true compliance abnormality by definition. Additionally, the detrusor pressure returns to baseline at the end of the contraction, significantly decreasing her risk of upper tract damage as the increased pressure is not sustained (Fig. 12.6).

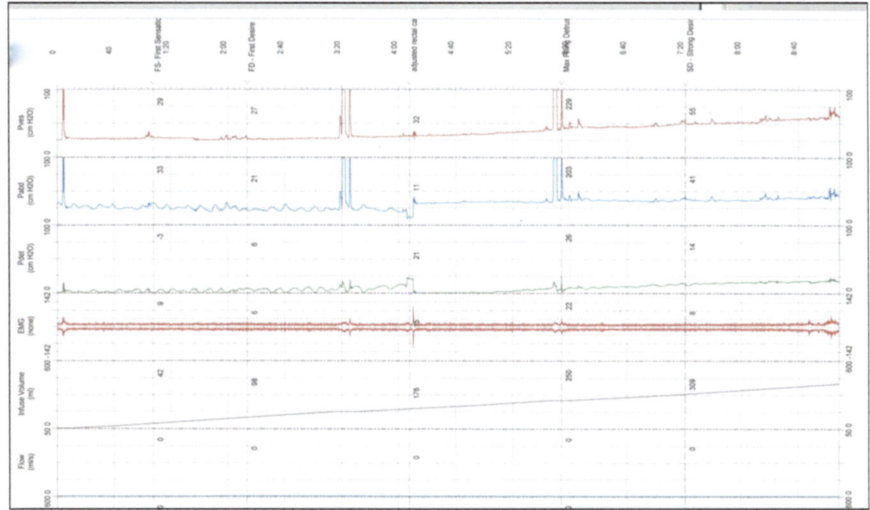

Fig. 12.5 Repeat urodynamics at 3 months with conservative management

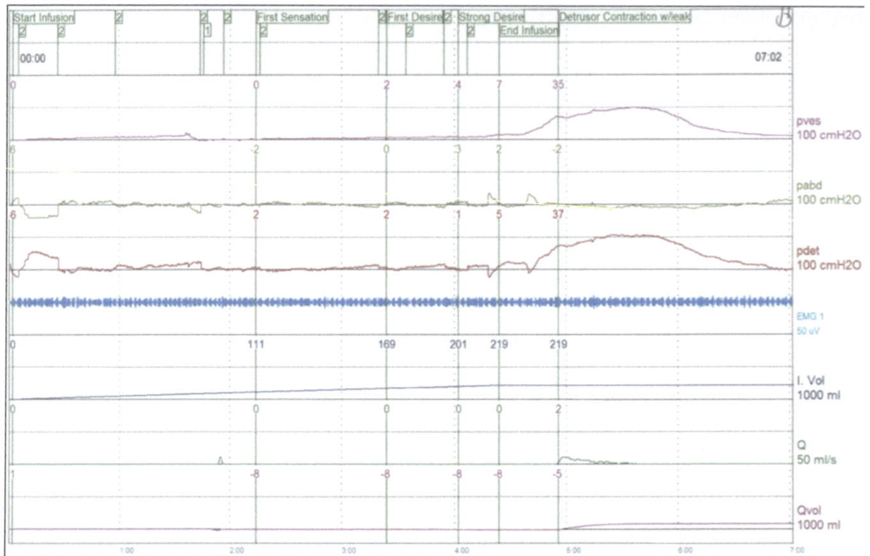

Fig. 12.6 C6 spinal cord injury status post-augmentation cystoplasty with a terminal involuntary detrusor contraction and normal compliance

Case #4

A 36-year-old female underwent pelvic radiation for cervical cancer 2 years ago. She is referred for multiple episodes of pyelonephritis requiring hospitalization. She complains of mixed urinary incontinence and on renal ultrasound she is found to have severe bilateral hydronephrosis. Her urodynamics are shown in Fig. 12.7. There is a sustained, tonic compliance abnormality with Pdet reaching 129 cm H_2O with subsequent IDC noted during the filling phase. There is no demonstrable stress incontinence at a volume of 385 cc.

However, when evaluating the patient's clinical history, she states that she voids three times daily with large urine volumes. When reviewing her voiding diary, her volumes are approximately 500 cc with each void. This again demonstrates the importance of voiding diaries not only for patient counseling, but also to tailor the urodynamic study. If this study had been continued to 600 cc, detrusor overactivity or stress urinary incontinence may have been demonstrated.

Protection from further upper tract deterioration in this setting is vital. While she was initially placed on an aggressive CIC and anticholinergic regimen, her repeat renal ultrasound and urodynamics at 3 months showed no improvement due to poor patient compliance. While progression to injection of onabotulinum-toxinA would normally be a reasonable option due to the long-term effects on the detrusor muscle, patient compliance with CIC is still paramount. While CIC is also imperative in the setting of an augmentation cystoplasty, increasing the overall bladder capacity can certainly aid in protection of the upper tracts in a poorly compliant patient. After undergoing augmentation and extensive counseling on the importance of CIC, she had no further episodes of pyelonephritis and her mixed urinary incontinence was greatly improved at 6-month follow-up (Fig. 12.7).

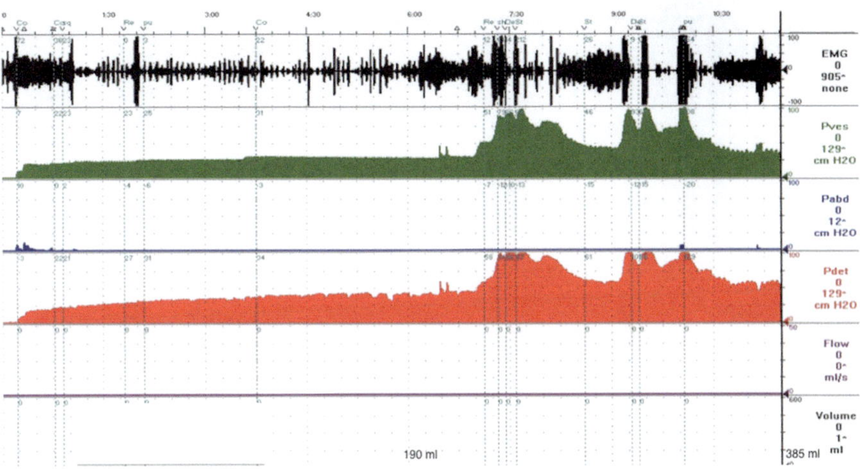

Fig. 12.7 Pelvic radiation for cervical cancer with abnormal compliance. Courtesy of Stephen Kraus

Case #5

A 17-year-old male with spina bifida presented for urologic evaluation. He has been managing his bladder by anticholinergics and CIC every 4 h. His urodynamic tracing, shown in Fig. 12.8, demonstrates a poorly compliant bladder with a small capacity, IDC with leak, and detrusor sphincter dyssynergia (DESD). The DLPP is 58 cm H_2O. When paired with the videourodynamics in Fig. 12.9, it is evident that he has an extremely small bladder capacity (150 cc), with right vesicoureteral reflux as well as a "spinning top" abnormality. This is often seen in DESD in which there is a dilated posterior urethra. Additionally, bladder neck narrowing is seen and may signify bladder neck dyssynergia.

Due to the patient's failure of conservative therapy and risk to upper tracts, he would be an excellent candidate for onabotulinum-toxinA or augmentation cystoplasty with a right ureteral reimplant (Figs. 12.8 and 12.9).

Case #6

A 73-year-old male presents with intermittent urinary urgency incontinence 1 year after a suprapontine cerebrovascular accident. His urodynamic tracing, shown in Fig. 12.10, demonstrates an involuntary bladder contraction, without a compliance abnormality. In other words, there is no distinct, continuous rise in detrusor pressure as volume increases. As previously mentioned, involuntary bladder contractions may be mistaken for abnormal compliance on urodynamics tracings. In this scenario, there are short, involuntary, phasic rises in detrusor pressure, which return to baseline storage pressure.

With this clinical picture, the patient can be managed with anticholinergics to minimize the symptoms of detrusor overactivity—timed toileting and daily trospium or darifenacin would be a good option for him due to his age (cognition concerns) and clinical history (Fig. 12.10).

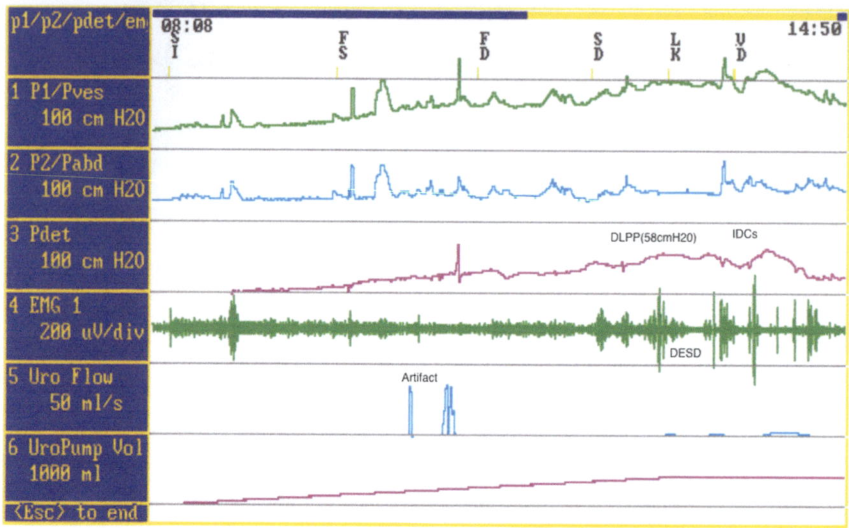

Fig. 12.8 Neurogenic bladder and abnormal compliance

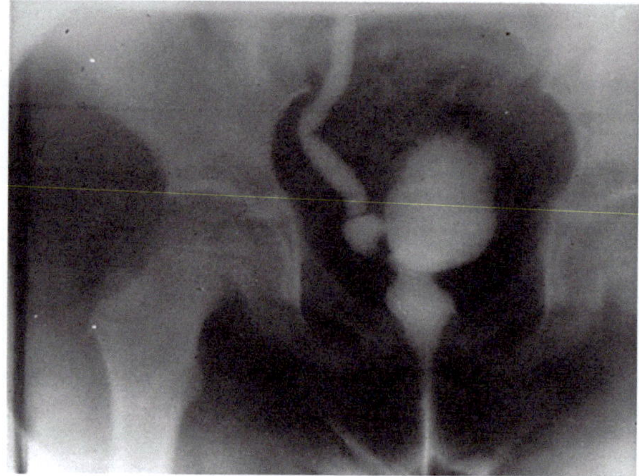

Fig. 12.9 Videourodynamics showing a "spinning top" abnormality, small bladder capacity, and right vesicoureteral reflux

Case #7

A 32-year-old female presents with complaints of urinary urgency and frequency and intermittent incontinence. She was recently diagnosed with multiple sclerosis (MS). Her urodynamics are shown below in Fig. 12.11. The tracing is consistent with several transient rises in detrusor pressure associated with increased external sphincteric activity. This patient is at less risk for upper tract damage compared to the previous patient with a tonic rise in detrusor pressure (case #1) because this

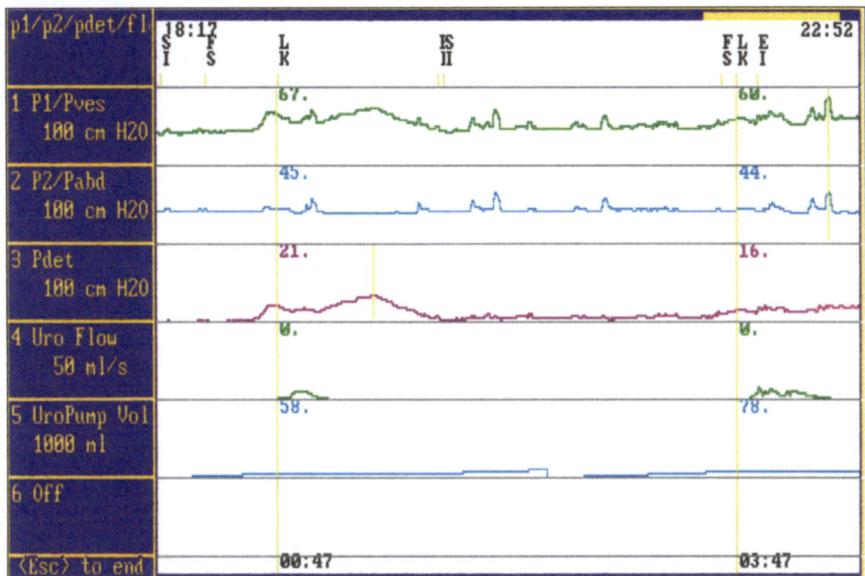

Fig. 12.10 Involuntary detrusor contraction without a true compliance abnormality

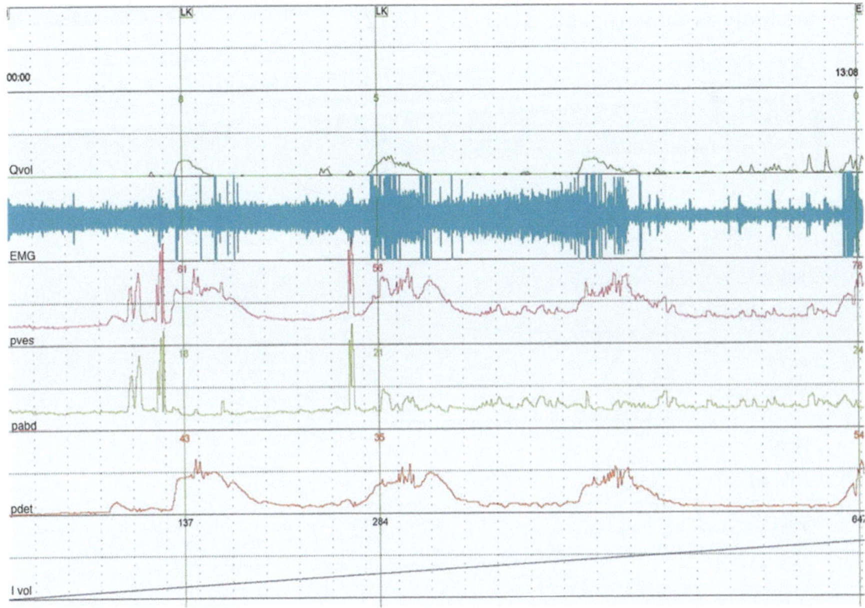

Fig. 12.11 Phasic detrusor contractions with leak. Involuntary contractions of short duration, "phasic contractions," are demonstrated

patient has only transient involuntary rises in detrusor pressure, as opposed to sustained, prolonged increased storage pressures. Her urodynamics are consistent with neurogenic detrusor overactivity with detrusor external sphincter dyssynergia.

She may be treated with daily anticholinergics as well, but her emptying ability must be monitored closely. Oftentimes, treatment of this condition results in increasing post-void residual urine and the need for CIC. Her urodynamics should be repeated with symptom changes as MS can be progressive (Fig. 12.11).

Case #8

A 55-year-old male presents with bothersome frequency, hesitancy, and nocturia. He has an American Urologic Symptom Score of 22. His prostate was estimated at 55 g on physical exam. Three years ago he was diagnosed with benign prostatic hyperplasia and was subsequently placed on combination therapy (tamsulosin and finasteride) but his symptoms have persisted. His urodynamic tracing is shown below in Fig. 12.12. This tracing demonstrates classic BOO—high pressure and low flow are clearly evident. There is a terminal compliance abnormality noted as Pdet changed near capacity due to BOO. This patient may benefit from treatment of the benign prostatic enlargement causing the BOO. As he has failed medical therapy, minimally invasive or standard transurethral techniques may be offered for this condition.

A similar high pressure, low flow tracing with or without a terminal compliance abnormality can also be seen in the setting of BOO in women secondary to pelvic organ prolapse or even iatrogenic BOO after a fascial or transvaginal mesh sling placement for stress urinary incontinence. Management would again be tailored at relieving the obstruction by either reducing the prolapse or performing a sling incision/urethrolysis for iatrogenic BOO (Fig. 12.12).

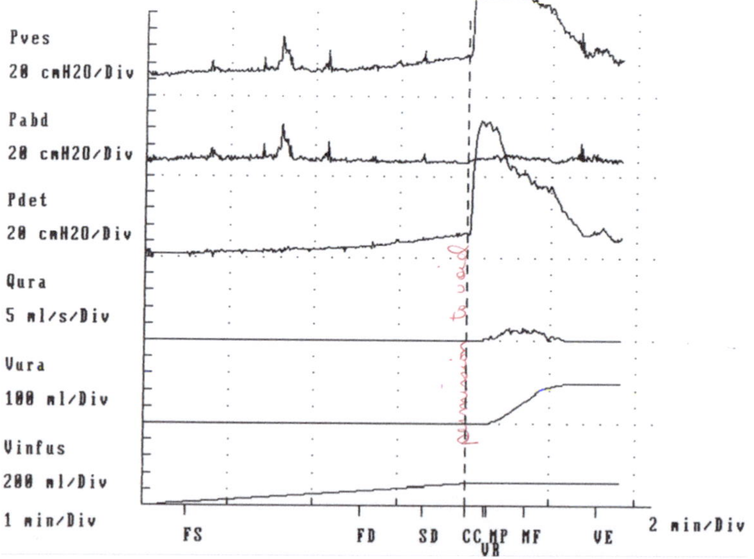

Fig. 12.12 Classic bladder outlet obstruction—high pressure, low flow

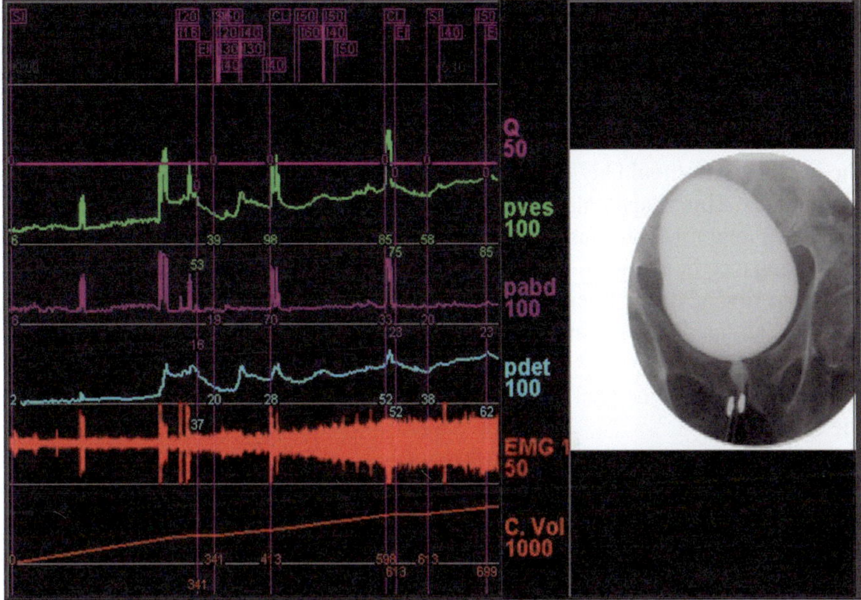

Fig. 12.13   Detrusor external sphincter dyssynergia. Courtesy of Stephen Kraus

Case #9

A 33-year-old quadriplegic male presents with persistent urinary incontinence. He has previously been managed with onabotulinum-toxinA injections of 300 units. He has received two separate sets of injections. The urodynamics in Fig. 12.13 show a lack of coordination between the detrusor muscle and the pelvic floor and external urethral sphincter. This is another case in which videourodynamics are beneficial. The fluoroscopic image demonstrates DESD with a "spinning top" abnormality—a dilated posterior urethra and narrow bladder neck. This patient has failed onabotulinum-toxinA injection therapy, and thus the next option would be an augmentation cystoplasty (Fig. 12.13).

Conclusion

Although there has been no agreed upon normative value for compliance, most sources cite that it lies somewhere between 10 and 20 ml/cm H_2O and can be calculated by evaluating the change in volume compared to the change in detrusor pressure at two given points. Normally, the bladder accommodates filling and stores urine at low pressures due to the viscoelastic properties of the bladder, but various pathologies can cause abnormalities in bladder compliance.

This chapter has discussed many conditions associated with abnormal compliance including cerebrovascular accident, BOO, SCI, transverse myelitis, multiple sclerosis, and pelvic surgery. It has touched upon situations that can be falsely interpreted as abnormal compliance. For example, IDC can mimic abnormal compliance. According to the ICS, when performing urodynamic studies for neuropathic lesions the infusion rate should be low in order to avoid producing an artificial compliance abnormality. This chapter also reviewed clinical scenarios in which videourodynamics can be important, such as to evaluate vesicoureteral reflux or DESD.

Compliance has proven to be a reproducible and reliable measurement to determine the risk of upper tract damage and, as such, a true compliance abnormality warrants an upper tract evaluation. Therefore, interpreting bladder compliance on an urodynamic tracing can provide invaluable information about a patient's voiding and also help guide medical and surgical treatment options as discussed throughout the chapter.

References

1. Abrams P, et al. The standardization of terminology in lower urinary tract function. Report from the standardization sub-committee of the International Continence Society; 2009.
2. Toppercer A, Tetreault JP. Compliance of the bladder: an attempt to establish normal values. Urology. 1979;14(2):204–5.
3. Weld K, Graney M, Dmochowski R. Differences in bladder compliance with time and associations of bladder management with compliance in spinal cord injured patients. J Urol. 2000;163: 1228–33.
4. Churchill BM, Gilmour PE, Williot P. Urodynamics. Pediatr Clin North Am. 1987;34:1133.
5. Nitti V. Cystometry and abdominal pressure monitoring. In: Nitti V, ed. Practical urodynamics. 1998; p. 38–51. Chapter 5.
6. McGuire EM, Woodside JR, Borden TA. Prognostic value of urodynamic testing in myelodysplastic children. J Urol. 1981;126:205.
7. Ghoniem G, Roach M, Lewis V, Harmon E. The value of leak pressure and bladder compliance in the urodynamic evaluation of meningomyelocele patients. J Urol. 1990;144:1440–2.
8. Nitti V. Urodynamic and video-urodynamic evaluation of the lower urinary tract. In: Wein, et al., editors. Campbell-Walsh urology. Saunders: 2011; 10th ed; p.1847–70. Chapter 62.
9. Blaivas J, Chancellor M, et al. Low bladder compliance. In: Blaivas J, Chancellor M, et al., editors. Atlas of urodynamics. 2007; p. 56–61. Chapter 6.

Chapter 13
Bladder Filling and Storage: "(Coarse) Sensation"

Ying H. Jura and Christopher K. Payne

Introduction

Adequate bladder sensation is essential for conscious bladder control; alterations in bladder sensation are important in certain pathologic conditions [1]. Classic examples of sensory disorders include increased sensation with bladder pain syndrome (BPS) and decreased sensation with neurogenic bladder disorders associated with peripheral neuropathies. Bladder sensation is assessed during filling cystometry.

Definitions of Normal and Abnormal Sensation

According to the International Continence Society (ICS) Terminology Committee, normal bladder sensation is evaluated by bladder volume at three defined points during filling cystometry and in relation to the patient's symptoms [2]. The three defined points are (1) first sensation of bladder filling, (2) first desire to void, and (3) strong desire to void (Table 13.1). Bladder sensation is increased if there is a consistent early first sensation of filling, desire to void, and/or strong desire to void that occurs at low bladder volume. Bladder sensation is reduced if bladder sensation is diminished throughout bladder filling. Bladder sensation may also be completely absent. During filling cystometry, the patient may also experience urgency, which is defined as a sudden compelling desire to void.

Y.H. Jura, MD (✉) • C.K. Payne, MD
Department of Urology, Stanford University School of Medicine, Stanford University,
300 Pasteur Drive, Stanford, CA 94305-5118, USA
e-mail: ying.jura@gmail.com; yjura@stanford.edu

© Springer Science+Business Media New York 2015
E.S. Rovner, M.E. Koski (eds.), *Rapid and Practical Interpretation
of Urodynamics*, DOI 10.1007/978-1-4939-1764-8_13

Table 13.1 International Continence Society terms for bladder sensation during filling cystometry

Normal bladder sensation	Can be judged by three defined points noted during filling cystometry and evaluated in relation to the bladder volume at that moment and in relation to the patient's symptomatic complaints
First sensation of bladder filling	Is the feeling the patient has, during filling cystometry, when he/she first becomes aware of the bladder filling
First desire to void	Is defined as the feeling, during filling cystometry, that would lead the patient to pass urine at the next convenient moment, but voiding can be delayed if necessary
Strong desire to void	Is defined, during filling cystometry, as a persistent desire to void without the fear of leakage
Increased bladder sensation	Is defined, during filling cystometry, as an early first sensation of bladder filling (or an early desire to void) and/or an early strong desire to void, which occurs at low bladder volume and which persists
Reduced bladder sensation	Is defined, during filling cystometry, as diminished sensation throughout bladder filling
Absent bladder sensation	Means that, during filling cystometry, the individual has no bladder sensation
Non-specific bladder sensations	During filling cystometry may make the individual aware of bladder filling, for example, abdominal fullness or vegetative symptoms
Bladder pain	During filling cystometry is a self-explanatory term and is an abnormal finding
Urgency	During filling cystometry is a sudden compelling desire to void

Compiled from Abrams P, et al. The standardization of terminology of lower urinary tract function: Report from the Standardisation Subcommittee of the International Continence Society. Neurourol Urodyn. 2002;21:261–74

How to Measure Sensation

Bladder sensation is measured during filling cystometry. Because sensation is inherently subjective, it requires communication between an attentive clinician and an alert, mentally competent patient [3].

While standardized ICS definitions exist for the various bladder sensations, ICS does not specify when and how these definitions should be communicated. Some clinicians simply ask the patient to report whatever they feel without any instruction. Others might instruct patients at the outset to report sensations and these sensations are described for the patients. Each clinician will communicate these definitions a little differently in order to achieve understanding among patients of different backgrounds. Due to the variability in the way information regarding bladder sensation is elicited, results can be difficult to reproduce across different laboratories.

Ideally, an ongoing conversation should be maintained between a clinician and patient throughout the study. The patient should be instructed to report when fluid in the bladder is first sensed. The patient is then asked to report occurrence of first desire to urinate followed by occurrence of strong desire to urinate. Finally, the patient should inform the clinician when restraining from urination is difficult to defer (urgency). The patient should also be queried as to what, if anything, is felt when any significant changes in detrusor pressure, like involuntary detrusor contractions, are noted. Many clinicians will provide everyday analogies in order to communicate to patients the differences among first desire, strong desire, and urgency. For example, first desire might be described as a sensation that would prompt a patient watching a good television show to go to the bathroom at the next commercial break while strong desire might prompt the patient to consider interrupting the show and walking to the bathroom and urgency is as a sensation that would prompt the patient to get up immediately and run to the bathroom.

Bladder sensation is subjective and a variety factors may affect the reliability of measurements of bladder sensation [4]. These factors may include patient anxiety, non-physiologic rate of bladder filling, and irritation from the catheter. Erdem and colleagues demonstrated the subjectivity of bladder sensation measurements by showing that a significant portion of adult men who were prepped for a urodynamics study, including catheter insertion, and told that the study had commenced reported first sensation of bladder filling (83 %), first desire to void (80 %), and strong desire to void (25 %) despite lack of bladder distension with air or fluid [5]. To investigate the impact of catheter placement on perceptions of bladder filling, another study was performed where the catheters were taped to the penile skin but not inserted [6]. Even without catheter insertion, about half of patients reported first sensation and a quarter of patients reported first desire, although no patients reported strong desire. When the catheter was then inserted but no filling occurred in the next phase of the study, a much greater portion of patients reported first sensation (87 %) and first desire (73 %), and some patients reported strong desire (18 %). This suggested that catheter placement contributes to the perception of bladder filling but other factors also play a role. The same study performed in a group of children, however, found that they were significantly less prone to reporting sensations of bladder filling without actual bladder filling [7]. Thus, sensations reported by children during urodynamic studies may be more reliable than those reported by adults. In terms of rate of bladder filling, there is conflicting data as to whether it affects bladder sensation [8–10].

One proposal to make assessment of bladder sensation more reproducible involves the use of an electronic keypad that allows patients to rate sensations of bladder filling between 0 (none) to 4 (desperate) [4]. Patients can choose their starting point and go up and down on the scale as they wish throughout the test without any prompting from the clinician. The investigators found this method promising in providing reliable and repeatable results with a statistically significant increase in bladder volume at each urge level.

Normal Sensation

Studies of normal volunteers have found a consistent pattern in patients' reports of bladder sensations [8, 11]. These studies were performed in men and women aged 18–30. In all patients, first sensation of bladder filling was followed by first desire

Table 13.2 Mean volumes for bladder sensation during filling from healthy volunteers; age (years), volume (ml)

	Men ($n=18$)	Women ($n=32$)
Age	22 ± 3	21 ± 2
First sensation of filling	222.5 ± 151	175.5 ± 95.5
First desire to void	325 ± 140.5	272 ± 106
Strong desire to void	453 ± 93.5	429 ± 153

Data adapted from Wyndaele and Wachter [8]

to void, and then followed by strong desire to void. Patients describe first sensation of filling as a vague sensation derived from fluid inflow that waxed and waned and was located in the lower pelvis. Patients did not recognize this sensation from their normal daily lives. First desire and strong desire to void were recognized as they are described by the ICS. Patients identified first desire to void as being a sensation familiar from daily life that is localized to the lower abdomen. It became gradually stronger during filling. Strong desire to void was described as a constant, almost uncomfortable sensation located in the perineal region or urethra.

Although sensation is typically part of a complete urodynamic study there has been little investigation of the clinical relevance of this information, the optimal means of eliciting the information, and the test–retest reliability of the assessments. Research has found a significant increase in volume between each sensation (see Table 13.2) [8, 11]. While volumes at which each sensation occurred varied widely among individuals and average volumes were significantly different between male and female patients, they occurred at a fairly constant percentage of total bladder volume. First sensation of bladder filling occurs at an average of 40 % of maximal cystometric capacity while strong desire to void occurs at an average 70 % of maximal cystometric capacity [12].

Cold receptors have been identified in the feline and human bladders [13]. Cold sensation is lacking in patients who have undergone cystectomy and enterocystoplasty [14]. While Bors described cold sensation as being felt in the skin rather than the bladder, other experts report the sensation as felt in the bladder rather than the urethra or skin [13]. In some laboratories, room temperature fluid is used to perform urodynamic studies instead of warmed, body temperature fluid (as a matter of convenience). While the clinical significance of intact cool sensation is currently unknown, it seems reasonable to ask if the patient feels an infusion of something cool into the bladder as another test of sensation if room temperature fluid is used.

Conditions of Altered Sensation

Sensation maybe altered in a number of different conditions. The following is a list of some of these conditions:

Increased Bladder Sensation

- Interstitial cystitis/bladder pain syndrome (IC/BPS) and other pelvic pain syndromes
- Infection

Reduced or Absent Bladder Sensation

- Sensory neurogenic bladder
- Diabetic cystopathy

Mixed Disorder of Bladder Sensation

- Idiopathic overactive bladder

Interstitial Cystitis/Bladder Pain Syndrome

The Society for Urodynamics, Female Pelvic Medicine and Urogenital Reconstruction (SUFU) defines IC/BPS as an unpleasant sensation (pain, pressure, discomfort) perceived to be related to the urinary bladder, associated with lower urinary tract symptoms of more than 6 weeks duration, in the absence of infection or other identifiable causes [15]. Since the pathophysiology is unknown and vast majority of patients diagnosed with IC/BPS have no identifiable pathologic abnormality of the bladder it is best considered to be a disorder of bladder sensation [16].

Urgency is a commonly reported symptom in both IC/BPS and OAB [17]. A comparative study found that urgency is reported by 81 % of patients diagnosed with IC/BPS and 91 % of patients with OAB [18]. The same proportion of patients in both groups (60 %) indicated that the urgency occurred "suddenly" instead of more gradually over a period of minutes or hours. In IC/BPS, however, the urgency was primarily reported as due to pain, pressure, or discomfort, whereas in OAB the urgency was more commonly due to fear of leakage. A survey of 180 IC/BPS patients from the Events Preceding Interstitial Cystitis cohort found that 65 % of patients endorsed urge to urinate in order to relieve pain whereas 21 % endorsed urge to urinate due to fear of incontinence [19].

Historically, urodynamic studies were included as part of the diagnostic criteria for interstitial cystitis. In the original National Institute of Diabetes and Digestive and Kidney Disease (NIDDK) criteria, the inclusion criteria and exclusion criteria included (1) cystometric bladder capacity greater than 350 ml, (2) absence of intense urgency during cystometry at a bladder volume of 150 ml, or less and (3) presence of detrusor overactivity [20]. These criteria were intended to produce homogeneous populations for clinical research but were based only on expert opinion, and there is no evidence that any urodynamic findings have adequate sensitivity or specificity for IC/BPS. The 2011 American Urological Association Guidelines for IC/BPS recommends that urodynamics be considered if the diagnosis of IC/BPS is in doubt but this test is not necessary for making the diagnosis in uncomplicated presentations. Urodynamic studies may be helpful by identifying patients with significant detrusor overactivity, urethral or bladder neck obstruction, and urethral diverticula and other conditions that might lead to specific therapies. How selectively urodynamics should be used in the work-up of IC/BPS remains controversial among experts [20, 21].

Urodynamic studies comparing IC/BPS patient to normal patients have found that IC/BPS patients have a first desire to void at a significantly lower volume and tolerated a lower maximal cystometric capacity [22]. Patients described bladder filling as painful. In several studies, the average first sensation was around 100 ± 50 ml and maximal cystometric capacity was found to be around 200 ± 100 ml [22–25]. The presence of Hunner's ulcers is associated with increased bladder sensation and reduced cystometric capacity [24, 25]. As noted previously, bladder sensation measurements on urodynamics, however, are not necessary for diagnosis or management of IC/PBS; there is no evidence that measuring volumes on an urodynamic study is additive to assessing bladder function with a bladder diary.

Patients diagnosed with other pelvic pain syndromes may also exhibit increased bladder sensation. A study of men with chronic prostatitis or prostadynia without evidence of prostatic infection found that over 60 % of patients have low volume at first sensation (<150 ml) and first desire to void (300 ml) [26].

Infection

Infection is known to affect bladder sensation in the acute setting and even after the infection has resolved. A study comparing sensation during cystometry in non-neurologic patients with normal urine culture and those with positive urine culture but no symptoms of cystitis found that the infected group had a significantly lower volume of first and strong desires without detrusor overactivity [27]. There is also evidence that repeated infections may produce a persistent hypersensitivity in the bladder. Arya and colleagues performed a case–control study comparing filling cystometry data from women with a history of recurrent urinary tract infections (defined as three or more culture documented urinary tract infections in the previous 12 months) to women with stress urinary incontinence but no history of urinary tract infections [28]. Cystometry was obtained over a month after the last documented urinary tract infection in the women with a history of recurrent urinary tract infections. The investigators found significantly lower volumes for strong desires to void and maximal cystometric capacity, without evidence of detrusor overactivity, in the women with recurrent urinary tract infections.

Sensory Neurogenic Bladder Disorders

Neurogenic bladder disorders may arise from spinal cord injury, myelodysplasia, cerebrovascular accidents, multiple sclerosis, and localized peripheral nerve injuries, as well as many other neurologic diseases and conditions. Many of these patients have impaired sensation—diminished, altered, or absence of first sensation, first desire to void, and/or strong desire to void. Understanding the abnormality of sensation can be just as important as understanding the motor abnormality in developing a treatment plan for patients with neurogenic bladder.

In a study of neuropathic (majority with spinal cord injuries and myelodysplasia) and non-neuropathic patients, 71 % of neuropathic patients had impaired sensation as compared to 30 % of non-neuropathic patients [12]. Forty percent of neuropathic patients had absent sensation compared to 3 % of non-neuropathic patients. Of non-neuropathic patients who had two or more absent sensations, on further neurologic testing, about a third of the patients were discovered to have a neuropathology, including diabetic polyneuropathy, multiple sclerosis, and peripheral neuropathy after multiple pelvic surgery. Neurogenic bladder patients who have impaired bladder sensation along with detrusor overactivity need to be monitored particularly closely to avoid development of upper tract complications (Tracing 1).

Diabetic Cystopathy

Diabetic cystopathy has been classically defined as a peripheral and autonomic neuropathy that first affects sensory afferent pathways causing insidious onset of impaired bladder sensation that leads to a gradual increase in the time interval between voiding [29]. The loss of bladder sensation parallels a loss of peripheral sensation in the hands and feet. This may progress to bladder distension and, ultimately, decompensation. The typical urodynamic findings include impaired bladder sensation, increased compliance, and increased cystometric capacity. If untreated this can produce a secondary myogenic injury and urinary retention.

The most common form of lower urinary tract dysfunction in patients with diabetes, however, is not "classic" diabetic cystopathy but detrusor overactivity [29]. The pathophysiology of detrusor overactivity in diabetes is not fully elucidated. The underlying mechanism could also include impairment of bladder sensation, similar to "classic" diabetic cystopathy. We observe that such patients often lack early sensations during urodynamic studies and have sudden low volume urgency, detrusor overactivity, and urge incontinence. One might hypothesize normal bladder sensation is required to suppress the micro-instabilities of the bladder and prevent them from becoming urodynamically detectable involuntary detrusor contractions.

A retrospective review of video urodynamics results from patients with diabetes and persistent lower urinary tract symptoms and urinary incontinence found the first sensation of filling to occur on average around 300 ml and the mean bladder capacity to be almost 500 ml [30]. Twenty-six percent of patients in this study had documented peripheral neuropathy. Another study of diabetic patients with lower urinary tract symptoms found that first sensation occurred at >250 ml in 21 % of patients and maximal cystometric capacity of >600 ml in 25 % of patients [31].

Idiopathic Overactive Bladder

The ICS defines idiopathic OAB as a syndrome of urgency, with or without urge incontinence, usually with frequency and nocturia. Although urodynamic studies have typically been used in OAB patients to determine the presence or absence of detrusor overactivity there may also be alterations in bladder sensation in OAB. There appears to be a mixed population including patients with normal, decreased, and increased sensation.

A number of published reports have shown that detrusor overactivity is demonstrable in 50–75 % of patients with OAB [17]. A study comparing perceptions of bladder fullness in patients with detrusor overactivity and those without found that those with detrusor overactivity experienced sensations of fullness at significantly lower volumes [32]. One hypothesis is that these patients have normal bladder sensation and that the urgency they experience at low bladder volumes is the result of a normal response to involuntary detrusor contractions (Tracing 2). Neuromodulation by afferent stimulation of the pudendal nerve in patients with idiopathic OAB has been shown to result in elimination or delay of involuntary detrusor contractions along with an increased volume at which different levels of urgency are sensed during urodynamics [4].

There is a small portion of OAB patients who do not sense or only minimally sense involuntary detrusor contractions. In one study 3 % of neurologically intact patients were not aware of involuntary detrusor contractions on urodynamics [33]. Such patients may be more prone to leakage because the inability to sense involuntary detrusor contractions precludes an adequate voluntary or reflexive contraction of the pelvic floor in response (Tracing 3).

As previously stated, while urgency in patients with OAB is usually associated with involuntary detrusor contractions, there is evidence that at least 25–50 % of patients who experience urgency with filling do not have involuntary detrusor contractions on office urodynamics [17, 34]. These patients may have increased bladder sensation if involuntary detrusor contractions are truly absent. Another possibility is that involuntary detrusor contractions are present but not detected by office urodynamics. In a prospective randomized crossover study of 106 women with OAB with or without incontinence, office videourodynamics detected involuntary detrusor contractions in 66 % of patients [34]. Of the women without detrusor overactivity on office urodynamics, 59.5 % of these patients had detrusor overactivity on ambulatory monitoring. In 45 % of patients with detrusor overactivity on ambulatory monitoring only, the detrusor activity resulted in incontinence. One may hypothesize that in this last group, decreased bladder sensation may explain their inability to abort involuntary bladder contractions through recruitment of the pelvic floor musculature before leakage occurs (Tracing 4).

Idiopathic overactive bladder represents a complex heterogeneous population in terms of disorders of bladder sensation. Normal versus decreased bladder sensation may be part of what differentiates between patients with OAB dry and OAB wet.

Insensate Incontinence

True insensate incontinence is often secondary to neuropathies and cognitive disorders [35]. Imaging studies in healthy volunteers show that frontal lobes and various midbrain structures are important in the conscious recognition of afferent bladder signals [36]. Insensate incontinence has been most commonly studied in the elderly. Research in the elderly has found that those with urge incontinence and reduced sensation have the greatest cognitive impairment and brain scans have shown significantly poor global cortical perfusion. Such patients should still have a basic

Table 13.3 Evaluation of patient with complaints of insensate incontinence

Does patient have cognitive impairment or neuropathy?	Yes	No
Differential	• Consider true insensate incontinence	• Bladder outlet obstruction • Fistula • Functional incontinence • Post-void dribbling • Urethral diverticulum • Vaginal voiding
Work-up	• History and exam to rule out reversible causes of UI (DIAPPERS) – *Delirium* – *Infection* – *Atrophic vaginitis* – *Pharmaceuticals* – *Psychologic disorders* – *Excessive urine output* – *Restricted mobility* – *Stool impaction* • UA—rule out infection • PVR—rule out overflow	• History and exam • UA • PVR • Bladder diary with pyridium • Further studies pending results of bladder diary
Treatment	• Timed voiding for neuropathies • Prompted voiding for cognitive impairment	• Based on etiology

work-up to rule out reversible causes of incontinence including infection, impaction, etc. When no reversible cause is identified the treatment is usually based on timed and prompted voiding (Table 13.3).

In practice, clinicians often encounter in the office cognitively intact patients without any neurologic disorders who report symptomatic incontinence without any associated sensation. The differential in these patients should include functional incontinence, overflow from obstruction, post-void dribbling, vaginal voiding, and fistulas. The diagnosis can often be made with the history and physical exam alone. When this history is not clear and continuous leakage is not identified on exam the most helpful test to elucidate the problem in this situation, however, is not urodynamics but a home bladder diary. Patients are prescribed pyridium, which will help the patient verify urinary leakage and determine exactly when it is occurring. They can correlate the leakage with the detailed record of timing and activities surrounding incontinence episodes.

Summary

Adequate bladder sensation is important for normal bladder function. Important disorders of bladder sensation exist including IC/PBS and neurogenic bladder. Obtaining objective, reproducible measurements of bladder sensation on urodynamic studies is challenging and the clinical significance of this information is often unclear.

The key points on this topic include:

- Normal bladder function is evaluated at three points during fill cystometry: (1) First sensation of filling (2) First desire to void. (3) Strong desire to void. These points were defined by the ICS based on expert opinion.
- Because bladder sensation is subjective, it requires a dialogue between an attentive clinician and an alert, mentally competent patient.
- Due to the variability in the way clinicians elicit information regarding bladder sensation and how patients interpret these questions, results can be difficult to reproduce across laboratories and among patients.
- Studies in normal subjects show that volumes at which each sensation occurs at a fairly constant percentage of total bladder volume. First sensation of bladder filling occurs at an average of 40 % of maximal cystometric capacity while strong desire to void occurs at an average 70 % of maximal cystometric capacity.
- Neurogenic bladder patients who have impaired bladder sensation along with detrusor overactivity need to be monitored particularly closely to avoid development of upper tract complications.

Our major knowledge deficits include:

- How do we make measurements of bladder sensation more standardized and reproducible?
- What should the role of urodynamic studies be in the diagnosis and management of IC/BPS?
- Does idiopathic OAB include a mixed population in terms of bladder sensation—normal, increase, versus decreased?
- What is the role of bladder sensation in detrusor overactivity and urgency urinary incontinence?

References

1. Wyndaele J, De Wachter S. The sensory bladder (1): an update on the different sensations described in the lower urinary tract and the physiological mechanisms behind them. Neurourol Urodyn. 2008;27(4):274–8.
2. Abrams P, Cardozo L, Fall M, Griffiths D, Rosier P, Ulmsten U, et al. The standardisation of terminology of lower urinary tract function: report from the Standardisation Sub-committee of the International Continence Society. Neurourol Urodyn. 2002;21(2):167–78.
3. Nitti VW. Urodynamic and video-urodynamic evaluation of the lower urinary tract. In: Wein AJ, Kavoussi LR, Novick AC, Partin AW, Peters CA, editors. Campbell-Walsh urology. 10th ed. Philadelphia: Elsevier Saunders; 2011. p. 1847.
4. Oliver S, Fowler C, Mundy A, Craggs M. Measuring the sensations of urge and bladder filling during cystometry in urge incontinence and the effects of neuromodulation. Neurourol Urodyn. 2003;22(1):7–16.
5. Erdem E, Akbay E, Doruk E, Cayan S, Acar D, Ulusoy E. How reliable are bladder perceptions during cystometry? Neurourol Urodyn. 2004;23(4):306–9. discussion 10.
6. Erdem E, Tunckiran A, Acar D, Kanik EA, Akbay E, Ulusoy E. Is catheter cause of subjectivity in sensations perceived during filling cystometry? Urology. 2005;66(5):1000–3. discussion 1003–4.

7. Erdem E, Ulger S, Kanik AE. Comparison of bladder perceptions during cystometry in pediatric and adult patients. Urology. 2009;73(1):79–82.
8. Wyndaele JJ, Wachter SD. Cystometrical sensory data from a normal population: comparison of two groups of young healthy volunteers examined with 5 years interval. Eur Urol. 2002;42(1):34–8.
9. Robertson AS. Behaviour of the human bladder during natural filling: the Newcastle experience of ambulatory monitoring and conventional artificial filling cystometry. Scand J Urol Nephrol Suppl. 1999;201:19–24.
10. Sorensen SS, Nielsen JB, Norgaard JP, Knudsen LM, Djurhuus JC. Changes in bladder volumes with repetition of water cystometry. Urol Res. 1984;12(4):205–8.
11. Wyndaele JJ. The normal pattern of perception of bladder filling during cystometry studied in 38 young healthy volunteers. J Urol. 1998;160(2):479–81.
12. Wyndaele JJ. Is impaired perception of bladder filling during cystometry a sign of neuropathy? Br J Urol. 1993;71(3):270–3.
13. Tammela TL, Hellstrom PA, Kontturi MJ. Cold sensation and bladder instability in patients with outflow obstruction due to benign prostatic hyperplasia. Br J Urol. 1992;70(4):404–7.
14. Hellstrom PA, Tammela TL, Kontturi MJ, Lukkarinen OA. The bladder cooling test for urodynamic assessment: analysis of 400 examinations. Br J Urol. 1991;67(3):275–9.
15. Hanno PM, Burks DA, Clemens JQ, Dmochowski RR, Erickson D, FitzGerald MP, et al. AUA guideline for the diagnosis and treatment of interstitial cystitis/bladder pain syndrome. J Urol. 2011;185(6):2162–70.
16. Leiby BE, Landis JR, Propert KJ, Tomaszewski JE, Interstitial Cystitis Data Base Study Group. Discovery of morphological subgroups that correlate with severity of symptoms in interstitial cystitis: a proposed biopsy classification system. J Urol. 2007;177(1):142–8.
17. Elliott CS, Payne CK. Interstitial cystitis and the overlap with overactive bladder. Curr Urol Rep. 2012;13(5):319–26.
18. Clemens JQ, Bogart LM, Liu K, Pham C, Suttorp M, Berry SH. Perceptions of "urgency" in women with interstitial cystitis/bladder pain syndrome or overactive bladder. Neurourol Urodyn. 2011;30(3):402–5.
19. Greenberg P, Brown J, Yates T, Brown V, Langenberg P, Warren JW. Voiding urges perceived by patients with interstitial cystitis/painful bladder syndrome. Neurourol Urodyn. 2008;27(4): 287–90.
20. Blaivas JG. Urodynamics for the evaluation of painful bladder syndrome/interstitial cystitis. J Urol. 2010;184(1):16–7.
21. Payne C. Urodynamics for the evaluation of painful bladder syndrome/interstitial cystitis. J Urol. 2010;184(1):15–6.
22. Ness TJ, Powell-Boone T, Cannon R, Lloyd LK, Fillingim RB. Psychophysical evidence of hypersensitivity in subjects with interstitial cystitis. J Urol. 2005;173(6):1983–7.
23. Teichman JM, Nielsen-Omeis BJ, McIver BD. Modified urodynamics for interstitial cystitis. Tech Urol. 1997;3(2):65–8.
24. Nigro DA, Wein AJ, Foy M, Parsons CL, Williams M, Nyberg Jr LM, et al. Associations among cystoscopic and urodynamic findings for women enrolled in the Interstitial Cystitis Data Base (ICDB) study. Urology. 1997;49(5A Suppl):86–92.
25. Kuo HC. Urodynamic results of intravesical heparin therapy for women with frequency urgency syndrome and interstitial cystitis. J Formos Med Assoc. 2001;100(5):309–14.
26. Theodorou C, Konidaris D, Moutzouris G, Becopoulos T. The urodynamic profile of prostatodynia. BJU Int. 1999;84(4):461–3.
27. Wyndaele JJ. A clinical study of subjective sensations during bladder filling. Int Urogynecol J. 1991;2(4):215.
28. Arya LA, Northington GM, Asfaw T, Harvie H, Malykhina A. Evidence of bladder oversensitivity in the absence of an infection in premenopausal women with a history of recurrent urinary tract infections. BJU Int. 2012;110(2):247–51.
29. Wein AJ, Dmochowski RR. Neuromuscular dysfunction of the lower urinary tract. In: Campbell MF, Kavoussi LR, Novick AC, Partin AW, Peters CA, Walsh PC, et al., editors. MD consult 2012. Campbell-Walsh urology. 10th ed. Philadelphia: Elsevier Saunders; 2012. p. 1909–46.

30. Kaplan SA, Te AE, Blaivas JG. Urodynamic findings in patients with diabetic cystopathy. J Urol. 1995;153(2):342–4.
31. Bansal R, Agarwal MM, Modi M, Mandal AK, Singh SK. Urodynamic profile of diabetic patients with lower urinary tract symptoms: association of diabetic cystopathy with autonomic and peripheral neuropathy. Urology. 2011;77(3):699–705.
32. Wyndaele JJ. Is the lower urinary tract sensation different in patients with bladder instability? Prog Urol. 1992;2(2):220–5.
33. Romanzi LJ, Groutz A, Heritz DM, Blaivas JG. Involuntary detrusor contractions: correlation of urodynamic data to clinical categories. Neurourol Urodyn. 2001;20(3):249–57.
34. Radley SC, Rosario DJ, Chapple CR, Farkas AG. Conventional and ambulatory urodynamic findings in women with symptoms suggestive of bladder overactivity. J Urol. 2001;166(6): 2253–8.
35. Griffiths DJ, McCracken PN, Harrison GM, Gormley EA, Moore K, Hooper R, et al. Cerebral aetiology of urinary urge incontinence in elderly people. Age Ageing. 1994;23(3):246–50.
36. Pettersen R, Stein R, Wyller TB. Post-stroke urinary incontinence with impaired awareness of the need to void: clinical and urodynamic features. BJU Int. 2007;99(5):1073–7.

Chapter 14
Bladder Filling and Storage: "(Involuntary) Contractions"

Chong Choe and Kathleen C. Kobashi

Urodynamics (UDS) is the dynamic study of the storage and evacuation of urine. Its role is to provide the clinician with information about a patient's lower urinary tract function. Ideally, the patient's symptoms are reproduced during the study to provide objective measurements which correlate with the patient's symptoms. UDS should be considered as an adjunct to a detailed history and physical exam to better characterize the clinical picture and facilitate optimal treatment planning. An important portion of the UDS is the bladder filling and storage phase. Involuntary detrusor contractions (IDCs) may occur during this portion of the study and may provide insight into the pathophysiology of the patient's complaints. This chapter will focus on the different UDS manifestations of IDCs by investigating the UDS tracings of neurogenic and idiopathic detrusor overactivity, stress-induced overactivity, phasic overactivity, detrusor overactivity incontinence, detrusor after-contractions (DAC), and terminal detrusor overactivity.

The International Urogynecological Association (IUGA)/International Continence Society (ICS) joint report on the terminology for female pelvic floor dysfunction was published in 2010 [1]. It contains terminology for common urodynamic terms and observations and it is recommended that clinicians performing UDS consider using the current IUGA/ICS terminology in order to maintain consistency. It defines *detrusor overactivity (DO)* as the *"occurrence of involuntary detrusor contractions during filling cystometry. These contractions, which may be spontaneous or provoked, produce a wave form on the cystometrogram of variable duration and amplitude."* (see Fig. 14.1a) *Urgency* (urinary) is defined as the *"complaint of a sudden, compelling desire to pass urine which is difficult to defer."* It is important to note that urgency is a symptom and may or may not be represented by

C. Choe, MD (✉) • K.C. Kobashi, MD
Division of Urology and Renal Transplantation, Department of Urology, Virginia Mason
Medical Center, C7-Uro, 1100 9th Ave, Seattle, WA 98101, USA
e-mail: Jaychong.choe@vmmc.org

© Springer Science+Business Media New York 2015
E.S. Rovner, M.E. Koski (eds.), *Rapid and Practical Interpretation of Urodynamics*, DOI 10.1007/978-1-4939-1764-8_14

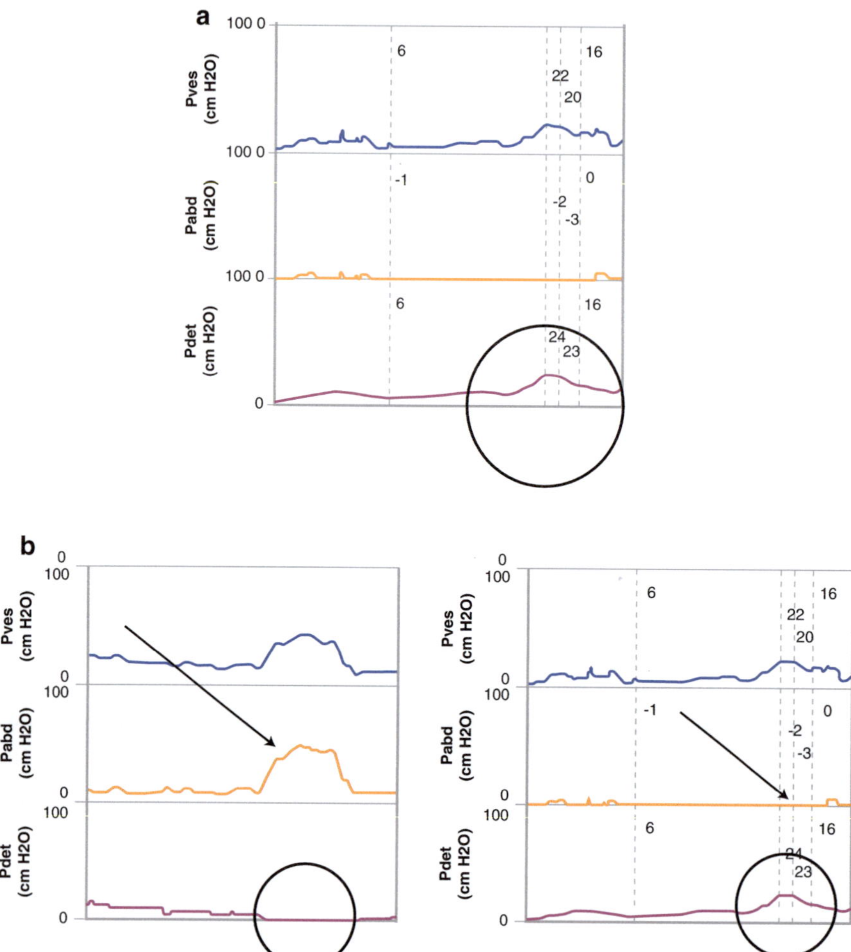

Fig. 14.1 (**a**) This is an example of detrusor overactivity (highlighted by the *circle*) during the filling cystometrogram. The P_{det} tracing is calculated using P_{ves} and P_{abd} values as explained in (**b**). (**b**) Using the equation $\mathbf{P_{det} = P_{ves} - P_{abd}}$, the calculated P_{det} (*circled*) in the figure on the left is zero since the rise in P_{ves} is associated with a rise in P_{abd} (highlighted by the *arrow*). This can be seen, as in this case, due to a Valsalva maneuver which causes a slow controlled rise in the P_{abd} and P_{ves} tracings for the duration of the maneuver. Conversely, the calculated P_{det} (*circled*) in the figure on the right represents a true increase in detrusor pressure since the rise in P_{ves} is not associated with a rise in P_{abd} (highlighted by the *arrow*). In other words, the increase in P_{det} is independent of any intraabdominal pressure activity.

findings of DO on UDS. In fact, it is well established that up to 50 % of patients with urgency incontinence do not demonstrate DO on UDS tracings [2].

Vesical pressure (P_{ves}) is the *measured* pressure inside the bladder. It is measured with a pressure transducer catheter placed into the bladder. Abdominal pressure (P_{abd}) is the *measured* pressure inside the abdomen. It is usually measured with a pressure transducer catheter placed into the rectum. Detrusor pressure (P_{det}) is a *calculated* value of the difference between P_{ves} and P_{abd} such that $\mathbf{P_{det} = P_{ves} - P_{abd}}$ (Fig. 14.1b). P_{det}, though a completely derived number, represents the true value of the pressure generated by the bladder and is distinguished from changes in the pressure tracings due to increased abdominal pressure such as that seen with coughing or straining. From a clinical perspective, evaluating the value of P_{det} is important, as documented by McGuire, due to the potentially deleterious effects on the upper tracts when the detrusor pressure (P_{det}) during filling or voiding is sustained above 40 cm H_2O [3].

The normal micturition cycle involves passive low-pressure filling of the bladder and a coordinated detrusor contraction coupled with urinary sphincter relaxation for the evacuation of urine. A normally functioning bladder stores urine at low pressures as a result of the bladder's viscoelastic properties and compliance. Filling cystometry provides information regarding bladder sensation, bladder capacity, detrusor activity, and bladder compliance. In addition, it is during this phase of the urodynamic study that the bladder outlet can be assessed for weakness (stress urinary incontinence). The two phases of UDS include the filling/storage phase and voiding phase (Fig. 14.2). Detrusor activity is normal during the voiding phase as the bladder contracts to expel urine. Detrusor activity should not be present during the filling and/or the storage phases and when seen is considered involuntary and is referred to as DO. DO can occur spontaneously or as a result of provocation. Provocative maneuvers such as coughing (Fig. 14.3) and Valsalva maneuvers are performed during the storage phase to assess for SUI. These provocative maneuvers can also provoke DO in a phenomenon described as stress-induced DO which will be covered later in the chapter.

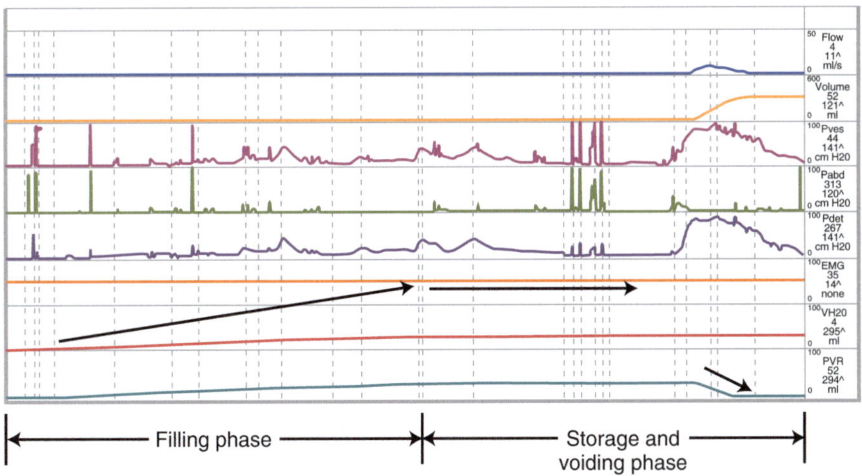

Fig. 14.2 The *filling phase* is indicated by the steady increase in volume in the bladder as it is being filled. The storage phase can be identified by a stable volume in the bladder. The voiding phase begins when the patient is given permission to void. Note that in this instance, the patient is able to void successfully. There is an increase in flow with a concomitant decrease in the post void residual (PVR) volume

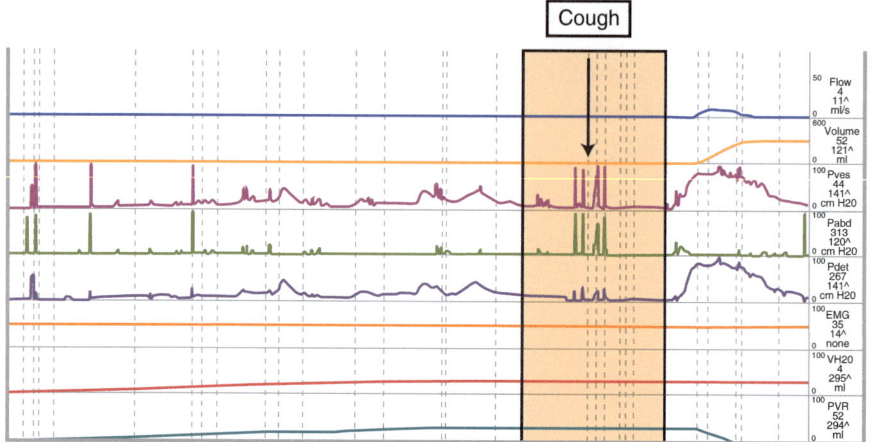

Fig. 14.3 Provocative maneuvers such as coughing (indicated by the arrow) result in increases in P_{ves} and P_{abd}. The P_{det} value is the calculated value determined by the difference in the measured P_{ves} and P_{abd} such that $\mathbf{P_{det} = P_{ves} - P_{abd}}$. In the case of a cough, P_{det} is negligible as there is no pressure coming from the detrusor itself. Acute increases in the P_{det} lead during provocative maneuvers such as coughing represent artifact and should not be misinterpreted as detrusor overactivity

The smooth muscle fibers of the bladder can exhibit spontaneous action potentials, a phenomenon thought to be the cause of phasic detrusor activity [4]. According to the 2002 ICS standardization of terminology [5], *phasic detrusor overactivity (PDO)* is defined as *a characteristic waveform, and may or may not lead to urinary incontinence.* Although the contour of the characteristic waveform is not specified, as the name suggests one would expect cyclical increases and decreases in the P_{det} tracing (Fig. 14.4).

Neurogenic detrusor overactivity (NDO) replaces the old terminology "detrusor hyperreflexia" and is defined as DO in a patient with a neurologic condition (Fig. 14.5) [1].

Idiopathic detrusor overactivity (IDO) (Fig. 14.6) replaces the old term "detrusor instability" and is the term used when there is no identifiable neurological cause for the DO. It is important to note that NDO and IDO may look identical on UDS. These terms are strictly defined by the patient's neurologic status and not by the presence of IDCs on the UDS tracings.

A causative relationship between SUI and DO has been suspected but never confirmed. Hindmarsh et al. proposed that proximal urethral underactivity with falls in the urethral closure pressure below 30 cm H_2O was often associated with DO. They suggested that DO may originate from stimuli to the bladder outlet [6]. Jung et al. measured the urethral perfusion pressure and isovolumetric bladder pressure in the anesthetized rat and concluded that the activation of urethral afferents by urethral perfusion can modulate the micturition reflex. They further speculated

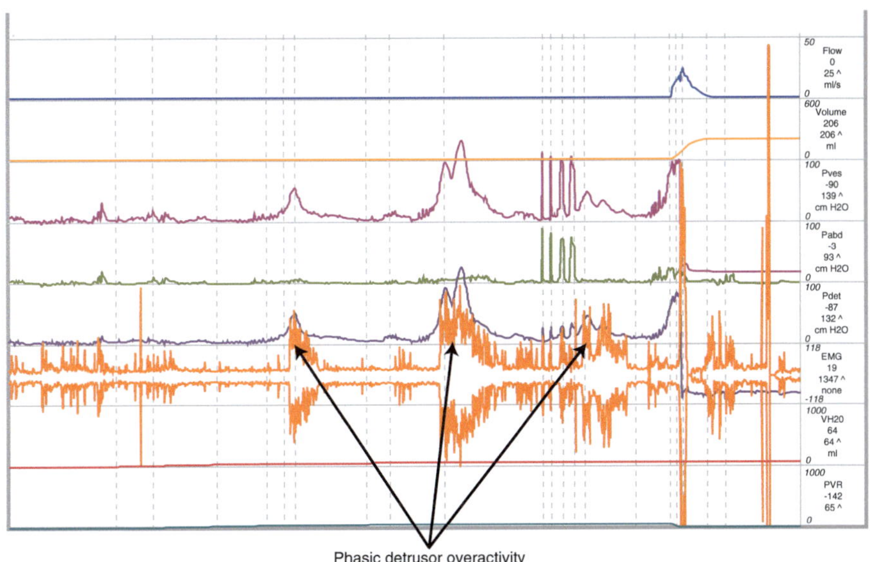

Fig. 14.4 This UDS demonstrates the "waveforms" in the P_{det} tracing with phasic DO. There is no standardization regarding the characteristics of the "waveform," but is generally recognized as cyclical increases and decreases in P_{det}. Note that the P_{abd} is silent suggesting that the increases in P_{det} are due to contractions arising in the bladder

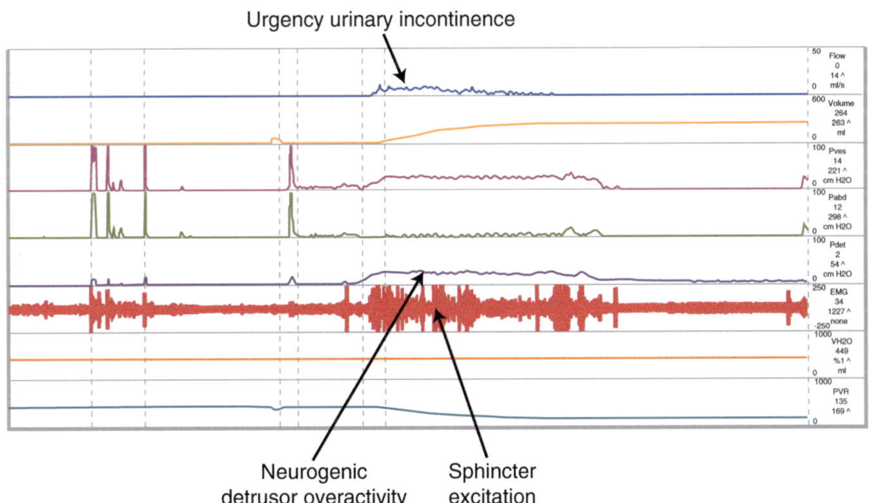

Fig. 14.5 This patient, who is recovering from a cerebral vascular accident, has NDO during the *storage phase* with associated UUI. It is important to highlight that the NDO occurred during the *storage phase* and not during the voiding phase. The compensatory EMG recruitment could be erroneously labeled as detrusor sphincter dyssynergia (DSD) which may occur during the *voiding phase* in patients with neurologic pathology

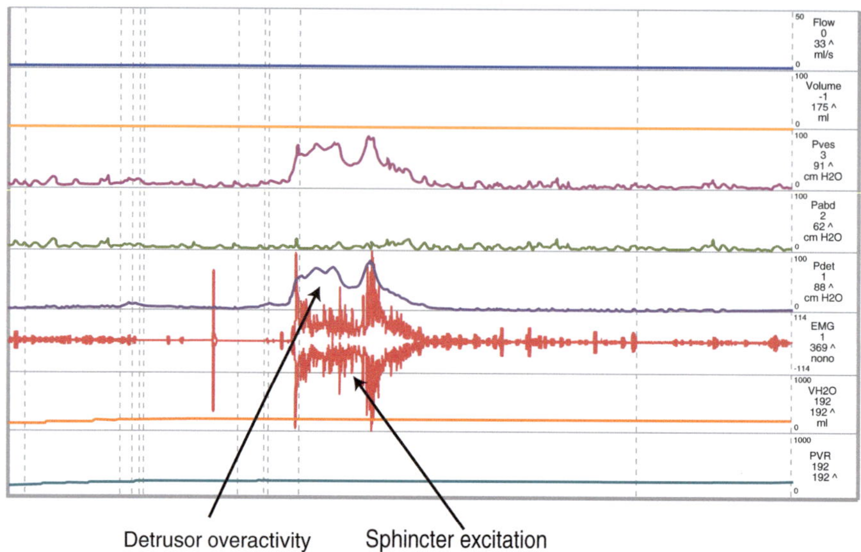

Fig. 14.6 This patient has no known neurologic disease. The detrusor overactivity is therefore referred to as idiopathic detrusor overactivity (IDO). It is important to reiterate that NDO and IDO P_{det} tracings can appear identical. The only difference between NDO and IDO is the patient's history of an associated neurologic disease. Conversely, if a patient is described as having NDO, it is implicit that he/she has an underlying neurologic disease. Again, note the compensatory EMG recruitment to prevent UUI

that the theoretical urethral-detrusor facilitative reflex or "stress-induced DO" could be a result of an incompetent bladder neck which allowed urine to reach the proximal urethra [7–9]. Interestingly, some women with mixed urinary incontinence (MUI) have resolution of urgency following surgical correction of SUI while other women may conversely develop de novo urgency after anti-incontinence surgery [10]. Unfortunately, current diagnostic methodology does not provide the means to accurately determine which patients with MUI would be best served with initial management of their SUI versus treatment of their urgency symptoms. SUI and DO can also potentially coexist as independent mechanisms which may explain the contradictory results reported in the literature evaluating the effects of pharmacotherapy and/or surgery in women with MUI. Although defining the predominant subjective component is important in the assessment of women with MUI, symptom analysis may not always be the most accurate diagnostic tool. The findings of stress-induced DO (Fig. 14.7) may help the clinician to better understand the patient's picture and ultimately guide the patient and the clinician in their discussions regarding treatment.

There are two measureable leak point pressures according to the IUGA/ICS joint report on urodynamic terminology are the *detrusor leak point pressure (DLPP)* and *abdominal leak point pressure (ALPP)*. DLPP is defined as *the lowest detrusor*

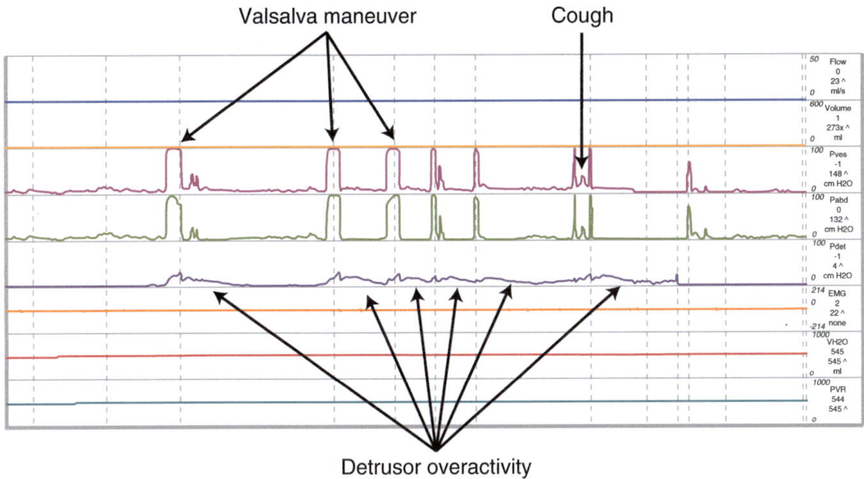

Fig. 14.7 Stress-induced DO occurs following episodes of provocative maneuvers (Valsalva and cough)

pressure at which leakage is observed in the absence of increased abdominal pressure or a detrusor contraction. ALPP is defined as the *lowest value of intentionally increased intravesical pressure (P_{ves}) that provokes urinary leakage in the absence of a detrusor contraction.* ALPP can be elicited during coughing (cough LPP) or Valsalva maneuver (Valsalva LPP). A group recently investigated incontinence that occurred with DO (Fig. 14.8), the pressure at which leakage occurred, and its possible association with subjective severity of urgency and UUI. They noted that subjective symptom severity and bother from urgency and UUI measured by validated questionnaires were greater in patients with urodynamic evidence of DO incontinence than those with urgency incontinence without DO [11]. They also found that patients with subjective MUI (UUI+SUI) leaked at a lower mean detrusor pressure than those who had pure UUI (19.6 cm H_2O vs 31.2 cm H_2O, respectively, $p=0.004$). The clinical relevance of the detrusor pressure at which patients leak with UUI remains undefined.

Terminal DO (TDO) is defined as *a single involuntary detrusor contraction occurring at cystometric capacity that cannot be suppressed and results in incontinence usually resulting in bladder emptying (voiding).* Investigators from France evaluated the demographics, urodynamic findings, and sphincter behavior in 166 women with a diagnosis of DO. They found that the incidence of PDO (Fig. 14.9) and TDO (Fig. 14.10) was similar at 46.9 and 53.1 % respectively. The PDO group were younger (52±19) than the TDO group (63±16) ($p=0.0003$), and TDO occurred more frequently than PDO with increase in age ($p=0.006$). The frequency of neurologic disease in the TDO group was high (60.5 %) in the pre and peri-menopausal age groups (45–74 years) and remained elevated in the other age groups (45.8 %) [12]. Other studies support the finding that TDO is related to aging

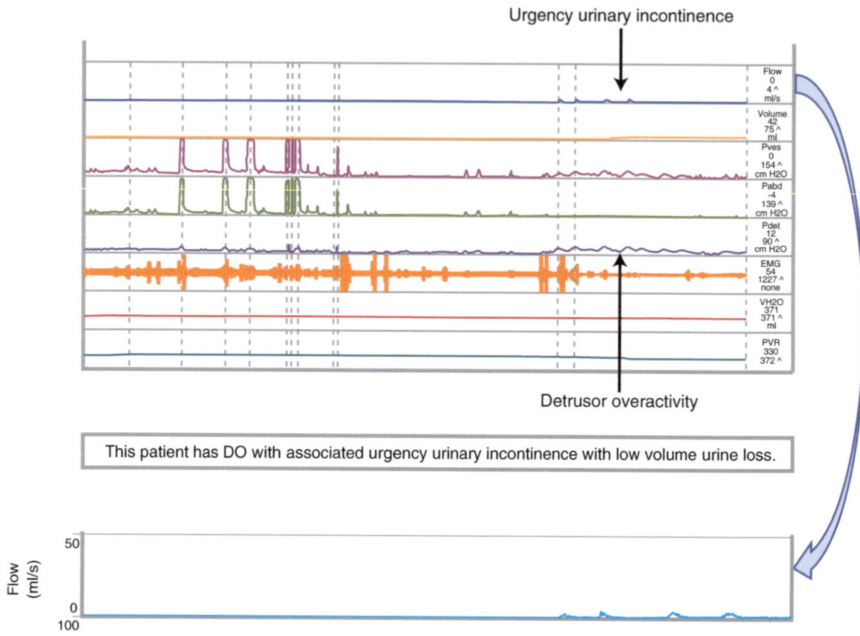

Fig. 14.8 This patient has DO with associated urgency urinary incontinence with low volume urine loss

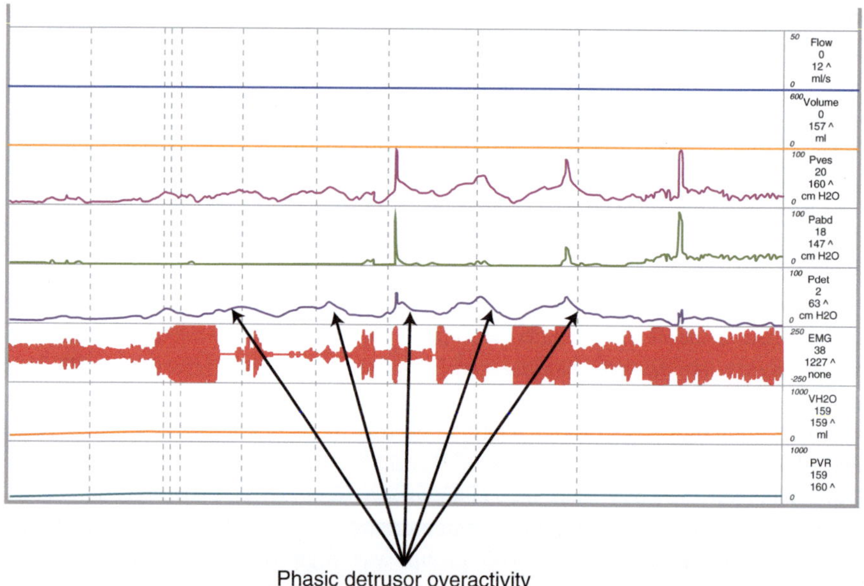

Fig. 14.9 UDS tracing shows phasic DO

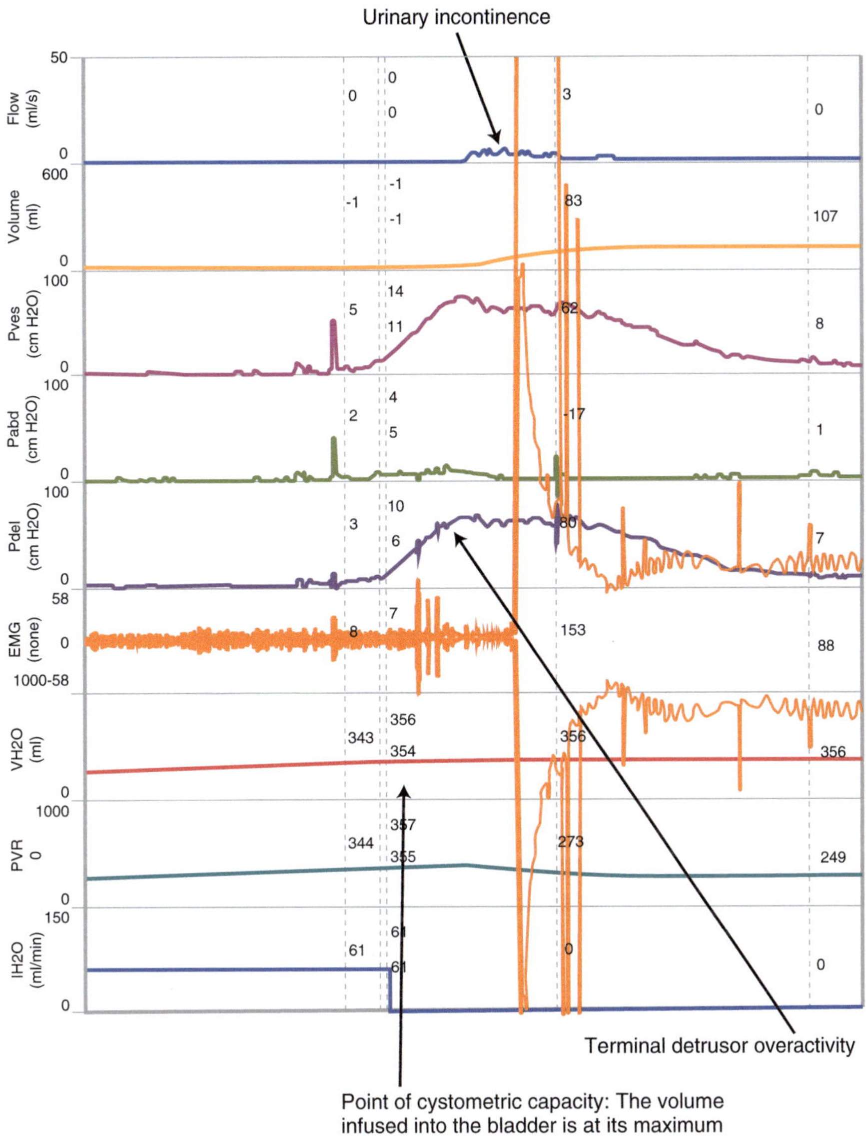

Fig. 14.10 This patient has terminal DO defined as a *single involuntary detrusor contraction occurring at cystometric capacity, which cannot be suppressed, and results in incontinence* [1]

and occurs particularly frequently in elderly patients with neurological conditions such as cerebrovascular accidents (CVA) [13–15].

A sudden increase in detrusor pressure after cessation of voiding and in the absence of flow has been referred to as a detrusor after contraction (DAC). There are various opinions on the causes of DAC. Some believed DAC may be an artifact in the P_{det} measurement when the sensor directly contacts the bladder wall [16]. Others performed cystometric evaluations using three pressure transducers (two microtip transducers and one external fluid-filled pressure transducer) and observed that in 50 % of the recordings of DAC, the increase in P_{det} was present in all three transducers [17]. Consequently, they concluded DAC was a true detrusor contraction. A different interpretation of DAC was proposed by Vereecken and colleagues. They noted that in 59 of 65 patients with DAC, the DAC was preceded by a contraction of the anal or urethral sphincter seen as a burst of activity in the EMG. They theorized that DAC developed from the sudden cessation of the outflow of urine either by voluntary or involuntary interruption of the urethral sphincter causing an acute rise in the P_{det} [18]. Although this urodynamic observation is not new and was first reported back in the early 1930s [19], only a few studies have been published which focus on DAC over the past 60 years. To date, no conclusive explanation of its significance or clinical importance has been established.

The goal of UDS is to reproduce the patient's symptoms and to determine the potential cause of these symptoms by urodynamic measurements or observations. In this chapter of "bladder filling and storage; (involuntary) contractions," the goal was to identify IDCs during the filling and storage phases of UDS. Learning to identify the presence of DO during UDS is important. However, its interpretation in the context of the patient's symptoms and condition, for example identifying high storage pressure ($P_{det} > 40$ cm H_2O) and recognizing its deleterious effects on the upper tracts, is far more important in order to better characterize the clinical picture and facilitate optimal treatment planning.

References

1. Haylen BT, et al. An International Urogynecological Association (IUGA)/International Continence Society (ICS) joint report on the terminology for female pelvic floor dysfunction. Neurourol Urodyn. 2010;29(1):4–20.
2. Chaliha C, Khullar V. Mixed incontinence. Urology. 2004;63(3 Suppl 1):51–7.
3. McGuire EJ, et al. Prognostic value of urodynamic testing in myelodysplastic patients. J Urol. 1981;126(2):205–9.
4. Buckner SA, et al. Spontaneous phasic activity of the pig urinary bladder smooth muscle: characteristics and sensitivity to potassium channel modulators. Br J Pharmacol. 2002;135(3): 639–48.
5. Abrams P, et al. The standardisation of terminology of lower urinary tract function: report from the Standardisation Sub-committee of the International Continence Society. Neurourol Urodyn. 2002;21(2):167–78.
6. Hindmarsh JR, Gosling PT, Deane AM. Bladder instability. Is the primary defect in the urethra? Br J Urol. 1983;55(6):648–51.
7. Ostergard DR. The neurological control of micturition and integral voiding reflexes. Obstet Gynecol Surv. 1979;34(6):417–23.
8. Jung SY, et al. Urethral afferent nerve activity affects the micturition reflex; implication for the relationship between stress incontinence and detrusor instability. J Urol. 1999;162(1):204–12.
9. Bump RC, et al. Mixed urinary incontinence symptoms: urodynamic findings, incontinence severity, and treatment response. Obstet Gynecol. 2003;102(1):76–83.

10. Webster GD, Kreder KJ. Voiding dysfunction following cystourethropexy: its evaluation and management. J Urol. 1990;144(3):670–3.
11. Smith AL, et al. Detrusor overactivity leak point pressure in women with urgency incontinence. Int Urogynecol J. 2012;23(4):443–6.
12. Valentini FA, et al. Phasic or terminal detrusor overactivity in women: age, urodynamic findings and sphincter behavior relationships. Int Braz J Urol. 2011;37(6):773–80.
13. Guralnick ML, et al. Objective differences between overactive bladder patients with and without urodynamically proven detrusor overactivity. Int Urogynecol J. 2010;21(3):325–9.
14. Kessler TM, Madersbacher H. [Urodynamic phenomena in the aging bladder]. Urologe A. 2004;43(5):542–6.
15. Geirsson G, Fall M, Lindstrom S. Subtypes of overactive bladder in old age. Age Ageing. 1993;22(2):125–31.
16. Pesce F, Rubilotta E. Detrusor after-contraction: is this important? Curr Urol Rep. 2004;5(5): 353–8.
17. Hoebeke PB, et al. The after-contraction in paediatric urodynamics. Br J Urol. 1996;78(5): 780–2.
18. Vereecken RL. The after-contraction: a true detrusor contraction or a late dyssynergic urethral sphincter contraction? BJU Int. 2000;85(3):246–8.
19. Beattie J. The neurology of micturition. Can Med Assoc J. 1930;23(1):71–5.

Chapter 15
Bladder Filling and Storage: "Continence: Stress Incontinence"

Anne M. Suskind and J. Quentin Clemens

Introduction

Stress urinary incontinence (SUI) is diagnosed based on the presence of characteristic symptoms and signs. The symptoms of SUI include "the *complaint* of involuntary leakage on effort or exertion, or on sneezing or coughing," while the signs are represented by "the *observation* of involuntary leakage from the urethra, synchronous with exertion/effort, or sneezing or coughing" [1]. The urodynamic definition of SUI is "the finding of involuntary leakage during filling cystometry associated with increased intra-abdominal pressure in the absence of a detrusor contraction" [2].

Studies have demonstrated that urodynamics are not necessary in the evaluation of straightforward SUI, where symptoms and signs are highly correlated [3, 4]. There are; however, many situations where this is not the case, making urodynamics an important and often essential component to the clinical evaluation. Some examples where urodynamics may be helpful include scenarios where the diagnosis of SUI is questionable or where multiple treatment options exist. For example, urodynamics can be useful in differentiating between components of stress and urge urinary incontinence in a woman with vague complaints, leading to different treatment pathways based on the predominant urodynamic diagnosis. Urodynamics can also be used to determine the severity of SUI, potentially yielding important information regarding which treatment option would be optimal.

A.M. Suskind, MD, MS • J.Q. Clemens, MD, FACS, MSCI (✉)
Division of Neurourology and Pelvic Reconstructive Surgery, Department of Urology,
University of Michigan, A. Alfred Taubman Health Care Center,
1500 E. Medical Center Dr., SPC 5330, Ann Arbor, MI 48109, USA
e-mail: suskina@med.umich.edu; qclemens@med.umich.edu

© Springer Science+Business Media New York 2015
E.S. Rovner, M.E. Koski (eds.), *Rapid and Practical Interpretation
of Urodynamics*, DOI 10.1007/978-1-4939-1764-8_15

Assessment of Urethral Function

Before conducting a urodynamic examination for SUI, the clinician must have a good understanding of certain measurements that are used to assess urethral function, as recommended by the American Urological Association's Guidelines on urodynamics [2]. Abdominal leak point pressures (ALPPs) and urethral pressure measurements are used to measure urethral competency in such circumstances and will be discussed in this section.

Abdominal Leak Point Pressure

The ALPP is a dynamic measurement that is used to assess SUI. As defined by the International Continence Society, ALPP is the "intravesical pressure at which urine leakage occurs due to increased abdominal pressure in the absence of a detrusor contraction" [1]. In other words, the ALPP measures the "ability of the urethra to resist abdominal pressures as an expulsive force" [5]. Theoretically, lower ALPPs should correspond to more severe urinary incontinence; however, in practice lower ALPPs do not always correlate with symptom severity or treatment outcome [6]. It is important to record the lowest value of this pressure at the exact moment of leakage in order to get an accurate measurement [7].

The ALPP can either be induced by cough (cough leak point pressure, or CLPP) or by valsalva (valsalva leak point pressure, or VLPP). McGuire originally suggested first measuring VLPP and only measuring CLPP if the VLPP was negative, as CLPP is typically substantially higher [5]. Further studies have shown that CLPP is more sensitive than VLPP in eliciting urinary leakage [8, 9].

Different types of pressures (i.e., Pabd, Pves, Pdet) can be used to measure ALPPs [10, 11]; however the initial description by McGuire, who popularized the ALPP concept, utilized Pves [5]. More important than the type of measurement used is the notion that urodynamics should be performed in a consistent fashion, particularly when repeated measurements are being performed in an individual both over the course of a single study and over time. Furthermore, whichever type of measurement is chosen to assess ALPPs, this measurement should be consistently performed. For the purposes of this chapter, we will define ALPPs using the Pves catheter.

ALPP values can be used to quantify the severity of SUI, and this information can potentially be used to guide treatment selection. In particular, patients with very low ALPP values are often recommended to undergo autologous tissue pubovaginal slings rather than other procedures [12]. Some more recent publications, however, suggest that acceptable outcomes can be obtained with midurethral sling techniques, regardless of ALPP values [6]. In contemporary urologic practice, the utility of ALPP values in guiding patient treatment is largely based on individual practice preferences and experience. The AUA/society of urodynamics, female pelvic medicine and urogenital reconstruction (SUFU) guidelines on adult urodynamics support the use of VLPP to demonstrate urodynamic SUI and state that assessment of urethral function (VLPP/ALPP, CLPP, and MUCP) can be helpful in predicting outcomes with some types of therapy [2].

There are various technical components that can affect the ALPP measurement. Intravesical volume can affect the ALPP measurement if it is either too high or too low. If the volume is too low, the bladder may not leak, whereas if the volume is too high, it may induce an artifactual detrusor contraction that could change the interpretation of the study [5]. ALPPs were first described to be performed at a bladder volume of 150 mL [12], and have since been described at volumes of 200–300 mL [13].

Catheter size is another important consideration in the measurement of ALPP. A transurethral catheter can act to partially occlude the urethral lumen or even prevent leakage all-together, potentially distorting the value of the ALPP [9, 11]. While there is no standard catheter size recommended for urodynamic testing, it is generally agreed that smaller catheters have less occlusive potential and are generally preferred.

Urethral Pressure Measurements

Urethral pressure measurements are used to assess urethral competence and incontinence severity. Defined by Griffiths in 1985, urethral pressure is "the fluid pressure needed to just open a closed (collapsed) urethra" [14]. Historically, these measurements have been unstandardized and fraught with difficulties, making their value unclear [7, 15, 16]. While it is fully accepted that urethral pressure is an important and integral component to urinary continence, it remains challenging to measure and characterize this pressure in a reliable manner [15]. The urethral pressure profile (UPP), maximum urethral pressure (MUP), and maximum urethral closure pressure (MUCP) are sometimes used as part of the urodynamic evaluation for SUI and will be discussed below.

UPP is the graph of intraluminal pressure that is produced when urethral pressure is measured by a catheter along the entire length of the urethra. The maximum urethral pressure reading recorded on this graph is called the MUP, and the maximum difference between the MUP and the intravesical pressure is the MUCP [1], which is the most commonly used measurement of the urethra in current practice. MUCP has been assessed in multiple studies to determine whether or not it can be used to predict success among women undergoing anti-incontinence procedures, with mixed results [17, 18].

Similar to the measurement of ALPP, there are many technical considerations that must be considered when conducting and interpreting urethral pressure measurements. Among them is the catheter that is used to make the measurements. These catheters often have side holes (for fluid infusion) or a side-mounted transducer (for pressure measurements) that change the orientation of the catheter, potentially leading to misleading measurements. For example, a transducer that is facing the pubic symphysis may show a significantly higher MUCP than one facing the vaginal wall [19]. Urethral stiffness can also be problematic when obtaining accurate urethral pressure measurements. This is due to the fact that the urethral catheters do not directly measure urethral pressure, but rather they measure the normal stress component on the surface of the transducer. Stress, furthermore, is affected by the interaction between the urethral tissue and the transducer surface, and can be artificially high in a stiff urethra [15]. For these reasons, catheters should be as thin and flexible as possible.

How to Perform an Urodynamics Evaluation for SUI

Urodynamics should be performed in a thoughtful manner that is technically reproducible. As with any urodynamic study, there should be a clear clinical question that is driving the study. The first consideration for each study should be the position of the patient. In order to evaluate for SUI, the patient is commonly standing (for males) or sitting (for females). It is important to be able to simulate a situation that reproduces the patient's urinary incontinence during the examination, which can potentially be done in either position.

The technical qualities of the urethral catheter are another important consideration when performing urodynamics. Double-lumen catheters are standard equipment for the measurement of intravesical and intraurethral pressure. The double-lumen allows for simultaneous measurement and filling in a fill/void sequence without the need for re-catheterization [20]. The size of the catheter is another important consideration, as there is evidence to believe that flow can be reduced or altered by larger catheters. The International Consultation on Incontinence Committee on "Dynamic Testing" recommends the use of thinner (5–7 F) double-lumen catheters for filling and pressure recording [21].

The bladder should be filled via the bladder catheter to an appropriate volume to assess the ALPP. We recommend starting these provocative maneuvers at a volume of 150 mL and re-testing every 50–100 mL until SUI is elicited. A combination of cough and valsalva can be used to reproduce signs of urinary leakage. Fluoroscopy can be used to capture images during urinary leakage in order to evaluate the bladder neck and urethra.

Once ALPP maneuvers have been completed, the urethral pressure measurements can be performed. Typically they are conducted as the catheter is withdrawn from the bladder and urethra.

Use of Pabd Catheter

In most urodynamics studies both Pabd and Pves catheters are used. There are certain situations; however, when the use of a Pabd catheter may not be necessary. For example, in neurogenic patients the primary focus of the study is often on the filling phase and the use of Pabd adds time and inconvenience for the patient. Therefore, we tend to utilize a selective approach with use of Pabd and focus its use on patients where obtaining a calculated detrusor leak point pressure is a primary question.

Examples

Example 1

Clinical History: Forty-nine-year-old female with a neurogenic bladder has persistent urinary incontinence per urethra after an ileovesicostomy. The patient wears two to three large protective undergarments per day. It is unclear whether the etiology of her urinary incontinence is due to her bladder (detrusor overactivity) or to an incompetent bladder outlet (open bladder neck or intrinsic sphincter deficiency [ISD]) (Figs. 15.1, 15.2, and 15.3).

Commentary on Example 1: This tracing shows SUI with provocative maneuvers at a volume of 132 mL (Fig. 15.1). At this volume, the patient has a VLPP of 44 cm H_2O and a CLPP of 102 cm H_2O (Fig. 15.2). First sensation was noted at 18 mL. During filling, this tracing demonstrates normal compliance. Bladder capacity was 172 mL. There were no involuntary detrusor contractions. Fluoroscopy images showed an open bladder neck, both at rest and during leakage (Fig. 15.3). Contrast was noted to empty via the patient's ileovesicostomy into the collection bag at low pressures (20 cm H_2O).

The impression is that the patient has SUI secondary to ISD.

This study was able to determine the etiology of the patient's urinary incontinence. Due to her open bladder neck, which is a common finding among patients with neurogenic conditions, this condition needs to be addressed surgically. Options to surgically address the urethra include periurethral injection therapy, an occlusive autologous tissue sling, or bladder neck closure.

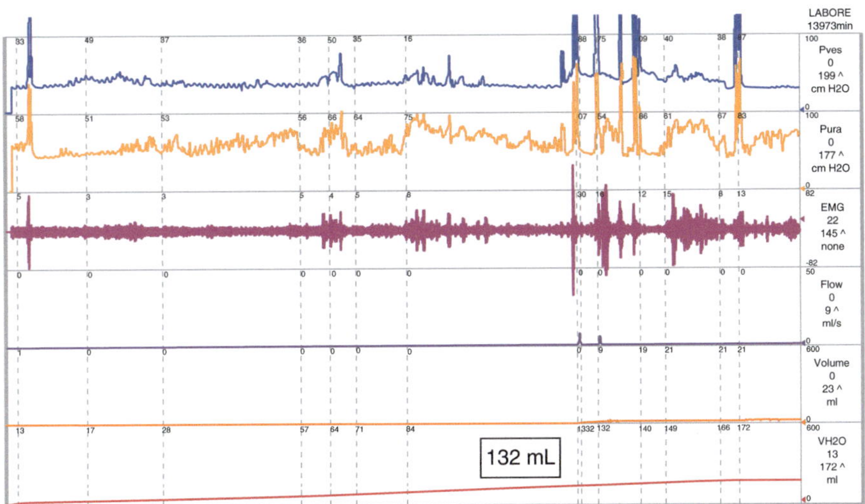

Fig. 15.1 Urodynamics tracing for Example 1

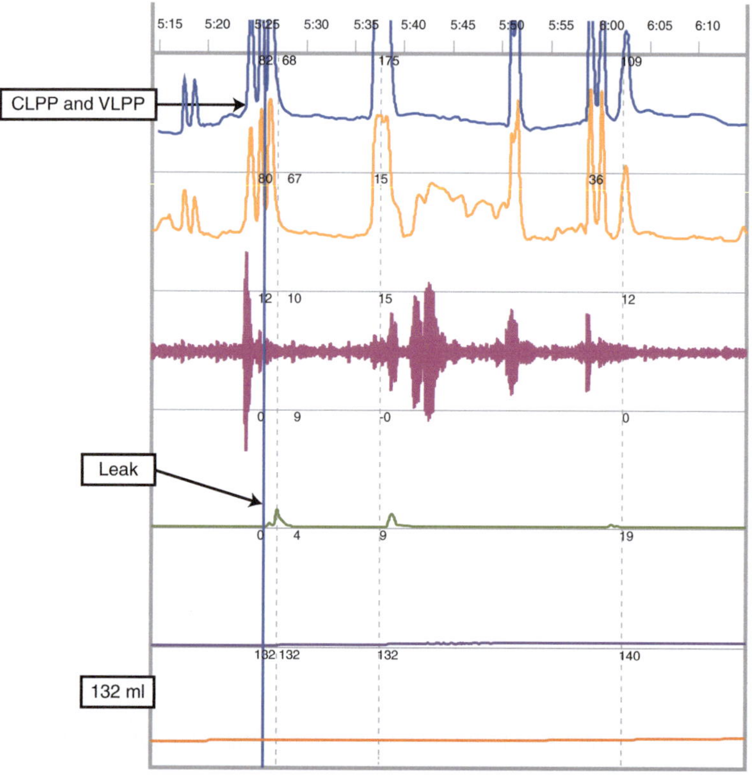

Fig. 15.2 Portion of urodynamics tracing for Example 1 showing SUI

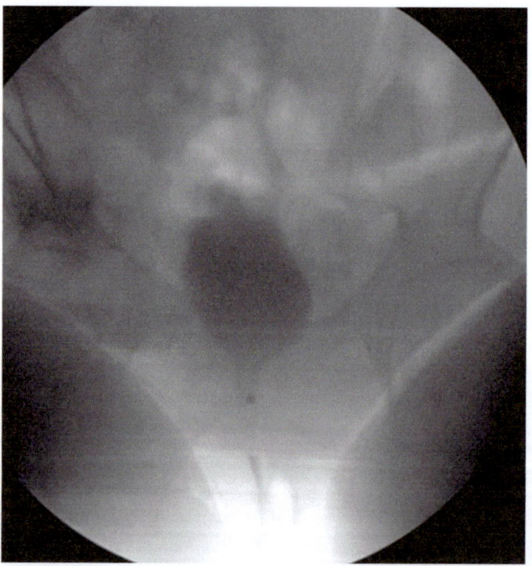

Fig. 15.3 Fluoroscopy image for Example 1 showing an open bladder neck during leakage of urine

The quality of this tracing is good. Of note, no abdominal catheter was used in this study. Often we choose not to use an abdominal catheter in the evaluation of neurogenic patients because the measurement of detrusor pressure (as opposed to vesical pressure) is frequently unnecessary to answer the clinical question, as in this case.

Example 2

Clinical History: Sixty-seven-year-old female with symptoms of mixed urinary incontinence. It is unclear from her history whether her symptoms are predominantly related to stress or urge urinary incontinence. The patient tried Imipramine without benefit and has a 24 h pad weight of 205 g (Figs. 15.4 and 15.5).

Commentary on Example 2: This tracing shows evidence of SUI (Fig. 15.4). First sensation is at 82 mL. Compliance is normal. Capacity is 344 mL. Stress maneuvers were performed at approximately 200 mL and again at 250 mL. These maneuvers demonstrated SUI with a VLPP of 80 cm H_2O at 266 mL. There were no involuntary detrusor contractions. Voiding was assessed with a pressure flow study. This demonstrated a normal bell-shaped flow curve with a peak flow rate of 23 mL/s and a maximum detrusor pressure of 33 cm H_2O. The patient emptied her bladder to completion. Fluoroscopy showed a smooth-walled bladder and a bladder neck that was closed at rest and opens during leakage and voiding (Fig. 15.5).

This patient has SUI.

The study was able to determine the predominant signs of SUI in a setting where the patient had indeterminate symptoms that did not allow us to differentiate between stress and urge urinary incontinence.

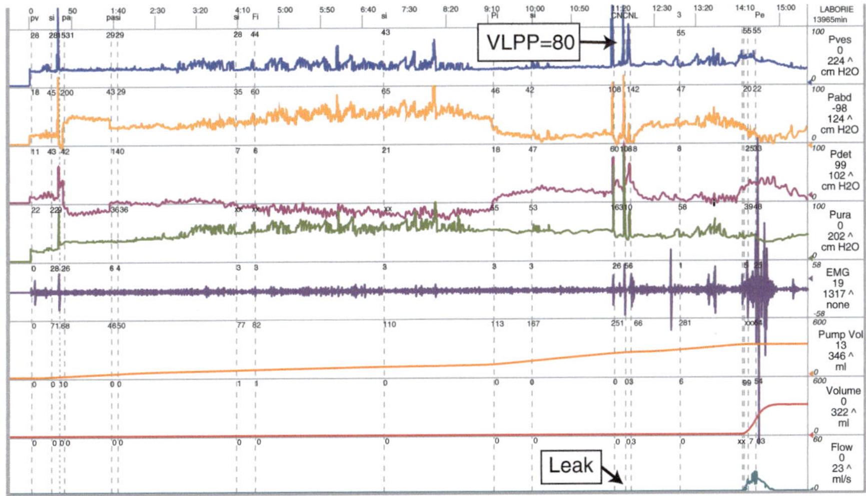

Fig. 15.4 Urodynamics tracing for Example 2

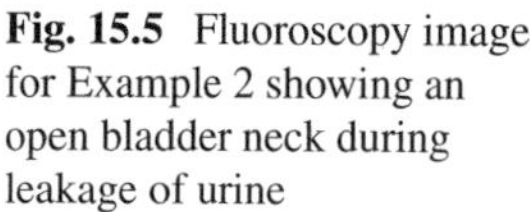

Fig. 15.5 Fluoroscopy image for Example 2 showing an open bladder neck during leakage of urine

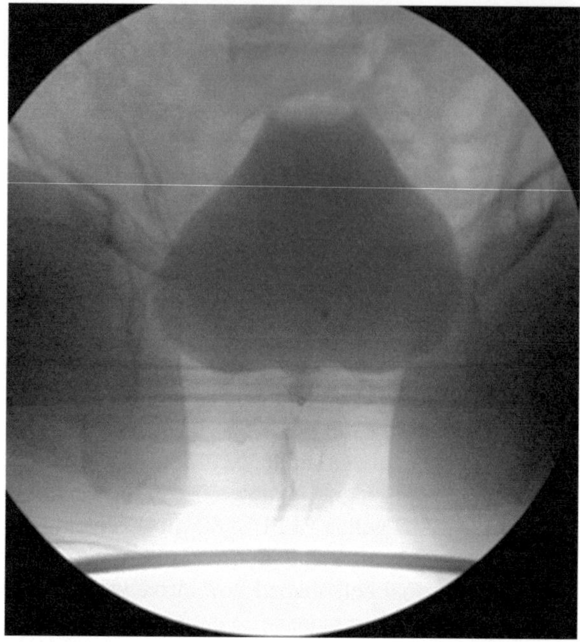

For the most part, the quality of this tracing is good. Of note, the catheter changed position about half-way through the study and was readjusted and re-zeroed, indicated by a sharp change in the tracing shown at 133 mL. This commonly occurs during urodynamic evaluations and it does not mean that the study has to be re-started.

Example 3

Clinical History: Sixty-nine-year-old male with history of myasthenia gravis and urinary incontinence. The patient has a history of a colectomy for colon cancer and has an ileostomy. The urodynamics study was performed in order determine the etiology of his urinary leakage (Figs. 15.6 and 15.7).

Commentary on Example 3: This tracing demonstrates SUI with provocative maneuvers at 74 mL and again at 279 and 306 mL (Fig. 15.6). The tracing shows a CLPP of 69 cm H_2O at 279 mL and a VLPP of 54 cm H_2O at 306 mL. As is often the case in male patients, leakage of urine was visualized at the meatus and on fluoroscopy, but was not captured on the urodynamic tracing. The patient reported no bladder sensation. Compliance was normal and bladder capacity was 306 mL. There was no evidence of detrusor overactivity. The patient was unable to void with the catheter in place, but was able to void for an uroflow examination with a maximum flow rate of 51 mL/s in a sawtooth pattern, indicative of valsalva voiding.

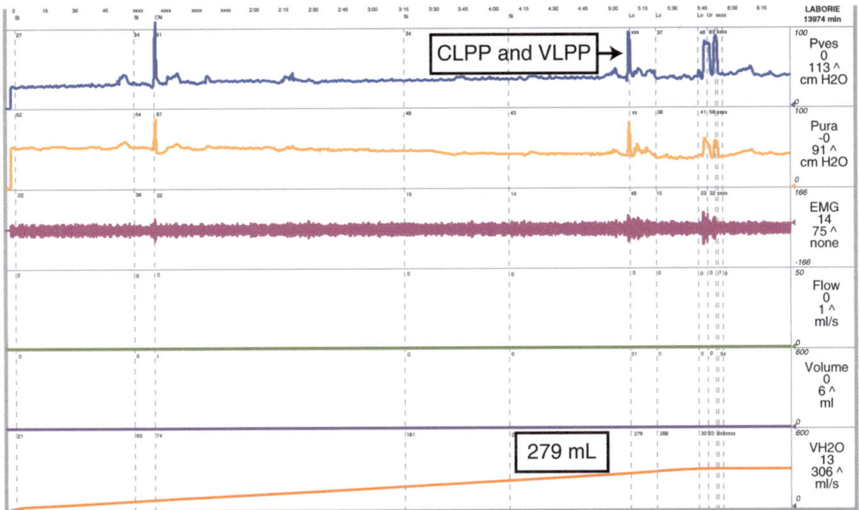

Fig. 15.6 Urodynamics tracing for Example 3

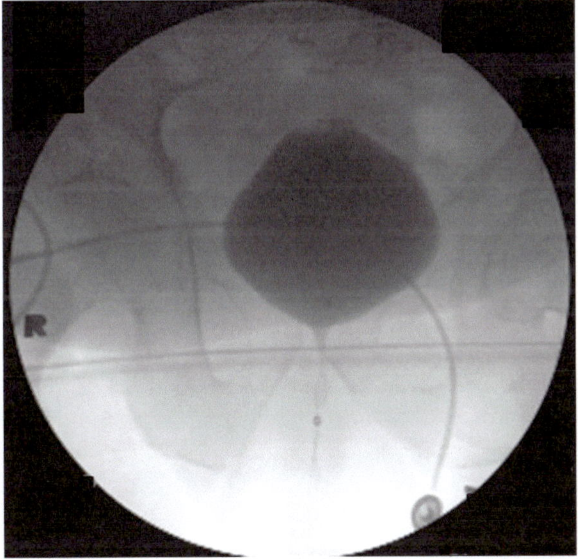

Fig. 15.7 Fluoroscopy image for Example 3 during leakage of urine

Fluoroscopy showed an open bladder neck at rest. The bladder wall was smooth and no vesicoureteral reflux was noted (Fig. 15.7).

This patient has SUI secondary to an open bladder neck and ISD. These findings are most likely attributable to his underlying myasthenia gravis or his prior colectomy.

This tracing was helpful to define the origin of the patient's SUI. Potential treatment options aimed at restoring the position and function of the bladder neck include a medication trial (e.g., imipramine, duloxetine), injectable therapy to the bladder neck, male sling, or artificial urinary sphincter placement.

The quality of this tracing is good. A rectal catheter was not used because of the patient's altered anatomy (i.e., colectomy). In this patient, we were able to obtain our clinical answer without the use of this catheter. Additionally, this patient was unable to void with the urethral catheter in place. This is a common occurrence, and in this case, the uroflow was able to give us adequate information.

Example 4

Clinical History: Sixty-one-year-old female with refractory urinary incontinence. She reports "difficulty delaying urination," especially when she stands up from a seated position. Twenty-four hour pad weight is >400 g. She has tried imipramine, an antimuscarinic, and estrogen cream in the past, all without any notable benefit. The patient also has a history of a "bladder suspension" that was performed approximately 20 years ago. It is unclear whether she has stress or urge predominant urinary incontinence (Figs. 15.8, 15.9, and 15.10).

Commentary on Example 4: This tracing shows stress maneuvers resulting in the demonstration of stress incontinence (Fig. 15.8). The patient had a VLPP of 106 cm H_2O at 198 mL and a CLPP of 147 cm H_2O at 236 mL. Interestingly, as shown in Fig. 15.9, the stress incontinence induced an involuntary detrusor contraction, resulting in the leakage of a larger amount of urine. Since a Pabd catheter was not used in this study, we can determine that this was an involuntary detrusor contraction based

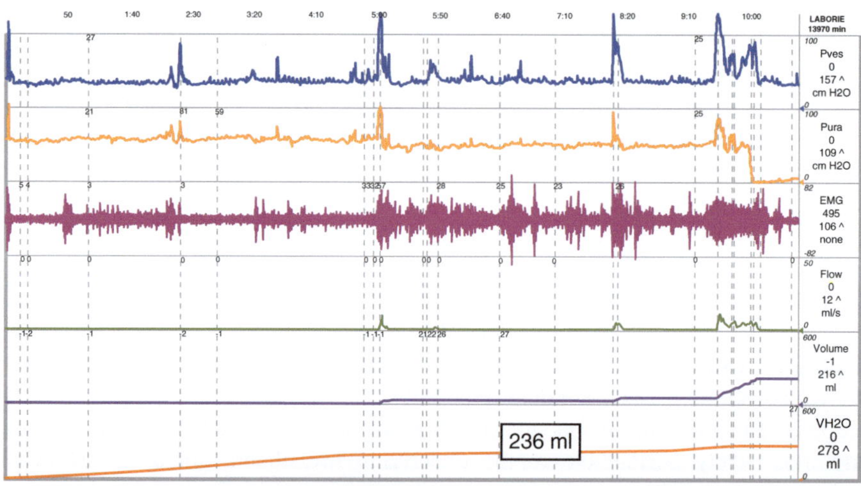

Fig. 15.8 Urodynamics tracing for Example 4

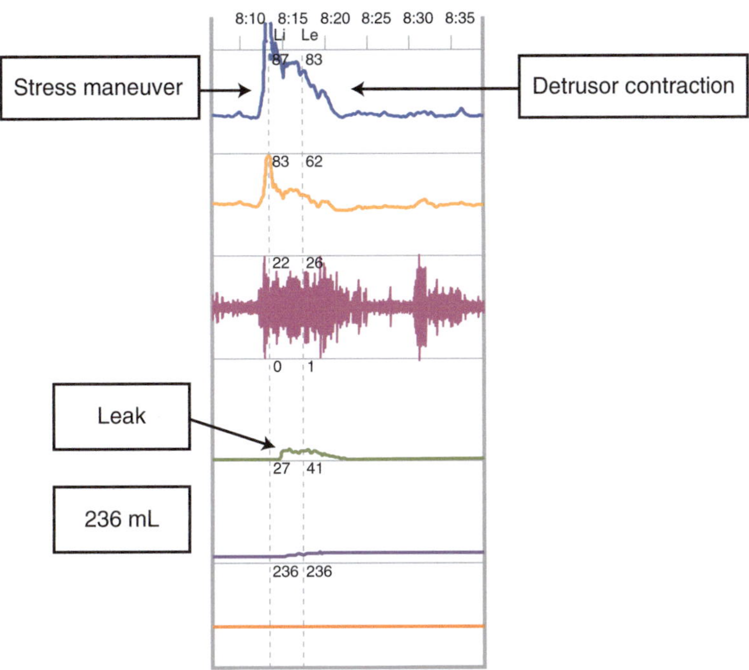

Fig. 15.9 Portion of urodynamics tracing for Example 4 showing a stress-induced detrusor contraction resulting in leakage of urine

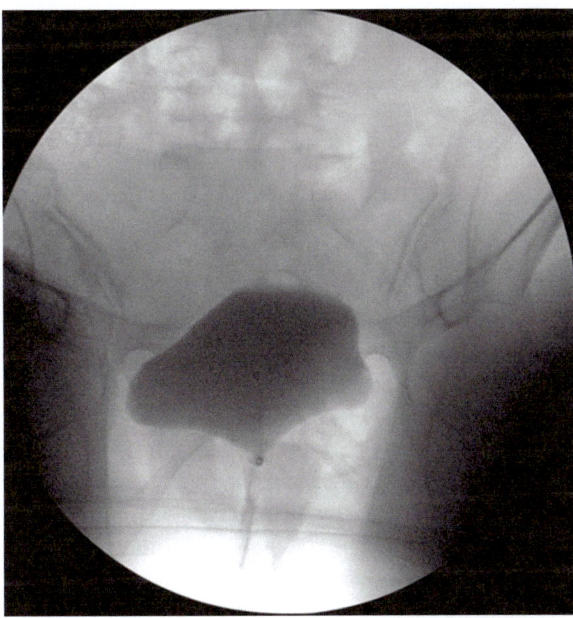

Fig. 15.10 Fluoroscopy image for Example 4 during leakage of urine

the patient's sensation of a bladder contraction during this point in the study. This point emphasizes the importance of being present during the urodynamics evaluation in order to correctly interpret the findings. Bladder compliance was normal. First sensation was almost immediate at 7 mL. Bladder capacity was 278 mL. Voiding resulted in a flow pattern that was flattened. Peak flow rate was 12 mL/s and maximum detrusor pressure during flow was 81 cm H_2O. Post-void residual was zero. Pelvic floor muscles relaxed during voiding. Fluoroscopy showed an open bladder neck during leakage of urine (Fig. 15.10).

The patient has stress-induced detrusor overactivity resulting in the leakage of urine.

This study was very helpful in determining the predominant etiology of the patient's mixed urinary incontinence. Due to this clear sequence of events (i.e., stress followed by urge incontinence), it is logical to first address the stress component. Options for addressing the stress component include pelvic floor physical therapy, urethral bulking agents, and midurethral or pubovaginal slings. Options for addressing the urge component include avoidance of fluid and food irritants, timed voiding, pelvic floor physical therapy, and antimuscarinic therapy.

This is a nice tracing that demonstrates a couple of key points. The first point is that it is very important for the clinician to be present during the urodynamic study in order to be able to appreciate the sequence of events, which was crucial in making the diagnosis in this case. Simply reading the tracing without knowledge of this timing in real time might lead to missing the stress component of the leakage, since this was not captured particularly well on the tracing. Another point is that the addition of fluoroscopy was helpful to be able to localize the timing of leakage to the stress maneuver or to the detrusor contraction in real time.

Example 5

Clinical History: Fifty-eight-year-old male with urinary incontinence status post-radical prostatectomy. The patient reports severe incontinence and uses 10–15 male pads per day (Figs. 15.11, 15.12, and 15.13).

Commentary on Example 5: This tracing demonstrates leakage with stress maneuvers at a volume of 150 mL (Fig. 15.11). As evidenced in the tracing, VLPP was 95 cm H_2O and CLLP was 229 cm H_2O at this volume (Fig. 15.12). Bladder compliance was normal, and capacity was 402 mL. There were no involuntary detrusor contractions. The patient was able to void to completion (post-void residual = 0) at a volume of 402 mL. Flow pattern was bell-shaped with a peak flow rate of 9 mL/s. Detrusor pressure at peak flow was 39 cm H_2O. Fluoroscopy shows a funnel pattern to the bladder neck, consistent with previous radical prostatectomy (Fig. 15.13).

This patient has SUI at relatively low volumes and with simple maneuvers.

Both the urodynamic tracing and the fluoroscopy were helpful during this study. The tracing documented severe SUI and the fluoroscopy indicated a normal bladder neck, i.e., no bladder neck stenosis. The most definitive surgical treatment for this

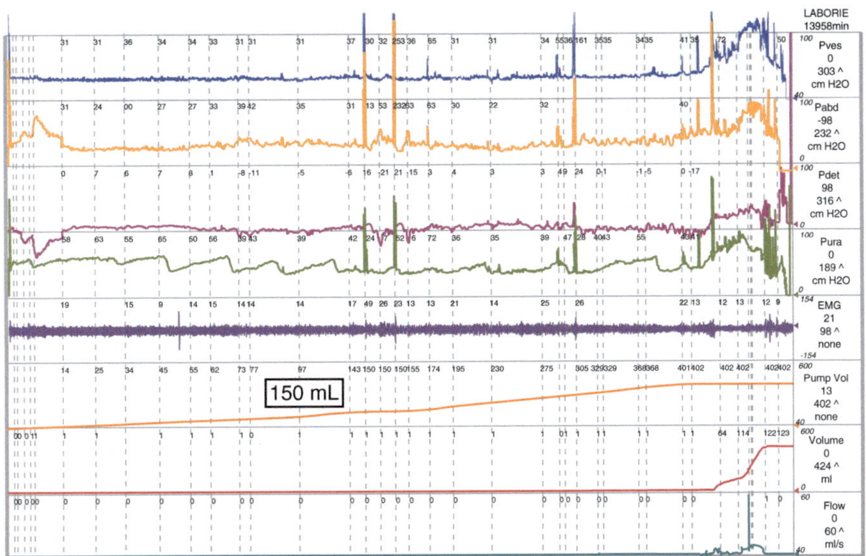

Fig. 15.11 Urodynamics tracing for Example 5

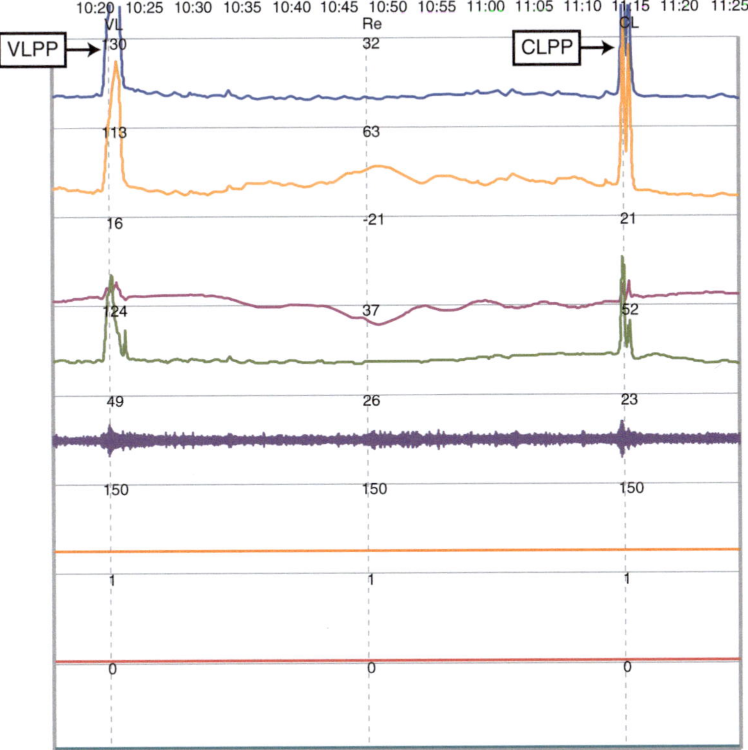

Fig. 15.12 Portion of urodynamics tracing for Example 5 showing SUI

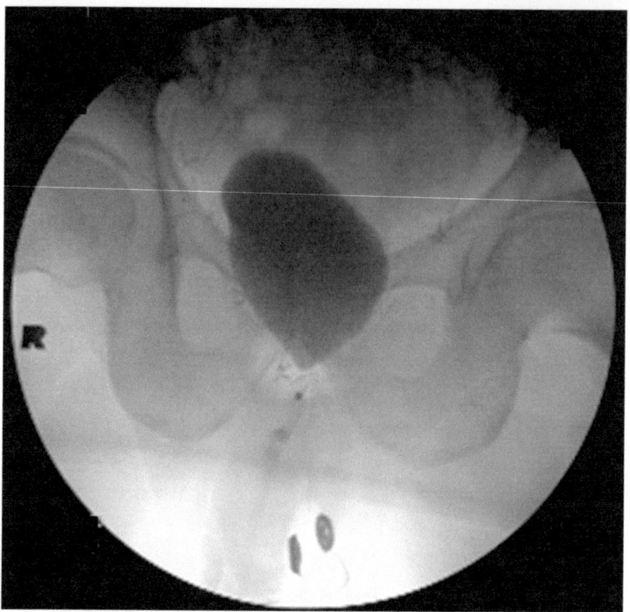

Fig. 15.13 Fluoroscopy image for Example 5 during leakage of urine

patient would be an artificial urinary sphincter due to the severity of his symptoms and low ALPPs.

This tracing is of good quality. Of note, as is often the case in male patients, the tracing does not pick up small amounts of leakage per urethra, due to the nature of the male anatomy. This is where it is useful to have fluoroscopy to visualize the leakage in the urethra and to be present for the test.

Example 6

Clinical History: Forty-three-year-old female with symptoms of SUI and urinary frequency. A uterine mass was palpated on vaginal exam (Figs. 15.14 and 15.15).

Commentary on Example 6: Leakage of urine with stress maneuvers was demonstrated at 140 mL (Fig. 15.14). The VLPP and CLLP were each 70 cm H_2O at this volume. The patient noted first sensation at 20 mL and reported first desire to void at 70 mL. She experienced a strong urge at 141 mL. Bladder capacity was determined to be 150 mL, as limited by this strong sense of urgency. Bladder compliance was normal. There are no involuntary bladder contractions. Fluoroscopy showed a mass pressing posteriorly on the bladder (Fig. 15.15). The voiding phase demonstrated a bell-shaped curve with a maximum flow of 23 mL/s and a post-void residual of 20 mL.

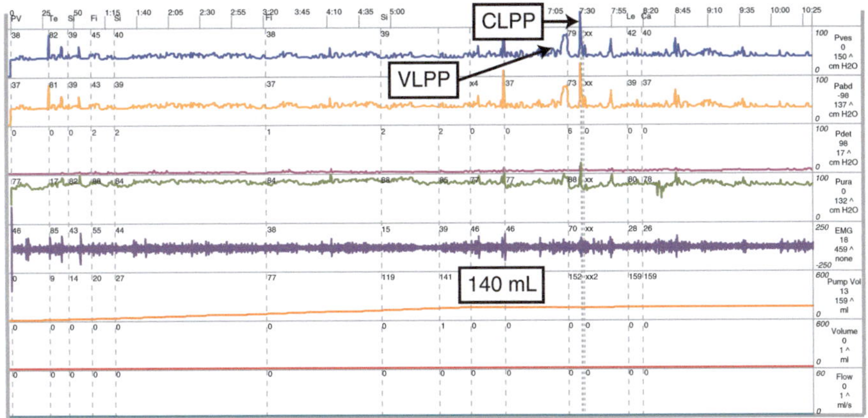

Fig. 15.14 Urodynamics tracing for Example 6

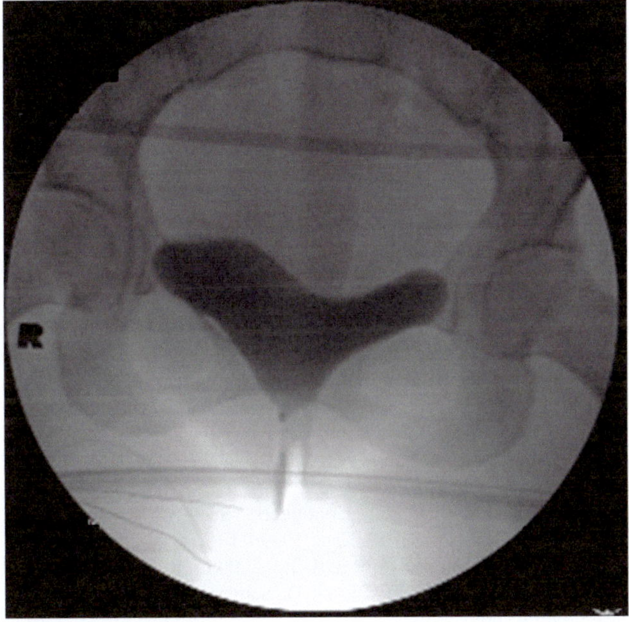

Fig. 15.15 Fluoroscopy image for Example 6

This patient has SUI and a small capacity bladder secondary to compression of the bladder from a uterine mass.

In terms of treating this patient, the first step is to work-up the uterine mass. Once this is addressed, appropriate treatment for the stress incontinence might include avoiding fluid and food irritants, timed voiding, urethral bulking agents, and a midurethral sling.

The tracing for this study is of good quality, but it is really the fluoroscopy that makes the diagnosis. This is an example of where fluoroscopy changes the interpretation of the study and is very valuable.

References

1. Abrams P, Cardozo L, Fall M, Griffiths D, Rosier P, Ulmsten U, et al. The standardisation of terminology in lower urinary tract function: report from the Standardisation Sub-Committee of the International Continence Society. Urology. 2003;61(1):37–49. Epub 2003/02/01.
2. Winters JC, Dmochowski RR, Goldman HB, Herndon CD, Kobashi KC, Kraus SR, et al. Urodynamic studies in adults: AUA/SUFU guideline. J Urol. 2012;188(6 Suppl):2464–72. Epub 2012/10/27.
3. Nager CW, Brubaker L, Litman HJ, Zyczynski HM, Varner RE, Amundsen C, et al. A randomized trial of urodynamic testing before stress-incontinence surgery. N Engl J Med. 2012;366(21):1987–97. Epub 2012/05/04.
4. van Leijsen SA, Kluivers KB, Mol BW, Broekhuis SR, Milani AL, Bongers MY, et al. Can preoperative urodynamic investigation be omitted in women with stress urinary incontinence? A non-inferiority randomized controlled trial. Neurourol Urodyn. 2012;31(7):1118–23. Epub 2012/04/11.
5. McGuire EJ, Cespedes RD, O'Connell HE. Leak-point pressures. Urol Clin North Am. 1996;23(2):253–62. Epub 1996/05/01.
6. Lemack GE. Urodynamic assessment of patients with stress incontinence: how effective are urethral pressure profilometry and abdominal leak point pressures at case selection and predicting outcome? Curr Opin Urol. 2004;14(6):307–11. Epub 2005/01/01.
7. Haylen BT, de Ridder D, Freeman RM, Swift SE, Berghmans B, Lee J, et al. An International Urogynecological Association (IUGA)/International Continence Society (ICS) joint report on the terminology for female pelvic floor dysfunction. Neurourol Urodyn. 2010;29(1):4–20. Epub 2009/11/27.
8. Peschers UM, Jundt K, Dimpfl T. Differences between cough and Valsalva leak-point pressure in stress incontinent women. Neurourol Urodyn. 2000;19(6):677–81. Epub 2000/11/09.
9. Turker P, Kilic G, Tarcan T. The presence of transurethral cystometry catheter and type of stress test affect the measurement of abdominal leak point pressure (ALPP) in women with stress urinary incontinence (SUI). Neurourol Urodyn. 2010;29(4):536–9. Epub 2009/08/21.
10. Stohrer M, Goepel M, Kondo A, Kramer G, Madersbacher H, Millard R, et al. The standardization of terminology in neurogenic lower urinary tract dysfunction: with suggestions for diagnostic procedures. International Continence Society Standardization Committee. Neurourol Urodyn. 1999;18(2):139–58. Epub 1999/03/19.
11. Lane TM, Shah PJ. Leak-point pressures. BJU Int. 2000;86(8):942–9. Epub 2000/11/09.
12. McGuire EJ, Fitzpatrick CC, Wan J, Bloom D, Sanvordenker J, Ritchey M, et al. Clinical assessment of urethral sphincter function. J Urol. 1993;150(5 Pt 1):1452–4. Epub 1993/11/01.
13. Faerber GJ, Vashi AR. Variations in Valsalva leak point pressure with increasing vesical volume. J Urol. 1998;159(6):1909–11. Epub 1998/05/23.
14. Griffiths D. The pressure within a collapsed tube, with special reference to urethral pressure. Phys Med Biol. 1985;30(9):951–63. Epub 1985/09/01.
15. Lose G, Griffiths D, Hosker G, Kulseng-Hanssen S, Perucchini D, Schafer W, et al. Standardisation of urethral pressure measurement: report from the Standardisation Sub-Committee of the International Continence Society. Neurourol Urodyn. 2002;21(3):258–60. Epub 2002/04/12.
16. Lose G. Urethral pressure measurement. Acta Obstet Gynecol Scand Suppl. 1997;166:39–42. Epub 1997/01/01.

17. Harris N, Swithinbank L, Hayek SA, Yang Q, Abrams P. Can maximum urethral closure pressure (MUCP) be used to predict outcome of surgical treatment of stress urinary incontinence? Neurourol Urodyn. 2011;30(8):1609–12. Epub 2011/07/23.
18. Kawasaki A, Wu JM, Amundsen CL, Weidner AC, Judd JP, Balk EM, et al. Do urodynamic parameters predict persistent postoperative stress incontinence after midurethral sling? A systematic review. Int Urogynecol J. 2012;23(7):813–22. Epub 2012/03/10.
19. Almeida FG, Bruschini H, Srougi M. Correlation between urethral sphincter activity and Valsalva leak point pressure at different bladder distentions: revisiting the urethral pressure profile. J Urol. 2005;174(4 Pt 1):1312–5. discussion 5–6. Epub 2005/09/08.
20. Schafer W, Abrams P, Liao L, Mattiasson A, Pesce F, Spangberg A, et al. Good urodynamic practices: uroflowmetry, filling cystometry, and pressure-flow studies. Neurourol Urodyn. 2002;21(3):261–74. Epub 2002/04/12.
21. Rosier PF, Gajewski JB, Sand PK, Szabo L, Capewell A, Hosker GL. Executive summary: The International Consultation on Incontinence 2008—Committee on: "Dynamic Testing"; for urinary incontinence and for fecal incontinence. Part 1: innovations in urodynamic techniques and urodynamic testing for signs and symptoms of urinary incontinence in female patients. Neurourol Urodyn. 2010;29(1):140–5. Epub 2009/08/21.

Chapter 16
Bladder Emptying: Contractility

Chasta Bacsu, Jack C. Hou, and Gary E. Lemack

Definition of Bladder Contractility

Bladder contractility is a term used to describe the strength of bladder detrusor muscle contractions [1, 2]. Since bladder contraction requires parasympathetic stimulation, the detrusor pressure depends on the inherent strength of the detrusor muscle itself, which can be affected by a variety of factors, and intact neural circuitry. Loss of either would clearly impact contractile strength and overall bladder function. *Normal detrusor function* is initiated by a drop in urethral pressure followed by a continuous detrusor contraction which leads to complete bladder emptying within a normal time span. For many women who void primarily by urethral relaxation, this contraction may be modest or even absent. *Detrusor underactivity* implies a detrusor contraction of reduced strength and/or duration resulting in prolonged voiding, and/or a failure to achieve complete bladder emptying. An *acontractile detrusor* identifies the condition where no detrusor contraction is noted, also typically associated with prolonged voids, incomplete emptying, or inability to void altogether. Examples of each of these conditions are demonstrated in urodynamic tracings shown in the remainder of the chapter.

Other factors, such as outlet resistance, can also greatly affect bladder contractility. Enhanced outlet resistance, in the setting of bladder outlet obstruction, will result in increased detrusor force for a variable period of time, followed potentially by a loss of force depending on the severity and duration of obstruction. Similarly diminished outlet resistance, for example in the setting of stress urinary incontinence, has been shown to result in lowered detrusor pressures during voiding.

C. Bacsu, MD, BSc • J.C. Hou, MD • G.E. Lemack, MD (✉)
Department of Urology, UT Southwestern Medical Center, Room JA5.130D,
5323 Harry Hines Blvd., Dallas, TX 75390-9110, USA
e-mail: gary.lemack@utsouthwestern.edu

© Springer Science+Business Media New York 2015
E.S. Rovner, M.E. Koski (eds.), *Rapid and Practical Interpretation of Urodynamics*, DOI 10.1007/978-1-4939-1764-8_16

The voiding phase of cystometry, also known as the pressure-flow study, measures the relationship between detrusor pressure and flow rate during voiding. While a low flow rate alone may be more likely to be associated with bladder outlet obstruction, this clearly is not always the case. Indeed, the primary purpose of the pressure-flow study is to differentiate bladder outlet obstruction from low flow due to detrusor underactivity or acontractility. Similarly, while uncommon, patients with relatively normal flow may have quite elevated detrusor pressures suggestive of obstruction, a diagnosis which can only be made during pressure-flow analysis [3, 4].

Assessment of Bladder Contractility

Measurement of detrusor contractility is commonly assessed by multichannel urodynamics during the pressure-flow study. Isovolumetric techniques to study detrusor contractility where the urinary stream is interrupted using balloon occlusion, inflatable penile cuffs or occlusive condom catheters are not commonly used as they can be uncomfortable, cumbersome, and may interfere with the normal desire to void. These tests are especially challenging in female patients [1, 2, 5]. Voluntary stopping of the urinary stream by contracting the urinary sphincter may not be reliable in measuring detrusor contractility [6]. Cystoscopic appearance (trabeculations, cellules) and radiological findings (bladder wall thickness) may provide indirect clues regarding bladder function and contractility, but again are non-specific findings.

Several formulas and nomograms based on pressure-flow studies have been developed to better quantify detrusor contractility [1]. Watts Factor (WF) is a calculation used to follow changes in contraction strength as the bladder empties. It is based on detrusor pressure (P_{det}), flow rate (Q), volume in the bladder (V), velocity of shortening of bladder circumference, and constant values ($a=25$ cm H_2O, $b=6$ mm/s) based on in vitro studies [7]. WF_{max} is proposed to represent maximal detrusor contractility and is calculated at maximal flow rate (Q_{max}) [8].

$$\mathrm{WF} = \left[\left(P_{det} + a \right)\left(V_{det} + b \right) - ab \right] / 2\pi; \text{ where } V_{det} = Q / 2\left[3\left(V + V_t \right) / 4\pi \right]^{2/3}$$

where V_t = volume of noncontracting bladder wall tissue [7].

Although some studies report WF and WF_{max}, no consensus has been made regarding normative values particularly in female patients [6, 8, 9]. A WF_{max} of <12 $\mu W/mm^2$ for males and <5 $\mu W/mm^2$ for postmenopausal females has been used in some studies to define detrusor underactivity [8, 10, 11]. Use of WF may not be suitable for practical use due to complexity of the calculation, poor reproducibility, and lack of standardized cutoff values [6, 8].

Schafer simplified the approach to classify contractile strength based on relationship of detrusor pressure and urine flow rates in men with bladder outlet obstruction [1, 12]. Bladder contractility index (BCI) is based on detrusor pressure at maximum flow rate (P_{det} @ Q_{max}) and maximum flow rate (Q_{max}):

$$BCI = P_{det} \; @ \; Q_{max} + 5Q_{max}$$

In men, BCI > 150 suggests strong contractility; BCI 100–150 suggests normal contractility and BCI < 100 suggests weak contractility [1, 3].

To address the limitation that BCI was based on men with BOO, Tan modified the BCI calculation and proposed a new formula of contraction strength for elderly women (mean age 70.1 years) with urge incontinence, known as the projected iso-volumetric detrusor pressure (*PIP*) [2]:

$$PIP = P_{det} \; @ \; Q_{max} + Q_{max}.$$

With this modified formula, normal contractility in this cohort was defined as PIP = 30–75 [2].

The relationship between detrusor contractility and urine flow in the form of a pressure versus flow rate (*p/Q*) plot can be helpful in the understanding of detrusor function and outflow obstruction [12]. In efforts to better clarify this relationship, further calculations such as passive urethral resistance relation (PURR), linear PURR, detrusor-adjusted mean PURR factor (DAMPF) have been proposed and can be helpful in the assessment of patients with outflow obstruction taking into account their detrusor contractility which could otherwise be overlooked [12].

Detrusor Underactivity

Detrusor underactivity is defined by the ICS as "detrusor contraction of reduced strength and/or duration, resulting in prolonged bladder emptying within a normal time span" [13]. It is unclear if bladder contractility diminishes with age, though the most recent data suggests that this may indeed be the case [14–18]. What is clear is that merely the presence of a weak detrusor contraction during voiding itself may not lead to a diagnosis of detrusor underactivity, since the definition implies some sequelae occur (altered or prolonged voiding) as a result of this urodynamic finding. Both myogenic failure and bladder wall ischemia have been proposed as underlying pathophysiological mechanisms responsible for detrusor underactivity [17, 19–21].

Causes and predisposing factors of detrusor underactivity include medications, psychogenic factors, neurologic conditions, end-stage BOO, extensive pelvic surgery, or idiopathic. Urodynamic studies are helpful to diagnosis detrusor underactivity and rule out other causes of voiding dysfunction [17]. Urodynamically, detrusor underactivity is commonly found in a low pressure/low flow state. It also may be diagnosed mistakenly in women who void primarily by urethral relaxation,

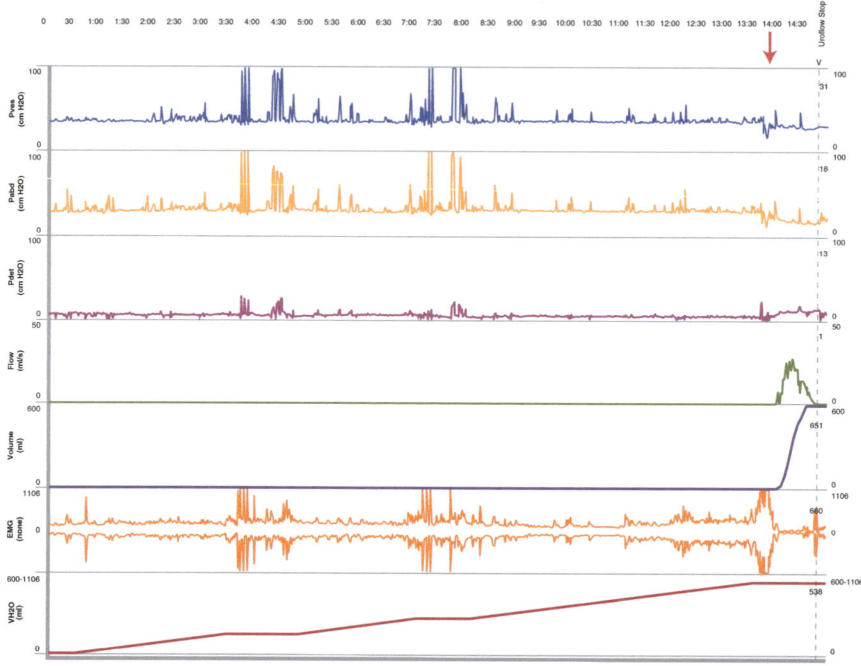

Fig. 16.1 Urodynamic tracing of urethral relaxation in a female. Note decreased EMG activity during voiding. Permission to void denoted by *red arrow*

in which case urinary flow rates may be normal, voiding is not prolonged, and as a result underactivity cannot be truly diagnosed even in the setting of a weak detrusor contraction. In a similar way, a weak detrusor contraction may be associated with intrinsic sphincteric deficiency (ISD) with both men and women, though the presence of relatively normal voiding in these instances argues against the diagnosis of detrusor underactivity, which implies an insufficient contraction. Again, it is important to stress that the urodynamic finding of a minimally contracting detrusor muscle may have no clinical relevance, particularly in women, who void efficiently and effectively by urethral relaxation or have chronically reduced outlet resistance due to ISD. Post-prostatectomy incontinence with compromised bladder outlet is another common situation where a relative detrusor underactivity occurs, in the absence voiding dysfunction or other sequelae.

Clinical scenario 1 (Fig. 16.1):

Urethral relaxation

A 69-year-old female with recurrent urinary tract infections but no bladder storage or emptying complaints. Her PVR is zero. Cystoscopy is unremarkable. She has no prior history of urologic pelvic surgery or neurological disease. Her urodynamics are interesting because the PFS demonstrates urethral relaxation. Note the decrease abdominal pressure and the lack of significant rise in either P_{ves} or P_{det}.

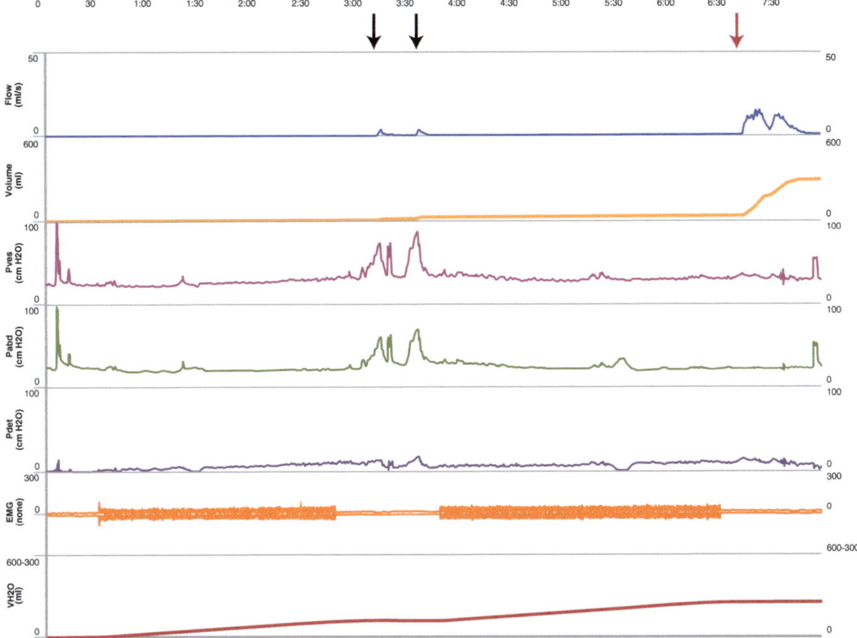

Fig. 16.2 Urodynamic tracing demonstrating low pressure voiding in a female with SUI. Note the presence of a compromised outlet due to SUI can result in lower voiding pressure. Stress urinary incontinence denoted by *black arrows*. Permission to void denoted by *red arrow*

Despite an apparent $P_{det}Q_{max}$ of only 13 cm H_2O (actual P_{det} value may be even lower due to drop in P_{abd}), she completely empties her bladder by urethral relaxation, voiding 651 mL, with a maximum flow rate of 27 mL/s and normal bell-shaped flow curve. This is due to urethral relaxation at the time of voiding—as detected by the diminished sphincteric activity noted on EMG monitoring.

Clinical scenario 2 (Fig. 16.2):

Reduced outlet resistance, low pressure voiding in woman with SUI

A 62-year-old female with symptomatic stress urinary incontinence. She reports voiding with a normal flow. She is noted to have SUI on her study at 114 mL with differential VLPP of approximately 39 cm denoted by first two arrows. The low VLPP is consistent with intrinsic sphincter dysfunction. Bladder compliance is normal and there was no evidence of detrusor overactivity. Her MCC was 251 mL.

During the PFS, the detrusor contraction is relatively weak, but adequate to allow her to empty her bladder to completion with a bimodal flow curve (Q_{max} 15 mL/s). The presence of a compromised bladder outlet has been associated with both lower valsalva leak point pressure (VLPP) and voiding pressures in women with SUI.

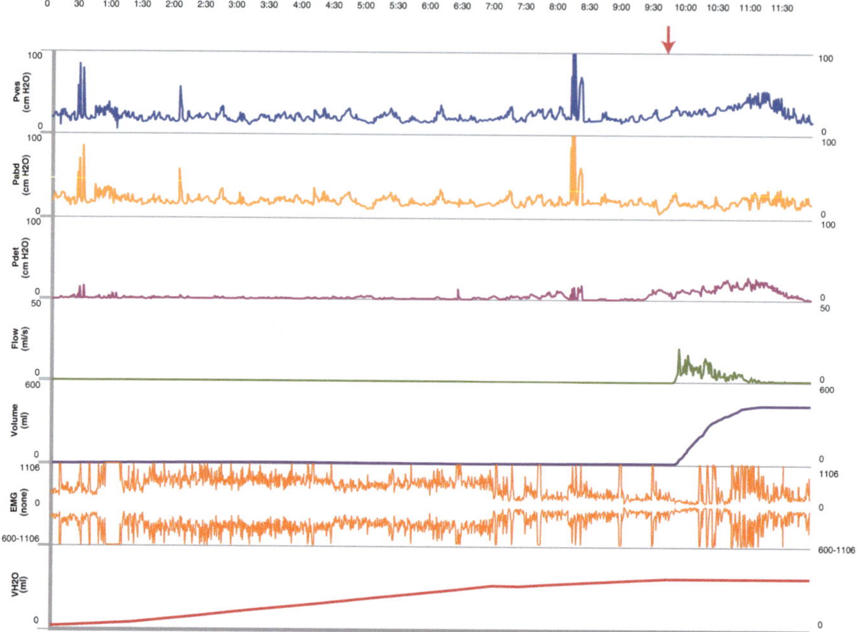

Fig. 16.3 Urodynamic tracing of a female with sensation of difficulty urinating due to detrusor underactivity. Permission to void denoted by *red arrow*

The quality of the UDS is good. A cough at the end of the study confirmed catheters were in appropriate position with adequate zeroing. Her voided volume was not marked on the tracing.

Clinical scenario 3 (Fig. 16.3):

Detrusor underactivity/Crede voiding

An 82-year-old female with recurrent UTIs, urinary frequency and sensation of difficulty emptying her bladder. First sensation is at 176 mL. No stress incontinence was seen with cough or Valsalva maneuver. MCC is 365 mL. Compliance is normal. No detrusor overactivity is noted. On pressure-flow component of study, the patient was noted to apply external pressure to her suprapubic region, or crede, to assist with voiding. She voids with a prolonged stream to completion without a residual volume, and a notably weak detrusor contraction.

EMG shows appropriate relaxation as voiding starts though increased EMG activity during void may reflect straining. In this case, due to the presence of abnormal voiding, the term detrusor underactivity should be applied.

The quality of this urodynamic tracing is fair. After permission to void (denoted by red arrow), a subtle rise in the P_{abd} is noted with crede maneuver which is also reflected in P_{ves} tracing. Q_{max} of 21 mL/s is not representative of her flow curve as she does a crede maneuver to achieve that reading. Average flow rate is considerably lower and more representative of her altered voiding function.

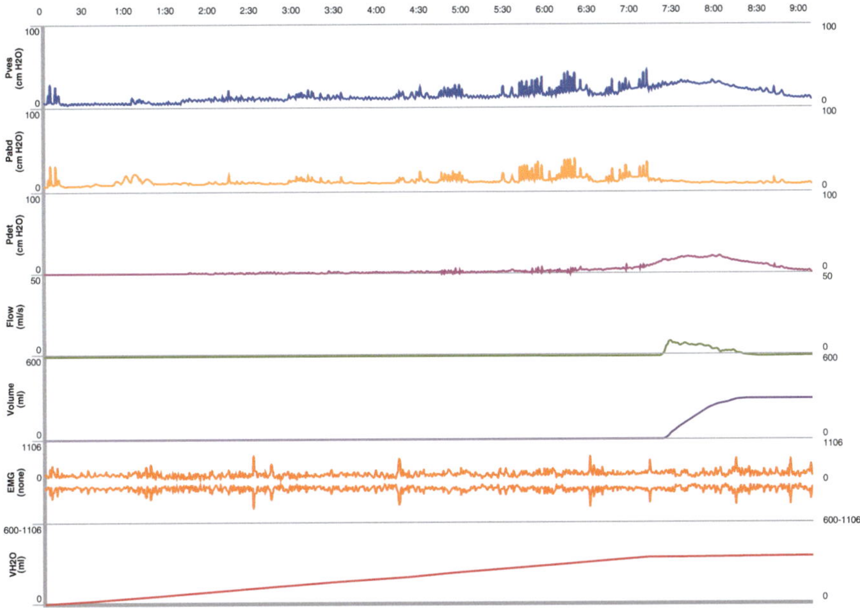

Fig. 16.4 Urodynamic tracing of a male who is 4 years post-radical prostatectomy with incomplete bladder emptying and elevated residual. The BCI is <100 consistent with detrusor underactivity. Permission to void given twice, and noted with increases in both abdominal and vesical catheters and corresponding small volume voids

Clinical scenario 4 (Fig. 16.4):

Idiopathic detrusor underactivity following radical prostatectomy

A 71-year-old man underwent a radical prostatectomy 4 years prior to the study. His PSA is still undetectable. He complains of a weak prolonged stream, urinary frequency, nocturia (3/night), and sensation of incomplete emptying over the past year. Cystoscopy was unremarkable. First sensation occurred at 103 mL. He experiences strong urge at 201 mL but is ultimately able to attain a normal MCC of 348 mL.

P_{det} does not rise substantially with his void, and a prolonged flow curve is noted. Q_{max} is 10 mL/s with $P_{det}Q_{max}$ of 14 cm H_2O. His BCI ($P_{det}Q_{max} + 5(Q_{max})$ is 64 (<100) which represents detrusor underactivity. He also was catheterized for 90 mL at the end of the study.

The quality of this tracing is fair. At the beginning of the study, P_{det} is below zero, which is physically implausible. Vesical and rectal catheter position should be assessed to insure accuracy in situations such as this. Often the catheters may be against the wall of the bladder or rectum and instilling more fluid (or releasing) in the rectal balloon or initiating bladder filling will move the pressure detector from the luminal wall and correct the problem. Prior to voiding, there are corresponding increases of P_{ves} and P_{abd} which represent patient movement and hiccups. It is important to annotate the study with findings such as this to facilitate interpretation.

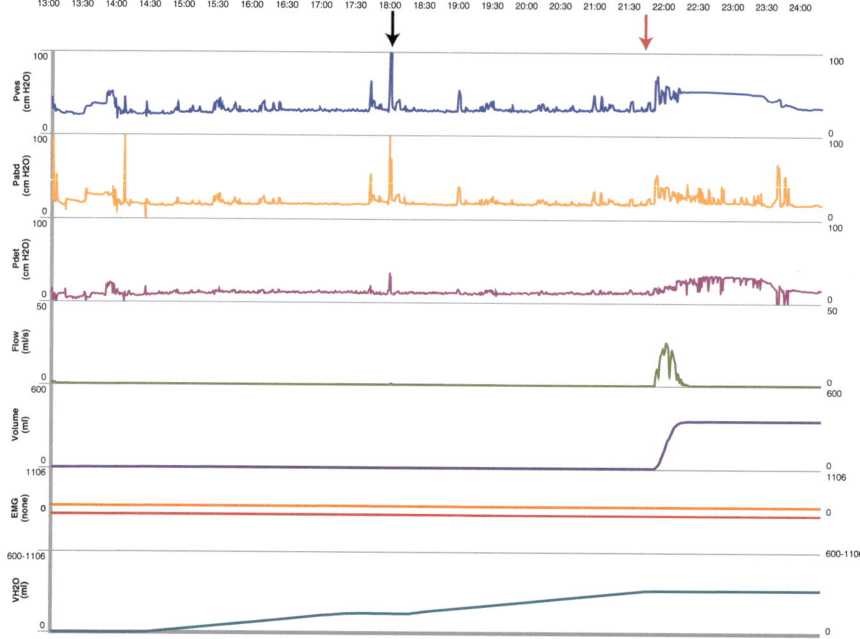

Fig. 16.5 Urodynamic tracing of a male with post-prostatectomy incontinence and relative detrusor hypocontractility. Similar to women with SUI, a compromised bladder outlet in a male can also be associated with low voiding pressures. Stress urinary incontinence denoted by *black arrow*. Permission to void denoted by *red arrow*

Clinical scenario 5 (Fig. 16.5):

Relative detrusor underactivity associated with sphincteric deficiency in man status-post radical prostatectomy.

A 68-year-old man 3 years out from radical retropubic prostatectomy is noted to have three pads per day leakage. Otherwise, he feels well, has had no bladder infections, and voids with a strong stream. In this urodynamic study, there is a reasonable bladder capacity (360 mL), an absence of detrusor overactivity during filling, stress incontinence (noted at first arrow), and a relatively weak detrusor contraction supplemented by straining. Since he empties to completion, and in the absence of a prolonged flow, this finding would not be consistent with the term "detrusor underactivity" but rather represents a reduced detrusor contraction, possibly related to loss of outlet resistance over time.

Treatments for Detrusor Underactivity

A limited understanding of causes and a dearth of effective treatments for detrusor underactivity suggests that further innovative research and treatment strategies are warranted [22]. Optimization of voiding in patients with detrusor underactivity is attempted by avoiding/treating constipation, discontinuing/limiting medications that can impact detrusor contractility, such as narcotics and medications with anticholinergic properties, and aggressive ambulation. Bethanechol and other parasympathomimetic agents have shown limited efficacy in clinical trials, and thus their use is largely discouraged [23, 24]. TURP in men with detrusor underactivity is controversial with lower success rates compared to those without detrusor underactivity, but may have a role in select patients by reducing outflow resistance or undiagnosed BOO after careful preoperative counseling [24–26]. Intermittent catheterization and indwelling catheterization are the remaining options for those with a symptomatic impaired bladder emptying secondary to underactivity.

Acontractile Detrusor

An acontractile detrusor is defined as "the detrusor cannot be observed to contract during urodynamic studies resulting in prolonged bladder emptying and/or a failure to achieve complete bladder emptying within a normal time span [13]." Detrusor acontractility may be a more severe form of detrusor underactivity, and is thought to be caused by the similar underlying pathophysiologic mechanisms in many instances. Neurogenic causes (i.e., sacral cord injury), fixed chronic obstruction (prolonged untreated benign prostatic growth), and functional causes (non-neurogenic neurogenic bladder/Hinman syndrome, non-relaxing pelvic floor) may all be associated with detrusor acontractility. As with detrusor underactivity, detrusor acontractility can be transient or permanent depending on the clinical circumstance. Also, the terminology implies not only to the finding of absent detrusor contraction, but to a resultant impact on voiding as well. In certain clinical scenarios, such as voiding by urethral relaxation, the detrusor contraction may be absent, but voiding remains normal.

Treatments for Detrusor Acontractility

The acontractile detrusor is typically managed by intermittent or indwelling catheterization (urethral or suprapubic), especially if due to a transient cause [27]. In cases of persistent detrusor acontractility, sacral neuromodulation (for non-obstructive causes), intravesical electrostimulation, latissimus dorsi detrusor myoplasty, or continent catheterizable channels have been utilized in differing clinical scenarios [27, 28].

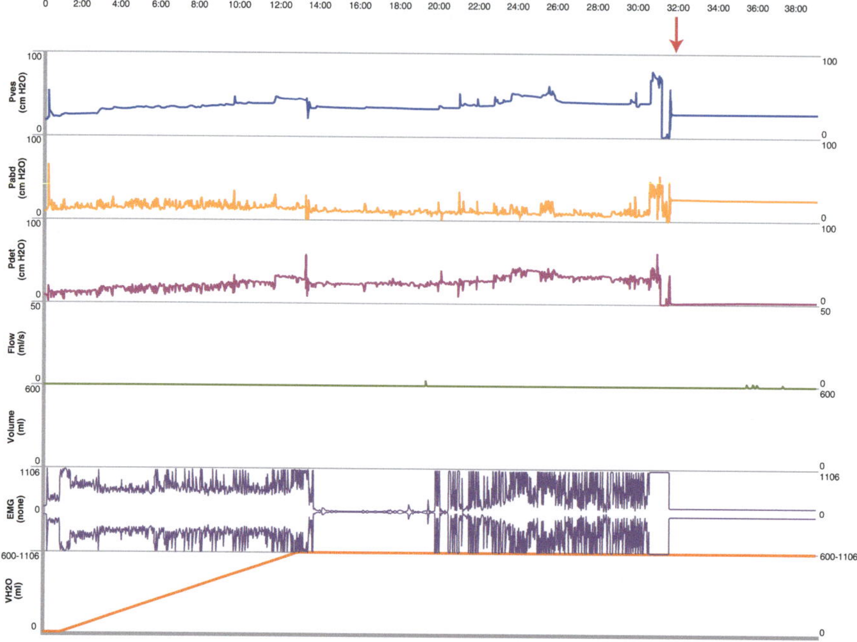

Fig. 16.6 Urodynamic tracing of a female with an acontractile detrusor and inability to void. Permission to void denoted by *red arrow*. Pressure transducers adjusted at this point

Clinical scenario 6 (Fig. 16.6):

Acontractile detrusor in a female

A 26-year-old female presents with complaints of bladder fullness without a typical desire/urge to void. She has noticed that if she tries to urinate the stream only dribbles and may take her several attempts to empty her bladder. She noticed that the stream has worsened with time over the course of 6–8 months. She has also had an increasing number of UTIs. She denies having a known neurological diagnosis but on further questioning reveals that she has experienced some visual changes, and occasional numbness and tingling in her left upper extremity. She has had no prior pregnancy, surgery, or neurological evaluation.

She was subsequently scheduled for urodynamics which revealed delayed first sensation (537 mL) and MCC of 733 mL. No incontinence was observed during filling. Despite having large MCC and desire, with permission, to void (at red arrow), she did not mount any detrusor contraction. An increase in vesical pressure is noted through this long filling curve suggestive of somewhat altered compliance. Given that this occurs over a volume of over 700 mL, the impact of this pressure change can be mitigated by an appropriate catheterization schedule. Urodynamic catheters were removed after the patient was unable to void with reasonable attempts of urination. After the catheter was removed, she only urinated 11 mL.

She has an acontractile bladder on UDS. The differential diagnosis of her acontractile bladder includes an undiagnosed neurologic condition, medication, or idiopathic causes such as Fowler's syndrome. She has been taught and will perform intermittent catheterization to empty her bladder. A neurological investigation revealed demyelinating lesions on CT suggesting multiple sclerosis.

This tracing is relatively poor quality as it is not perfectly zeroed, movement artifact is present, and the side scale has not been recalibrated to show the entire volume of fluid instilled. Since the patient could not void with the catheter in place a PFS could not be performed. However, detrusor acontractility is diagnosed during her attempt to void.

Clinical Scenario 7 (Fig. 16.7)

Acontractile detrusor in elderly male

A 72-year-old male with chronic history of difficulty voiding and post-void dribbling, which was never treated. Noted to have PVR of 650 mL. Urodynamic study shows large bladder capacity, delayed desire to void, a stable bladder during filling, normal compliance, and detrusor acontractility on attempt to void.

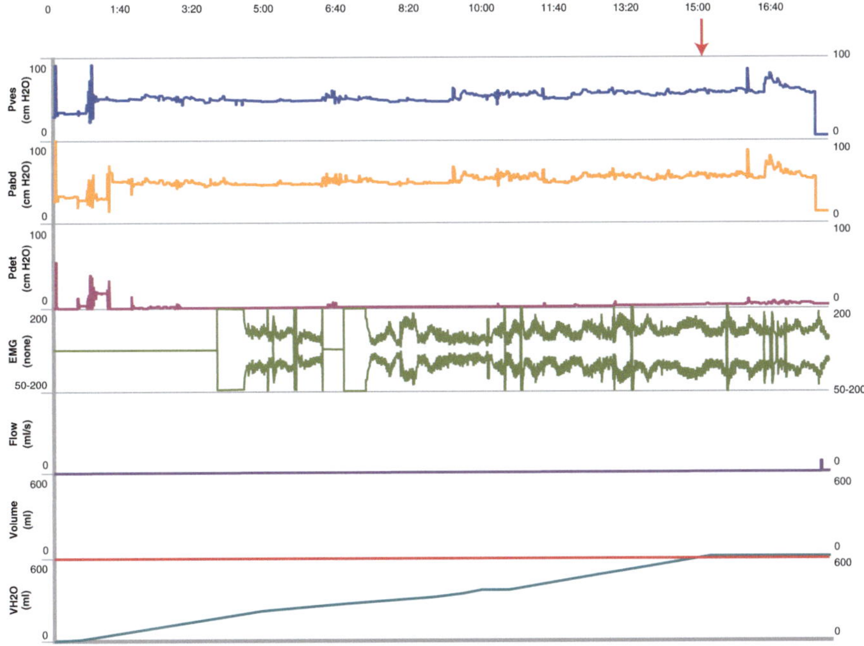

Fig. 16.7 Urodynamic tracing in an elderly male with large capacity bladder, delayed bladder sensation, and inability to urinate. Note no significant increase in detrusor pressure during voiding attempt. Permission to void denoted by *red arrow*

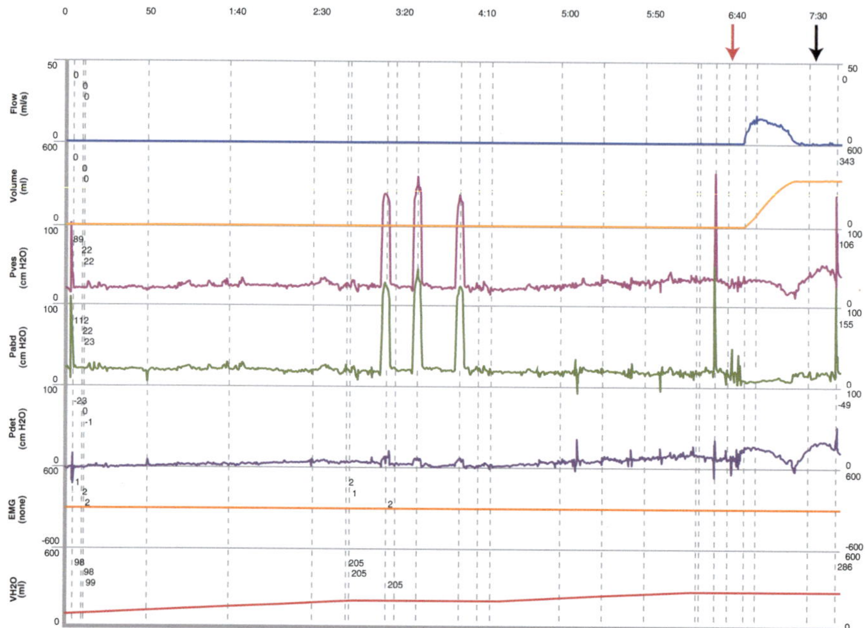

Fig. 16.8 Urodynamic tracing of a male with post-prostatectomy incontinence and low voiding detrusor pressure. Note the sustained detrusor contraction after he urinates. Permission to void denoted by *red arrow*. After contraction denoted by *black arrow*

Abnormal Detrusor Contractility

Clinical Scenario 8 (Fig. 16.8)

Detrusor after contraction

A 59-year-old man with post-prostatectomy incontinence. In this urodynamic study, note the sustained detrusor contraction after he urinates, denoted by second arrow. The detrusor after contractions may be an expression of sphincter contraction interrupting an incomplete detrusor contraction. It has been reported mostly in connection with urge incontinence and urge symptoms.

Clinical Scenario 9 (Fig. 16.9)

"Super Voider"

A 37-year-old male complains of dysuria and urinary frequency. His UDS tracing demonstrates high detrusor pressure (P_{det} 78 cm H_2O) while voiding and a high peak flow rate (Q_{max} 24 mL/s).

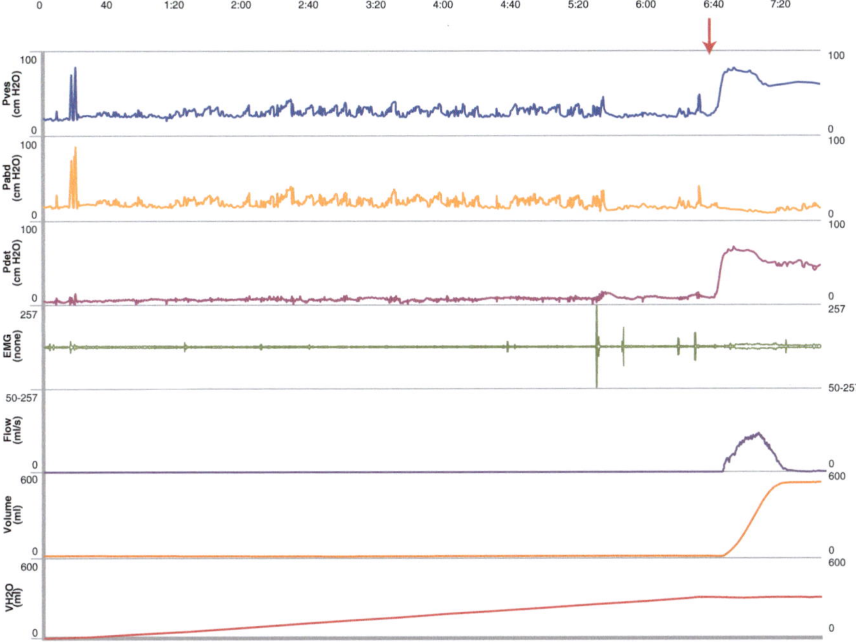

Fig. 16.9 Urodynamic tracing of a male voiding at high detrusor pressure and high flow rate. Permission to void denoted by *red arrow*

Detrusor Hyperactivity and Impaired Contractility

First described in 1987 [29], detrusor hyperactivity with impaired contractility (DHIC) is characterized on urodynamics by low-amplitude involuntary detrusor contractions during filling that are often associated with urethral relaxation, as well as impaired bladder emptying, and occurs predominantly in the elderly [30]. Presentation of DHIC can be variable and is often misdiagnosed. Females may be misdiagnosed with intrinsic sphincter deficiency (ISD), whereas males are more often misdiagnosed with bladder outlet obstruction (BOO); both of which may result in unnecessary surgery [30].

Treatment of DHIC can be challenging given the paradoxical nature of the voiding disorder [29]. Management strategies depend on the symptoms, degree of bother, and general health status in addition to urodynamic findings. Conservative measures of fluid restriction, pelvic floor exercises, and bladder retraining can provide satisfactory results in some patients [30]. In the presence of OAB predominant symptoms despite trial of conservative measures, low dose anticholinergics or a beta-3 agonist may be initiated with careful attention to post-void residuals (PVR) and related side effects for each type of medication; particularly cognitive

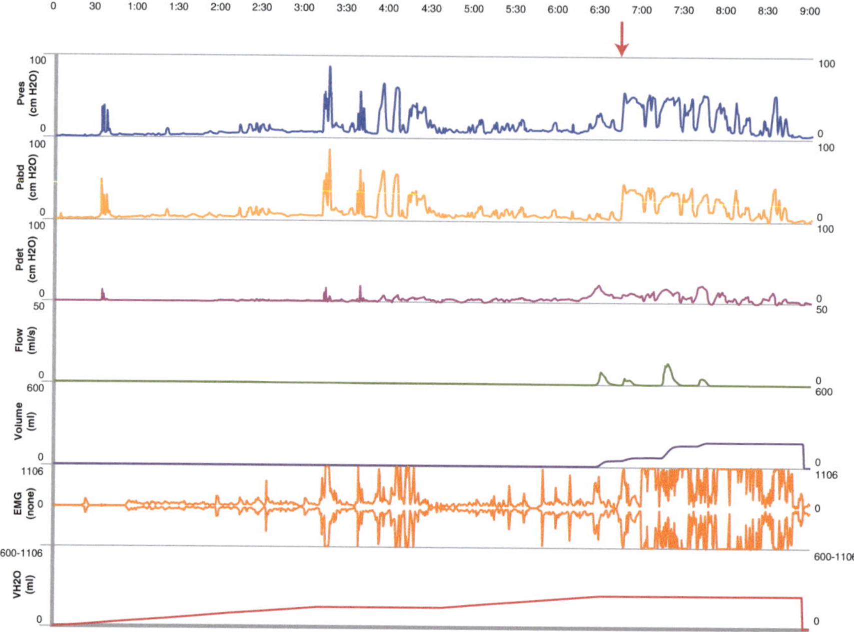

Fig. 16.10 Urodynamic tracing in an elderly female with detrusor hyperactivity and impaired contractility consistent with DHIC. Note terminal DO just prior to permission to void. Permission to void denoted by *red arrow*

impairment with anticholinergic use [30, 31]. If predominant symptoms are due to impaired bladder emptying, alpha blockers may help reduce outlet resistance and improve emptying particularly in male patients. Mixed symptoms can be safely managed with combination therapy of alpha blockers with anticholinergics or a beta-3 agonist. Intermittent catheterization (IC) is commonly employed to manage elevated PVR in DHIC [30]. Prompted voiding every 2 h can be beneficial for cognitively impaired and frail elderly. When all other approaches fail in the setting of high PVRs or large volume incontinence, protective incontinence devices and indwelling catheterization may be the only option.

Clinical Scenario 10 (Fig. 16.10):

DHIC in a female

A 73-year-old female complains of frequency, urge incontinence, and sensation of incomplete emptying. She has no prior history of GU surgery. Her past medical history is significant for diabetes and hypertension. She wears three thick incontinence pads per day.

Her urodynamics demonstrate reduced MCC of 245 mL. SUI was not seen with cough or valsalva during filling. She has urgency incontinence with terminal detrusor overactivity at 245 mL. After permission (denoted by red arrow), she voids primarily by straining and does not generate very high detrusor pressures. Q_{max} is

14 mL/s with an intermittent stream. Determination of P_{det} is especially challenging in the setting of valsalva voiding. She has a residual of 60 mL. This picture is suggestive of detrusor hyperactivity with impaired contractility.

The quality of this study is fair but the increases in P_{abd} from movement make interpretation challenging as it is not perfectly clear if incontinence episode is purely associated with an uninhibited detrusor contraction. It is best to have the clinician and an experienced urodynamics technician present at the time of urodynamics to increase the accuracy of diagnosis particularly when there is significant artifact present.

Clinical Scenario 11 (Fig. 16.11)

DHIC in a male

An 82-year-old male with history of prostate cancer treated by external beam radiation 10 years ago presents with urgency and urge incontinence. He has also had bladder cancer previously treated with intravesical instillations. He has been on tamsulosin for many years and finds mild improvement with it. He has tried multiple anticholinergics without any benefit. He wears eight pads per day and leaks throughout the day and night.

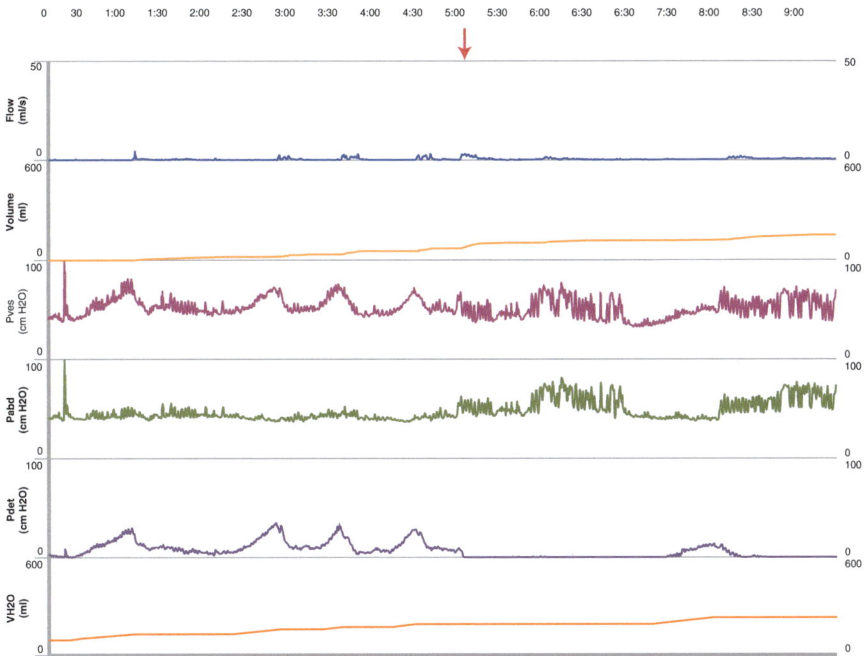

Fig. 16.11 Urodynamic tracing in an elderly male with combination of detrusor overactivity and impaired bladder emptying with no significant rise in detrusor pressure during voiding. This pattern is suggestive of DHIC. Permission to void denoted by *red arrow*

Urodynamics were performed as part of his investigation with a fill rate of 50 mL/s. He has phasic detrusor overactivity with small volume incontinence starting at 133 mL. MCC is estimated at 235 mL although may be less given his episodes of incontinence during the filling phase.

After permission (denoted by red arrow), he voided by straining with very a low-amplitude detrusor contraction. Flow curve is flattened and prolonged. PVR was 177 mL. This pattern is suggestive of detrusor hyperactivity impaired contractility and is consistent with his history.

The quality of this study is relatively poor. It could have been more appropriately zeroed so the P_{det} line would not be less than zero (negative) for the majority of the study. The clinician should have also decreased the rate to try to reduce the phasic detrusor contractions. Another flaw with this tracing is that the initial filling cystometrogram is missing. The interpreter recognizes this as the instilled volume does not start at zero.

Management of this patient is challenging as his predominant complaint is due to urgency/urge incontinence but he also empties his bladder very poorly. A TURP may not provide significant symptom relief in this setting, and generally should be avoided. Having failed medical management of urge incontinence, onabotulinumtoxinA injections could be considered and may be of some benefit to reduce his overactivity and leakage, though he would very likely require intermittent catheterization after such a treatment.

Valsalva Voiding

Valsalva voiding typically refers to the presence of straining or "muscular effort to initiate, maintain or improve the urinary stream [13]." Some series have further specified that valsalva voiding occurs when detrusor pressure (P_{det}) at time of bladder contraction is ≤ 10–15 cm H_2O when accompanied by abdominal straining to initiate micturition [32–34]. The flow pattern on uroflowmetry has a sawtooth pattern with a corresponding sawtooth pattern in the abdominal (P_{abd}) and vesical (P_{ves}) pressure tracers. Urodynamic studies of men with post-prostatectomy incontinence have found valsalva voiding in 30–53 % [35–37]. Valsalva voiding may occur in conjunction with BOO, detrusor underactivity, SUI, post-prostatectomy incontinence, and even in normal individuals [38]. In series of SUI females undergoing urodynamics preoperatively, 12–30 % had valsalva voiding [32, 34].

Clinical scenario 12 (Fig. 16.12):

Post-prostatectomy valsalva voider

A 63-year-old man post-radical prostatectomy complains of stress urinary incontinence and prolonged, weak stream. He does not have any UTIs. His PSA remains undetectable. Cystoscopy shows no bladder neck contracture.

He was assessed for SUI which was present at several points during filling (denoted by first arrow). His compliance appears to decrease slightly at the end of fill. He also has a low-amplitude detrusor contraction with urge incontinence at the

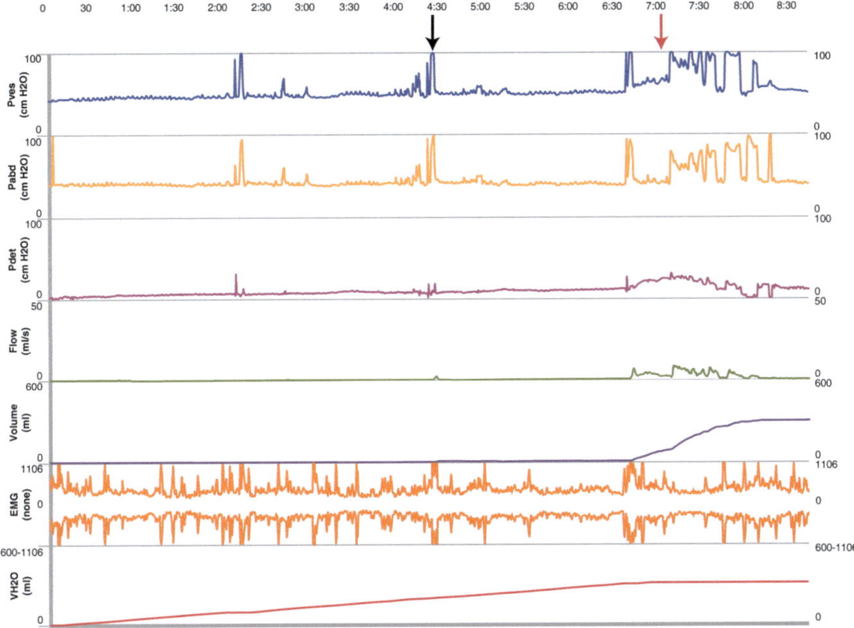

Fig. 16.12 Urodynamic tracing in a male who urinates with a valsalva voiding pattern. Stress urinary incontinence denoted by *black arrow*. Permission to void denoted by *red arrow*

end of fill (perhaps induced by valsalva). He then valsalva voids to empty his bladder (denoted by second arrow). This sawtooth pattern in P_{abd} and P_{ves} with an intermittent flow is characteristic of the valsalva voiding pattern. He voids to completion with no PVR. The quality of this tracing is good, free from significant artifact.

Clinical scenario 13 (Fig. 16.13):

Female who strains to empty

A 53-year-old female complains of frequency, a weak stream, and sensation of incomplete emptying. She has had a hysterectomy but denies other surgery. She denies history of UTIs or any known neurological disease.

Her urodynamics demonstrate first sensation at 99 mL. SUI was assessed and not demonstrated at 220 mL. Her MCC is slightly reduced at 272 mL. Compliance is normal. When she voids, she Valsalva voids with a characteristic sawtooth pattern. Her overall voiding time is prolonged and flow is intermittent. True P_{det} cannot be reliably assessed in the presence of valsalva voiding but it is clear that her detrusor pressures are not elevated. She voids 304 mL and does not have a PVR. EMG was not performed in this study. The quality of this study is adequate as it is nicely zeroed and free from significant artifact. The apparent and artifactual rises in detrusor pressure during voiding are a result of slightly unequal transmission in vesical and abdominal pressures (artifact).

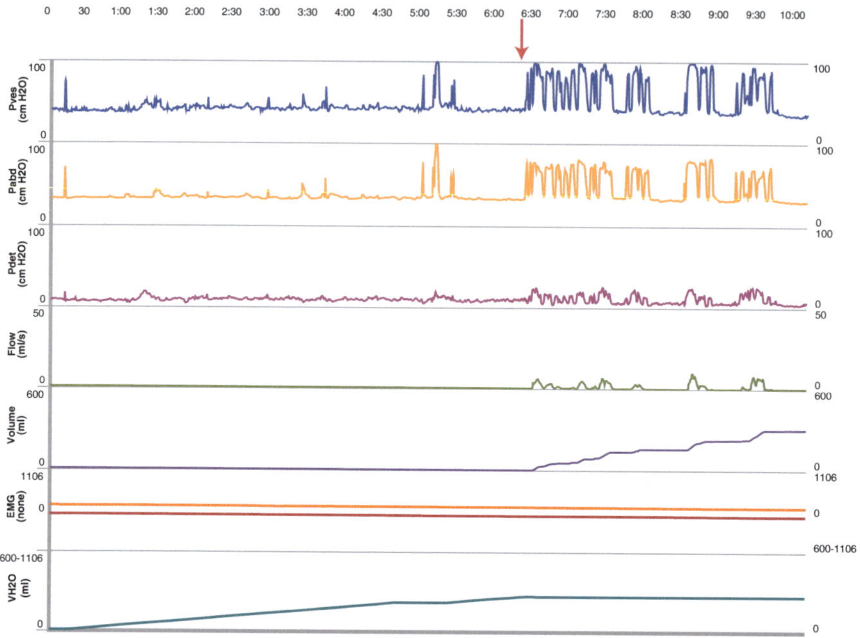

Fig. 16.13 Urodynamic tracing in a female with valsalva voiding. Note the characteristic saw-tooth pattern in P_{abd} and P_{ves}. Permission to void denoted by *red arrow*.

Voiding Dysfunction and Pelvic Floor Dysfunction

Voiding dysfunction secondary to pelvic floor dysfunction (PFD) (also referred to as dysfunctional voiding) can affect both men and women. Its exact incidence is unknown but is estimated to affect at least 2 % of adults [39]. It may manifest by symptoms of urgency, frequency, hesitancy, weak or intermittent stream, incomplete emptying, double voiding, incontinence, dysuria, constipation, and even recurrent urinary tract infections [39, 40]. Although dysfunctional voiding is most commonly seen in children, a number of patients with a long standing history of mixed lower urinary tract symptoms may not be diagnosed until adulthood [39–41]. PFD is thought to be a learned behavior which may date back to childhood toilet training [39, 40]. It can occur in combination with defecatory dysfunction/constipation, pelvic or genital pain, and sexual dysfunction [42]. Neurologic causes of dysfunctional voiding should often be excluded in patients given this diagnosis. Adults with dysfunctional voiding tend to have predominantly obstructive and irritative LUTS compared to children who more frequently present with recurrent UTI and incontinence [39].

The International Continence Society has attempted to standardize terminology and defined dysfunctional voiding as "an intermittent and/or fluctuating flow rate due to involuntary intermittent contractions of the peri-urethral striated muscle during voiding in neurologically normal individuals" [13, 43, 44]. Clues suggestive of dysfunctional voiding based on a clinical history of LUTS may include difficulty urinating in public places, needing special techniques to relax or concentrate in order to urinate, listening to running water or touching the genitalia to prompt voiding; intermittent voiding pattern on non-invasive flow; and free of neurologic or anatomic causes for voiding abnormality [39, 45]. In patients with dysfunctional voiding, the external urinary sphincter may contract during voiding on EMG or during fluoroscopy generally as a sign that the pelvic floor is non-relaxing. Unlike neurogenic patients who have true detrusor-external sphincter dyssynergia (DESD), EMG activity of the external urethral sphincter in non-neurogenic patients decreases just prior to the detrusor contraction followed by an increased EMG activity during detrusor contraction [39]. Behavior modification, physical therapy using techniques such as myofascial release or pelvic floor biofeedback and addressing other symptoms such as constipation may help alleviate symptoms [46]. Hinman's syndrome (non-neurogenic neurogenic bladder) is a severe form of dysfunctional voiding in which the external urinary sphincter contracts during voiding. It is usually diagnosed in childhood and if unrecognized, can result in a severely trabeculated, decompensated bladder and irreparable upper tract damage [39].

Fowler's Syndrome

Fowler's syndrome is a special category of voiding dysfunction characterized by urinary retention and abnormal inability of external urinary sphincter relaxation in young women without neurologic disease or clear attributable cause [47, 48]. This condition has most often been reported in women under 30 years of age with development of urinary retention of nearly or greater than 1 L urine without a strong urge to urinate [47–49]. The condition is diagnosed by needle electromyogram (EMG) of the external urinary sphincter which demonstrates repetitive complex discharges and decelerating bursts of EMG activity during voiding. Increased urethral closure pressure is also often seen [47]. The underlying etiology of Fowler's syndrome is unclear [48, 50]. A current hypothesized cause of Fowler's syndrome is a "hormone-sensitive channelopathy" resulting in increased activity of the external urethral sphincter [47]. Nearly 50 % of Fowler's syndrome patients also have polycystic ovaries [47, 49, 51]. Neurologic examination and investigation including MRI of the central nervous system is unremarkable. Attempts to identify predisposing psychological factors have been inconclusive [50]. In roughly 70 % of patients, the first episode of urinary retention may occur following a surgical procedure.

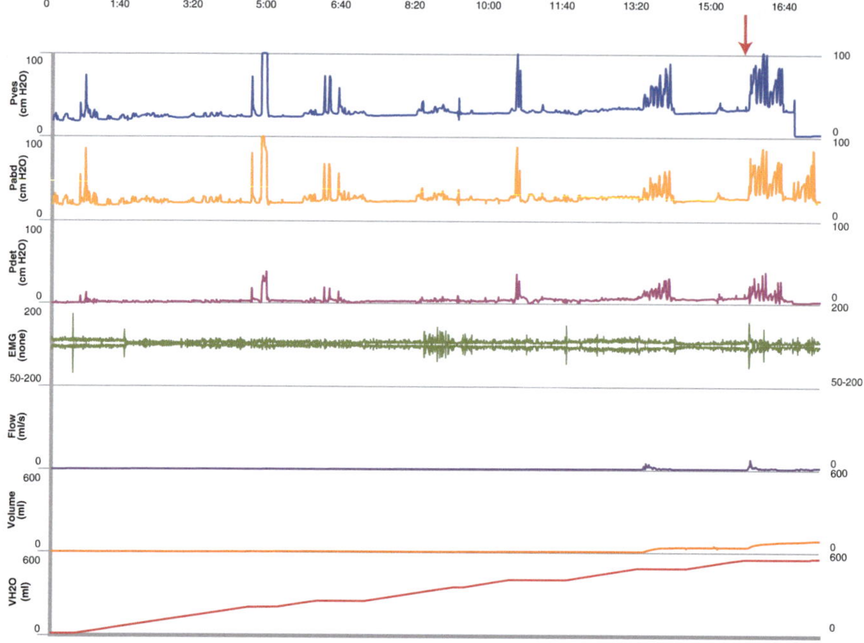

Fig. 16.14 Urodynamic tracing in a female with dysfunctional voiding. Note the presence of abdominal straining, elevated post-void residual, and increased EMG activity. It is not possible to determine if the increased EMG activity is due to the artifact of straining or due to pelvic floor contraction. Permission to void denoted by *red arrow*

Clinical scenario 14 (Fig. 16.14):

Difficulty voiding in female

A 28-year-old female noted to be in urinary retention of 1,500 mL 3 days after non-GU related surgery. She has no known neurological disease or symptoms. Her urodynamics demonstrated a MCC of 600 mL. She had normal compliance. She attempted to void (at red arrow) by abdominal straining and was unsuccessful leaving significant post-void residual. There was increased EMG activity in her attempts to void which could be either due to her straining or inadvertent recruitment of her pelvic floor muscles.

In patients who do not spontaneously recover their ability to void after first initiating intermittent catheterization, sacral neuromodulation can be offered. Women with urinary retention and diagnosis of Fowler's syndrome may have a higher likelihood of success with sacral neuromodulation compared to females retention [50]. Treatment of Fowler's syndrome using medications and onabotulinum toxin A injection has been largely unsuccessful [50].

Conclusion

Bladder contractility is a measure of detrusor muscle contractile strength and it can be affected by a variety of factors. Urodynamics is the only established tool used to evaluate bladder contractility and thus the overall bladder function. During assessment of the bladder contractility, flow rate must also be taken into consideration as outlet resistance can greatly affect bladder contractility. Understanding the relationship between bladder contractility and outlet resistance relation is of paramount importance. A careful analysis of the urodynamic tracing along with a thorough understanding of the clinical scenario can aid tremendously in a better understanding of the pathophysiology and help guide treatment recommendations.

References

1. Sullivan M, Yalla S. Functional studies to assess bladder contractility. J Urol Urogynakol. 2007;14(1):7–10.
2. Tan T, et al. Stop test or pressure-flow study? Measuring detrusor contractility in older females. Neurourol Urodyn. 2004;23:184–9.
3. Abrams P. Bladder outlet obstruction index, bladder contractility index, and bladder voiding efficiency: three simple indices to define bladder voiding function. BJU Int. 1999;84:14–5.
4. Gerstenberg TC, et al. High flow infravesical obstruction in men: symptomatology, urodynamics and the results of surgery. J Urol. 1982;127(5):943–5.
5. Griffiths C, Rix D, Macdonald A. Noninvasive measurement of bladder pressure by controlled inflation of a penile cuff. J Urol. 2002;167:1344–7.
6. Griffiths D. Detrusor contractility: order out of chaos. Scand J Urol Nephrol Suppl. 2004; 215:93–100.
7. Griffiths D, Constantinou C, Van Mastriqt R. Urinary bladder function and its control in healthy females. Am J Physiol. 1986;251:R225–30.
8. Sekido N. Bladder contractility and urethral resistance relation: what does a pressure-flow study tell us? Int J Urol. 2012;19:216–28.
9. Seki N, et al. Voiding dynamics in women with stress urinary incontinence and high-stage cystocele. Int J Urol. 2011;18(3):219–24.
10. Cucchi A, et al. Urodynamic findings suggesting two-stage development of idiopathic detrusor underactivity in adult men. Urology. 2007;70:75–9.
11. Cucchi A, Quaglini S, Rovereto B. Development of idiopathic detrusor underactivity in women: from isolated decrease in contraction velocity to obvious impairment of voiding function. Urology. 2008;71:844–8.
12. Schafer W. Analysis of bladder-outlet function with the linearized passive urethral resistance relation, linPURR, and a disease-specific approach for grading obstruction: from complex to simple. World J Urol. 1995;13:47–58.
13. Haylen B, et al. An International Urogynecological Association (IUGA)/International Continence Society (ICS) joint report on the terminology for female pelvic floor dysfunction. Neurourol Urodyn. 2010;29:4–20.
14. Maderbacher S, et al. The aging lower urinary tract: a comparative urodynamic study of men and women. Urology. 1998;51:206–12.
15. Gomes C, Arap S, Trigo-Rocha F. Voiding dysfunction and urodynamic abnormalities in elderly patients. Rev Hosp Clin Fac Med Sao Paulo. 2004;59:206–15.

16. Nordling J. The aging bladder: a significant but underestimated role in the development of lower urinary tract symptoms. Exp Gerontol. 2002;37:991–9.

17. Ababanel J, Marcus E-L. Impaired detrusor contractility in community-dwelling elderly presenting with lower urinary tract symptoms. Urology. 2007;69:436–40.

18. Prieto C, Sanchez D, Salinas C. Effect of aging on detrusor function in males. Arch Esp Urol. 1997;50:579–83.

19. Taylor J, Kuchel G. Detrusor underactivity: clinical features and pathogenesis of an underdiagnosed geriatric condition. J Am Geriatr Soc. 2006;54:1920–32.

20. Elbadawi A, Yalla S, Resnick N. Structural basis of geriatric voiding dysfucntion. II. Aging detrusor normal versus impaired contractility. J Urol. 1993;150:1657–67.

21. Griffiths D, et al. Cerebral control of the lower urinary tract: how age-related changes might predispose to urge incontinence. Neuroimage. 2009;47:981–6.

22. Anderssen K-E. Detrusor underactivity/underactive bladder: new research initiatives needed. J Urol. 2010;184:1829–30.

23. Krishnamoorthy S, Kekre N. Detrusor underactivity: to tone or not to tone the bladder? Indian J Urol. 2009;25:407–8.

24. Barendrecht M, et al. Is the use of parasympathomimetics for treating underactive urinary bladder evidence-based? BJU Int. 2007;99:749–52.

25. Ou R, et al. Urodynamically diagnosed detrusor hypocontractility: should transurethral resection of the prostate be contraindicated. Int Urol Nephrol. 2012;44:35–9.

26. Han D, et al. The efficacy of transurethral resection of the prostate in patients with weak bladder contractility index. Urology. 2008;71:657–61.

27. Ginsberg D. Bladder acontractility: detrusor myoplasty and other options. Nat Rev Urol. 2011;8:185–6.

28. Lombardi G, et al. Clinical efficacy of intravesical electrostimulation on incomplete spinal cord patients suffering from chronic neurogenic non-obstructive retention: a 15 year single centre retrospective study. Spinal Cord. 2013;51:232–7.

29. Resnick N, Yalla S. Detrusor hyperactivity with impaired contractile function. JAMA. 1987;257:2076–3081.

30. Yalla S, Sullivan M, Resnick N. Update on detrusor hyperactivity with impaired contractility. Curr Bladder Dysfunct Rep. 2007;2:191–6.

31. Lui S, Chan L, Tse V. Clinical outcome in patients with detrusor hyperactivity with impaired contractility (DHIC). BJU Int. 2011;107(supp):7.

32. Miller E, et al. Preoperative urodynamic function may predict voiding dysfunction in women undergoing pubovaginal sling. J Urol. 2003;169:2234–7.

33. Bhatia N, Bergeman A. Urodynamic predictability of voiding following incontinence surgery. Obstet Gynecol. 1984;63:85–91.

34. Pham K, et al. Preoperative Valsalva voiding increases the risk of urinary retention after midurethral sling placement. Int Urogynecol J. 2010;21:1243.

35. Chao R, Mayo M. Incontinence after radical prostatectomy: detrusor or sphincter causes. J Urol. 1995;154:16–8.

36. Han J, et al. Treatment of post-prostatectomy incontinence with male slings in patient with impaired detrusor contractility on urodynamics and/or who perform valsalva voiding. J Urol. 2011;185:1370–5.

37. Gomha M, Boone T. Voiding patterns in patients with post-prostatectomy incontinence: urodynamic and demographic analysis. J Urol. 2003;169:1766–9.

38. Miller E. Physiology of the lower urinary tract. Urol Clin North Am. 1996;23:171–6.

39. Groutz A, et al. Learned voiding dysfunction (Non-neurogenic, neurogenic bladder) among adults. Neurourol Urodyn. 2001;20:259–68.

40. Carlson K, Rome S, Nitti V. Dysfunctional voiding in women. J Urol. 2001;165:143–8.

41. Bower W, et al. Assessment of non-neurogenic incontinence and lower urinary tract symptoms in adolescents and young adults. Neurourol Urodyn. 2010;29:702–7.

42. Wang Y-C, Hart D, Mioduski J. Characteristics of patients seeking outpatient rehabilitation for pelvic-dysfunction. Phys Ther. 2012;92:1160–74.

43. Rosier P, et al. Developing evidence-based standards for diagnosis and management of lower urinary tract or pelvic floor dysfunction. Neurourol Urodyn. 2012;31:621–4.
44. Abrams P, et al. The standardisation of terminology in the lower urinary tract: report from the Standardisation Sub-Committee of the International Continence Society. Urology. 2003;61(1): 37–49.
45. Groutz A, Blavais J. Non-neurogenic female voiding dysfunction. Curr Opin Urol. 2002;12: 311–6.
46. Adelowo A, et al. Do symptoms of voiding dysfunction predict urinary retention? Female Pelvic Med Reconstr Surg. 2012;18:344–7.
47. DasGupta R, Fowler C. The management of female voiding dysfunction: Fowler's syndrome— a contemporary update. Curr Opin Urol. 2003;13:293–9.
48. Kavia R, et al. Urinary retention in women: its causes and management. BJU Int. 2006; 97:281–7.
49. Yande S, Joshi M. Bladder outlet obstruction in women. J Midlife Health. 2011;2:11–7.
50. De Ridder D, Ost D, Bruyninckx F. The presence of Fowler's syndrome predicts successful long-term outcome of sacral nerve stimulation in women with urinary retention. Eur Urol. 2007;51:229–34.
51. Fowler C, et al. Abnormal electromyographic activity of the urethral sphincter, voiding dysfunction, and polycystic ovaries: a new syndrome? BMJ. 1988;297:1436–8.

Chapter 17
Bladder Emptying:
Coordination of Bladder and Sphincters

Cory Harris, Philip P. Smith, and Angelo E. Gousse

Introduction

In order to accurately interpret an urodynamics study one must have a fundamental knowledge of the normal micturition cycle and the complex but intuitive coordination of urinary sphincters. The micturition cycle is composed of two phases (1) the bladder filling/urinary storage phase and (2) the voiding phase. Micturition is controlled by multiple reflex pathways that coordinate urethral and bladder function. These pathways maintain a reciprocal relationship between the urinary bladder and the urethral outlet. In general, bladder filling is under sympathetic control with increased sympathetic activity to the bladder neck and pudendal innervations to the external urinary sphincter (EUS). This activity negates parasympathetic input to the bladder and inhibits detrusor contraction. Voiding is normally accomplished by activation of the micturition reflex—which is the result of de-suppression of the pontine micturition center (PMC). During bladder filling, neurons within the PMC are turned off. However, at a critical level of bladder distention, the afferent activity

C. Harris, MD (✉)
Department of Urology, Memorial Hospital Miramar, South Broward Hospital District,
1951 SW 172 Avenue, Suite 305, Miramar, FL 33019, USA
e-mail: Cdharris07@gmail.com

P.P. Smith, MD
Department of Surgery, University of Connecticut Health Center, Farmington,
CT 06030, USA

Department of Urology, Connecticut Children's Medical Center, Hartford, CT 06106, USA

Center on Aging, University of Connecticut Health Center, Farmington, CT 06030, USA

A.E. Gousse, MD
Herbert Wertheim College of Medicine, Florida International University,
Memorial Hospital Miramar, South Broward Hospital District,
1951 SW 172 Avenue, Suite 305, Miramar, FL 33019, USA

© Springer Science+Business Media New York 2015
E.S. Rovner, M.E. Koski (eds.), *Rapid and Practical Interpretation
of Urodynamics*, DOI 10.1007/978-1-4939-1764-8_17

arising from the volume transduction process is sufficient to breach consciousness, resulting in the desire to urinate. A socially appropriate situation is sought, and at this point suppression of the PMC is released, thereby turning on the "hardwired" voiding reflex [1]. This reflex results in relaxation of the external urethral sphincter, contraction of the bladder due to parasympathetic stimulation with inhibition of sympathetic input, and suppression of the sacral guarding reflex. This same pattern of activity is elicited at lower, subthreshold volumes with voluntary voiding, a unique example of conscious control over an autonomic-mediated visceral process.

One is able to assess these concepts on urodynamics. During bladder filling, there is a gradual increase in sphincter electromyogram (EMG) activity. The voiding phase commences during urodynamics once permission is given to void. Once permission is given, just prior to voiding, the first recorded event is a sudden and complete relaxation of the striated sphincteric muscles, characterized by complete electrical silence of the EMG [2]. This is followed almost immediately by a rise in detrusor pressure as the bladder and proximal urethra become isobaric. The vesical neck and urethra open and voiding ensues. If a person wants to stop in the midst of voiding or to prevent voiding during an involuntary detrusor contraction, he or she contracts the striated sphincter, interrupting the stream and then, through a reflex mechanism, the detrusor contraction abates. The sphincter complex is also coordinated during sudden increases in abdominal pressure. During coughing or Valsalva maneuvers there is a reflex contraction of the sphincter manifested as an increase in EMG activity (Fig. 17.1).

Notice in Fig. 17.1, as bladder filling occurs EMG activity increases (increased somatic innervation to external sphincter) at the line annotated as "strong desire." Once the patient is given the command, permission to void (line titled "void"), EMG activity diminishes, a detrusor contraction is generated and voiding ensues (Fig. 17.2).

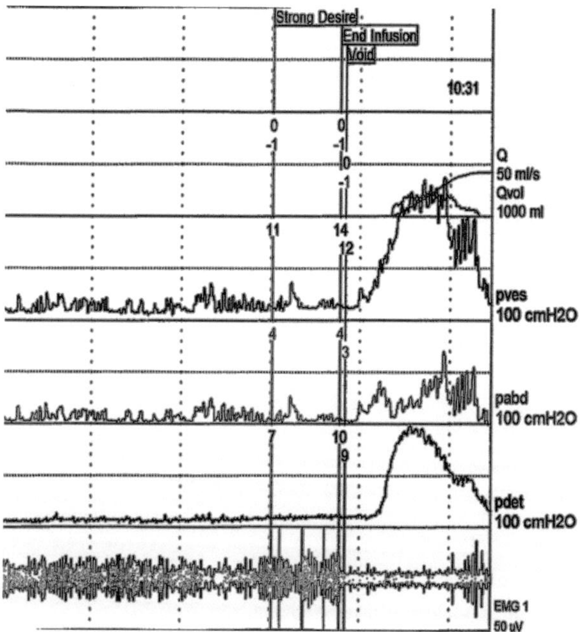

Fig. 17.1 Normal voiding pattern

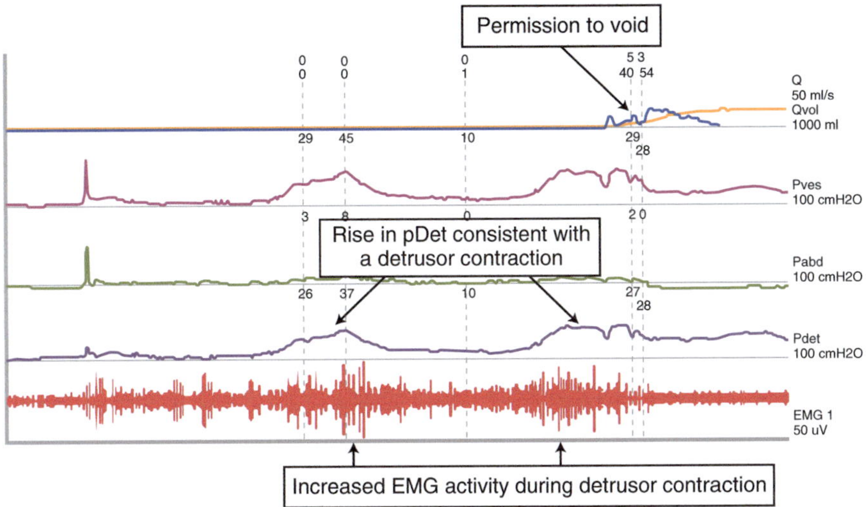

Fig. 17.2 Voluntary contraction of EUS

In Fig. 17.2 there is increased EMG activity during an involuntary detrusor contraction. Ordinarily the sphincter complex relaxes resulting in EMG quieting prior
to voiding. In some cases it is normal to see increased EMG activity during detrusor
contraction. Contracting the external sphincter (Kegels) during episodes of urgency
helps to suppress the detrusor contraction by decreasing parasympathetic activity to
the bladder. Once this happens, the detrusor contraction abates and urgency is
relieved. In Fig. 17.2, notice the increase in EMG activity during an involuntary
detrusor contraction. This results in increased urethral resistance with preserved
continence and the detrusor contraction is abated and filling continues until the next
involuntary detrusor contraction at which point contraction of pelvic floor occurs
again. In this scenario, sphincter contraction during detrusor contraction is a normal
response, however, in other situations this process can represent pathology.

Figure 17.3a, b was taken during the voiding phase of an urodynamics study
evaluating a 13-year-old female with persistent daytime and nighttime incontinence.
She has a history of chronic constipation and holding her urine. The patient's symptoms worsened with puberty. Patient is neurologically normal with no evidence of
occult spinal dysraphism on exam.

During this study, once the patient was given permission to void there is evidence
of increased EMG activity during voluntary detrusor contraction resulting in inter-
mittency of urinary flow. Involuntary contraction of the external urethral sphincter
during voiding in the absence of neurologic injury or disease is known as dysfunctional voiding. It has also been described as learned voiding dysfunction and by
some as non-neurogenic, neurogenic bladder [3]. Dysfunctional voiding, as defined
by the International Continence Society (ICS), is an intermittent and/or fluctuating
flow rate due to involuntary intermittent contractions of the periurethral striated
muscle during voiding, in neurologically normal subjects [4]. It can be difficult to
diagnose using surface EMG electrodes because of other factors that can produce

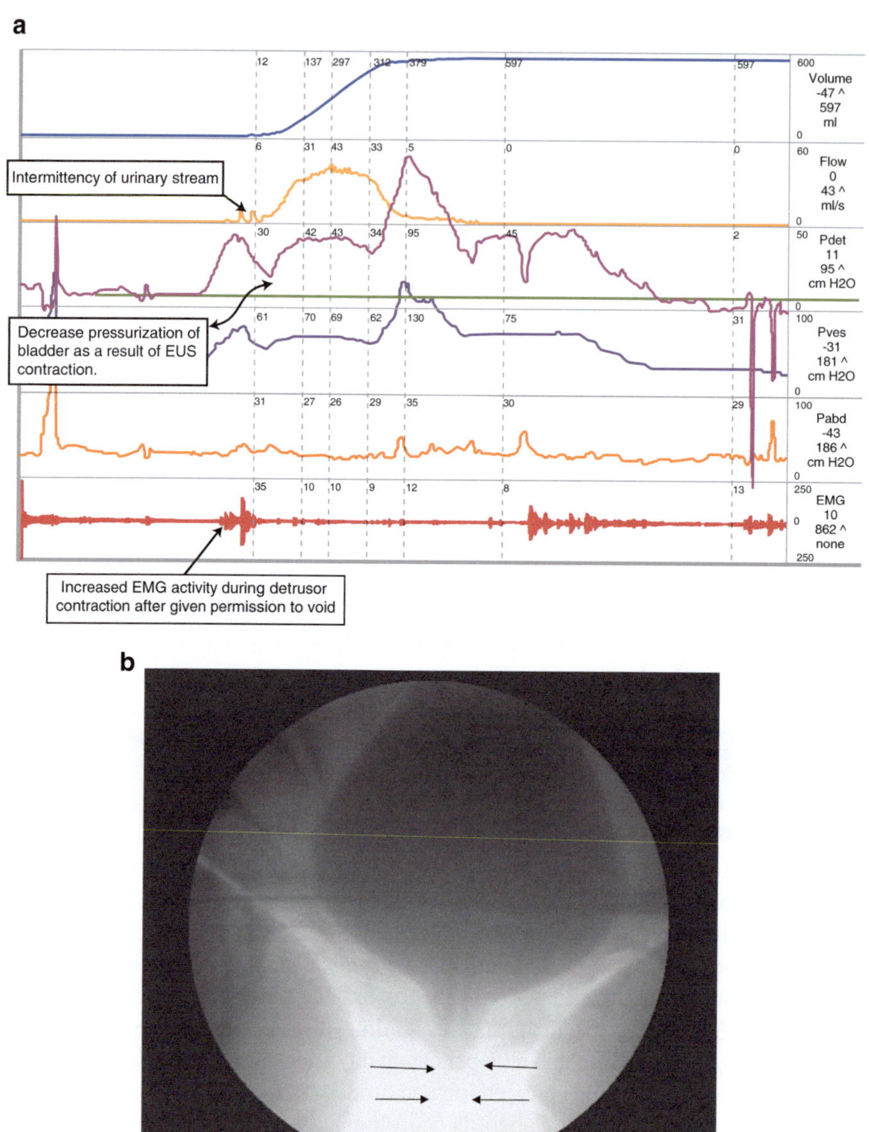

Fig. 17.3 (**a**) Increased EMG activity causing urethral obstruction. (**b**) Open bladder neck with poor flow past-urethral sphincter

increased EMG activity on a tracing, including attempts at augmenting bladder contractions by abdominal straining, movement, guarding reflex, and wet electrodes. Using fluoroscopy has proven invaluable in the diagnosis because one can see a dilation of the urethra to the level of the striated sphincter (spinning top urethra) and/or intermittent contractions of the striated sphincter. Figure 17.3b is the fluoroscopic image taken at time of EMG activation. As indicated by notched arrows the patient's bladder neck opens however there is minimal flow past EUS during this episode of sphincter activity (Fig. 17.3a, b).

The differences between the two studies are subtle but important. Once there is a conscious decision to void, the dominant reflex pathways are those responsible for bladder emptying. The fact that the patient's EUS complex activates during a conscious void is pathologic. The other difference is in Fig. 17.2 where there is a conscious contraction on the pelvic floor resulting in increased EMG activity (an adaptive mechanism to prevent incontinence) whereas in Fig. 17.3 this is a learned, involuntary activation of pelvic floor. One way to determine if increased EMG activity is voluntary versus involuntary is to simply ask to patient during event while the study is in progress (Fig. 17.4).

In Fig. 17.4, rises in abdominal pressure (as noted by notched horizontal arrows) are associated with increases in EMG activity (diagonal arrows). This is due in part by the guarding reflex. Increases in abdominal pressure lead to increased EMG activity to maintain continence in patients with an intact reflex arc.

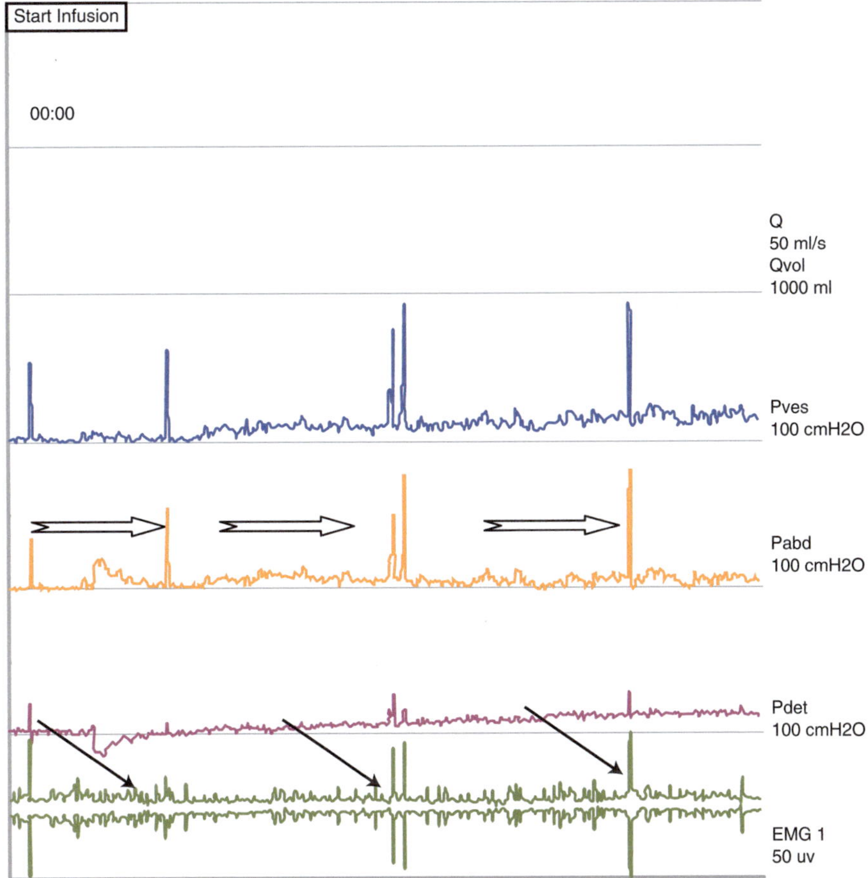

Fig. 17.4 Rise in EMG activity during increase in intra-abdominal pressure

Neurological conditions, lesions, or trauma can cause disturbances in urinary storage and voiding resulting in bladder dysfunction. Detrusor sphincter dyssynergia (DSD) is defined by the ICS as "the impaired coordination between detrusor and sphincter during voiding due to a neurologic abnormality (i.e., detrusor contraction synchronous with contraction of the urethral and/or periurethral striated muscles)" [4]. Neurological conditions more commonly resulting in DSD include: SCI, MS, spinal dysraphism and transverse myelitis. In the absence of a neurological abnormality, impaired coordination of bladder contraction and sphincter relaxation is more appropriately referred to as dysfunctional voiding or pelvic floor hyperactivity.

As noted previously, during normal voluntary micturition, once the threshold bladder distention is reached, PMC activation increases inhibiting spinal guarding reflexes and transmits excitatory signals to the bladder. The EUS relaxes with synergistic contraction of the detrusor as noted in Fig. 17.1.

DSD occurs in the setting of neurological abnormalities between the PMC and sacral spinal cord (Onuf's nucleus). This interruption is thought to result in failed inhibition of spinal guarding reflexes, and erroneous excitation of Onuf 's nucleus causing external urethral sphincter contraction to occur during detrusor contraction (Fig. 17.5).

Figure 17.5 is a tracing from a 34-year-old female with transverse myelitis. Notice the increased EMG activity during detrusor contraction. Diagnosis of DSD by EMG requires elevated EMG activity during detrusor contraction, in the absence of Valsalva and Crede maneuvers. These maneuvers would be detected as a rise in P_{abd}. Notice there is no rise in P_{abd}.

Figure 17.6a is a tracing from a 5-year-old male with a history of tethered cord who underwent urodynamics to assess voiding function. Notice with the rise in P_{abd} there is also increased EMG activity as discussed earlier. Also note during bladder contraction as noted by rise in P_{det} there is also increased EMG activity consistent with diagnosis of DSD (Fig. 17.6a, b).

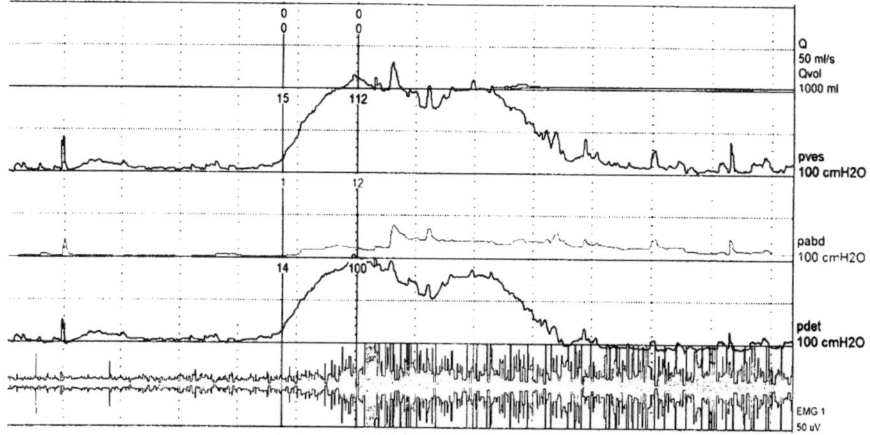

Fig. 17.5 Detrusor sphincter dyssynergia. An involuntary contraction of the striated sphincter that continues throughout the involuntary detrusor contraction

a

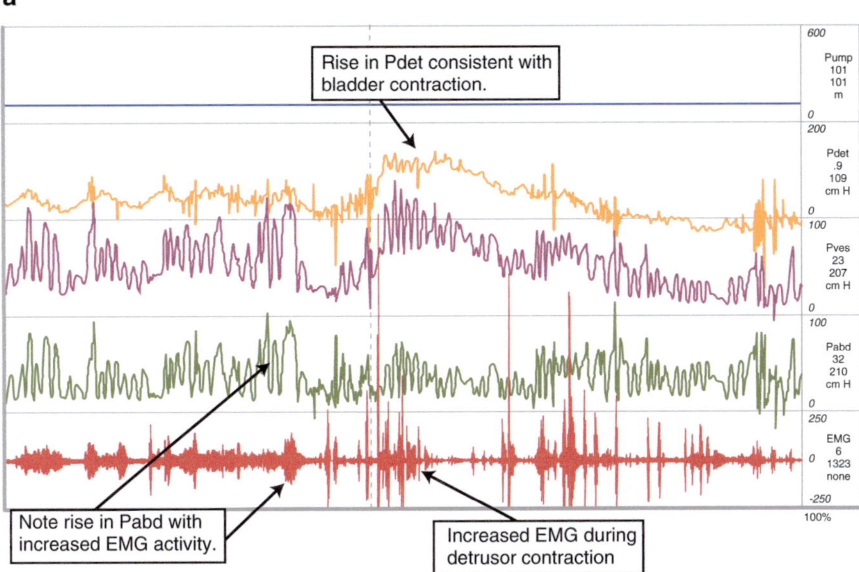

b

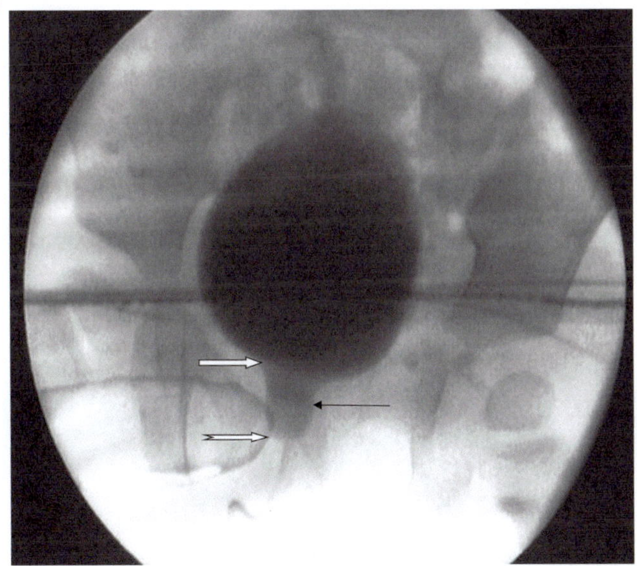

Fig. 17.6 (**a**) Increased EMG activity with Valsalva and during detrusor contraction. (**b**) X-ray image obtained at P_{detmax} revealing dilated posterior urethra and lack of contrast seen past area of sphincter consistent with diagnosis of DSD

In Fig. 17.6b, this patient has an open bladder neck (represented with solid white arrow) with a dilated posterior urethra (thin black arrow), however there is no contrast seen past the area of the EUS (notched white arrow). Pathology such as Parkinson's disease, dysfunctional voiding, and bladder outlet obstruction from urethral stricture and very rarely urethral atresia should be considered before the diagnosis of DESD, as they may have similar urodynamic findings.

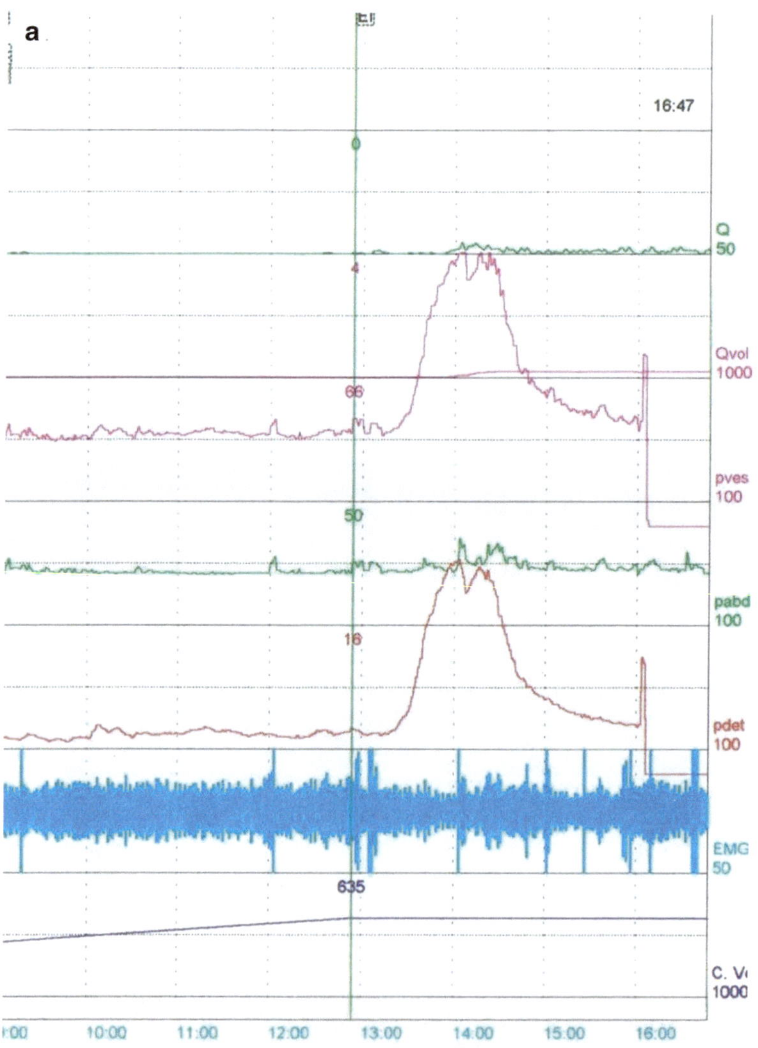

Fig. 17.7 (**a**) Urodynamic tracing of obstructive (high-pressure, low-flow) void pattern. (**b**) Fluoroscopic image during voiding phase demonstrating a closed bladder neck (*arrow*)

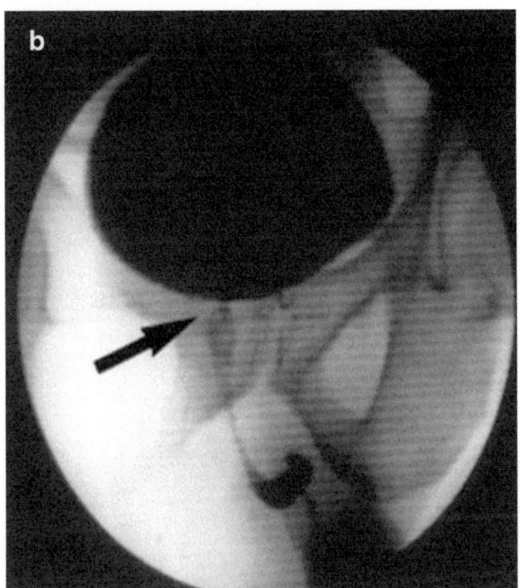

Fig. 17.7 (continued)

Primary Bladder Neck Obstruction

As was mentioned in the introduction, continence is maintained by both the bladder neck (or proximal sphincter), and the external urethral sphincter which is under sympathetic and pudendal control respectively. We have already discussed external sphincter pathology, and we will now review bladder neck pathology. In order to void successfully, the bladder neck must open. When the bladder neck fails to open adequately during voiding it results in obstruction to urinary flow (see Fig. 17.7a). In this tracing the patient clearly has an obstructed voiding pattern (high detrusor pressure with low urinary flow rate). This could be due to benign prostatic hyperplasia, urethral stricture or a variety of other pathologies in males. In females this tracing could represent obstruction from pelvic organ prolapse, urethral stricture, history of anti-incontinence surgery, or urethral diverticulum, among others. Notice there is no significant increase in EMG activity during void as seen in tracing with patient with DSD or dysfunctional voiding (the EMG only reflects changes in the EUS complex). In either sex, an important cause of these findings includes bladder neck obstruction: anatomic or functional (Fig. 17.7a).

The voiding phase of the micturition cycle is characterized by a coordinated decrease in outlet resistance, with opening of the bladder neck and relaxation of the EUS with a simultaneous increase in bladder pressure from detrusor contraction. The fluoroscopic image in Fig. 17.7b was taken during the voiding phase of the study. Notice there is no bladder neck funneling. The arrow demonstrates closed bladder neck.

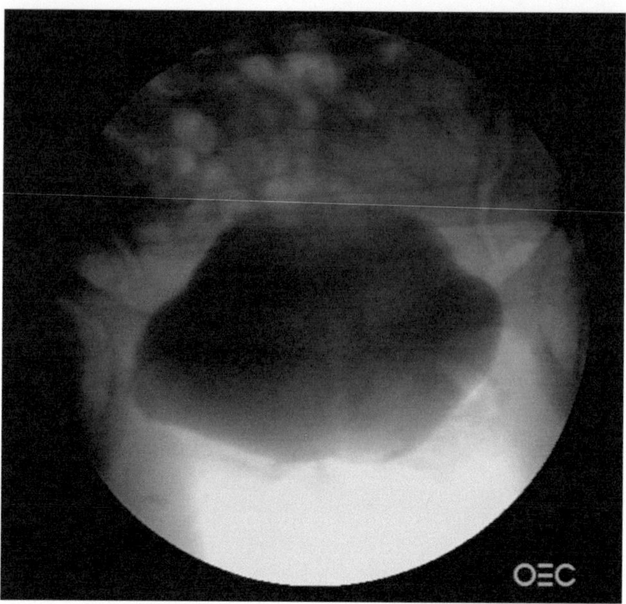

Fig. 17.8 Fluoroscopic image of closed bladder neck due to prior anti-incontinence procedure

These findings are consistent with diagnosis of primary bladder neck obstruction (PBNO). PBNO is a videourodynamic diagnosis, the hallmark of which is relative high-pressure, low-flow voiding with radiographic evidence of obstruction at the bladder neck with relaxation of the striated sphincter, and no evidence of distal obstruction [5]. Failure of the bladder neck to open with a detrusor contraction can only be diagnosed by simultaneous imaging of the bladder outlet during voiding. This process can be present in both women and men. The treatment options for men and women with PBNO are the same and include watchful waiting, pharmacotherapy with alpha-adrenergic blockade, or surgical intervention with endoscopic incision of bladder neck (Figs. 17.7b).

All urodynamics studies should be interpreted in context of the patient's history and physical. The tracing above is of 50-year-old female with irritative voiding symptoms after undergoing a mid-urethral sling for stress urinary incontinence. Although Figs. 17.7b and 17.8 have similar radiographic findings the etiology of these findings differs. The findings in Fig. 17.8 are likely related to the patient's history of anti-incontinence surgery resulting in obstruction at the bladder neck. The differential diagnosis of these findings includes bladder neck contracture from previous prostate surgery, urethral stricture, and enlarged prostate in male patients, as in Fig. 17.7b. In females, it includes prolapse repair with sub-urethral plication, history of anti-incontinence surgery and hyperactive pelvic floor as demonstrated in Fig. 17.8.

Figure 17.9 is a tracing from a 32-year-old nulliparous female with a 10-year history of frequency/urgency/urge incontinence. Prior efforts to treat "recurrent

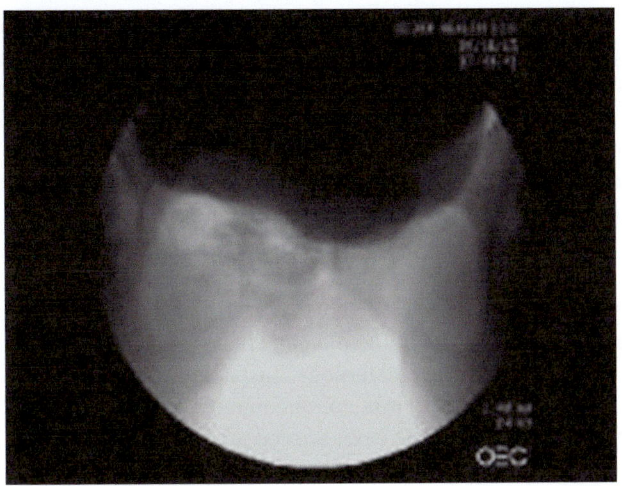

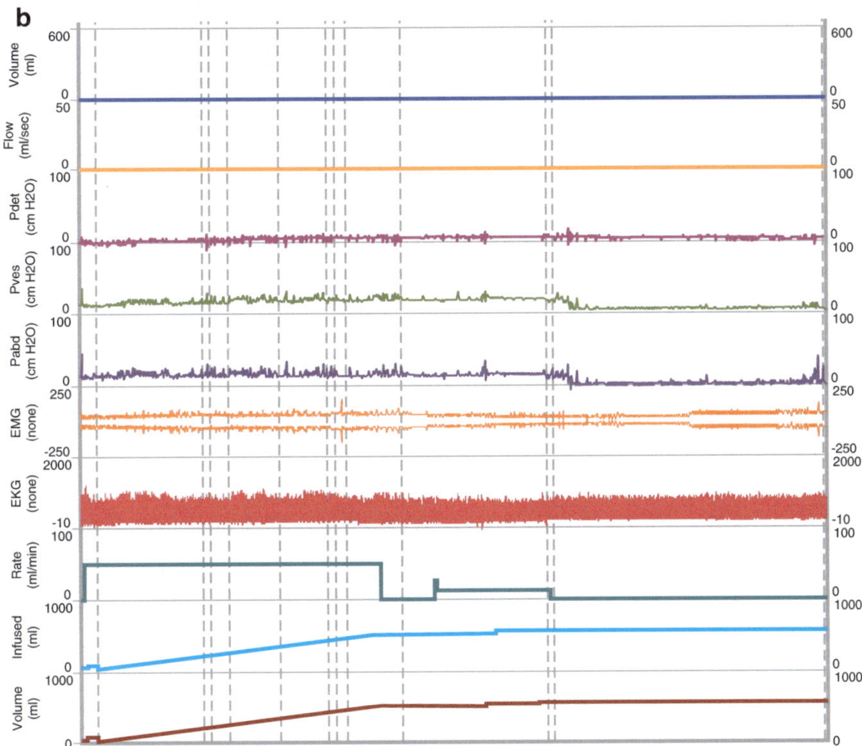

Fig. 17.9 (**a**) Radiographic image reveals closed bladder neck. (**b**) Urodynamic tracing demonstrating absence of detrusor or EMG activity during study

UTI" with antibiotics and irritative symptoms with antimuscarinics had not met with success. History was notable also for insertional dyspareunia preventing satisfactory intercourse. The patient is a college professor and an elite tri-athlete. Her examination was unremarkable other than a tense and tender pelvic floor that she was unable to noticeably relax once contracted, non-detectable bulbocavernosus reflex, and a normal neurologic examination. During the urodynamics study the patient was filled to supra-physiologic volumes and was unable to generate detrusor contraction under observation. There was no activation of EMG. The fluoroscopic images demonstrated a closed bladder neck throughout the study.

This study could have been labeled as non-diagnostic. However, evaluating this urodynamic study in context of the patient's history and exam points to symptoms revolving around pelvic floor pathology. In patients with pelvic floor symptoms due to poor muscular control, it is not uncommon to have difficulty voiding in an artificial environment. This has been termed a "bashful" or "shy" bladder. In this scenario, one must consider a diagnosis of detrusor underactivity.

The very fact that the patient is unable to void under observation, in conjunction with a consistent history and examination, leads to the potential diagnosis of pelvic floor dysfunction and the possibility therefore of an obstructive voiding dysfunction.

Normally, pre-conscious brain control areas prepare for the desire to void in response to increasing bladder afferent activity, in a process termed attentional biasing. The result of attentional biasing is normally a non-surprising and progressive desire to void. In this case, poor sensory function due to pelvic floor dysfunction may result in impaired biasing, resulting in a sudden and unexpected conscious emergence of the desire to void, creating the sensation of urgency [6].

Therapy in this case must be aimed at improving pelvic floor control and restoration of normal bladder volume sensations. Pelvic floor physical therapy and/or neuromodulation have had some benefit [7, 8].

References

1. Wein AJ, Novick AC, Alan P, Craig P, Kavoussi LR. Physiology and pharmacology of bladder and urethra. In: Campbell-Walsh urology. Philadelphia: Saunders/Elsevier; 2012. Chapter 60.
2. Blaivas J, et al. Atlas of urodynamics. 2nd ed. Malden: Blackwell Publishing; 1997. p. 11.
3. Hinman F. Nonneurogenic neurogenic bladder (the Hinman syndrome)—15 years later. J Urol. 1986;136:769–77.
4. Abrams P, Cardozo L, Fall M, et al. The standardisation of terminology of lower urinary tract function: report from the Standardisation Subcommittee of the International Continence Society. Neurourol Urodyn. 2002;21:167–78.
5. Nitti VW, Tu LM, Gitlin J. Diagnosing bladder outlet obstruction in women. J Urol. 1999;161:1535–40.
6. Smith PP, Wolfson LI, Kuchel GA, The Neurourology of Urinary Symptoms in Older Adults, Virtual Editions BJUI Online, BJU International, 2011 http://www.bjui.org/ContentFullItem.aspx?id=665&LinkTypeID=1&SectionType=1&title=The-Neurourology-of-Urinary-Symptoms-in-Older-Adults, DOI 10.1002/BJUIw-2011-010-web
7. Fitz F, Resnde A, Stupp L, et al. Biofeedback for the treatment of female pelvic floor muscle dysfunction: a systematic review and meta-analysis. Int Urogynecol J. 2012;23:1495–516.
8. Siegel S, et al. Sacral nerve stimulation for voiding dysfunction: one institution's 11-year experience. Neurourol Urodyn. 2007;26:19–28.

Chapter 18
Bladder Emptying: Complete Emptying

Alexander Gomelsky and Melissa R. Kaufman

Introduction

While the bladder may be considered by some to be an "unreliable witness [1]," its functions in the big picture are relatively straightforward. The bladder must complete two functions: the storage and emptying of urine. In reality, the ability to complete these tasks safely and efficiently requires the intimate coordination of numerous organs, supporting structures, and neurotransmitters, the description of which is far beyond the confines of this chapter. The goal of this chapter will be to focus on the emptying phase and what steps constitute complete emptying. The chapter will also illustrate some examples of incomplete emptying, their pathophysiology, and potential implications for the patient.

What Is Complete Emptying?

Interestingly, little information can be located regarding the exact definition of "complete emptying." This particular term is not covered in The Standardisation of Terminology of Lower Urinary Tract Function [2]; however, the "feeling of incomplete emptying" is mentioned as one of the post-micturition symptoms. It is described as "self-explanatory" and no additional details are given. Despite the lack of specific definition, it can be safely inferred that any definition of

A. Gomelsky, MD (✉)
Department of Urology, Louisiana State University Health – Shreveport,
1501 Kings Highway, Shreveport, LA 71130, USA
e-mail: agomel@lsuhsc.edu

M.R. Kaufman, MD, PhD
Department of Urologic Surgery, Vanderbilt University Medical Center, Nashville, TN, USA

© Springer Science+Business Media New York 2015
E.S. Rovner, M.E. Koski (eds.), *Rapid and Practical Interpretation of Urodynamics*, DOI 10.1007/978-1-4939-1764-8_18

"complete emptying" should include a low urinary post-void residual (PVR), defined as the volume of urine left in the bladder at the end of micturition [2]. Conversely, a high PVR typically indicates incomplete emptying.

It is important to note that an isolated elevated PVR is a poor surrogate for incomplete emptying. First, inhibition or attempts at emptying an incompletely full bladder may result in a high PVR. Second, the voided volume (VV) is often not taken into account (i.e., a large VV with an elevated PVR represents a different scenario than a small VV and elevated PVR). Third, PVR alone does not reflect the voiding mechanism (i.e., detrusor contraction, valsalva straining, pelvic relaxation) and any element of detrusor underactivity or bladder outlet obstruction (BOO). Thus, any examination of incomplete emptying should include not only the PVR, but also a measure of voiding such as a non-instrumented uroflowmetry (UF) or an intubated pressure-flow study (PFS).

What Constitutes an Elevated PVR?

Once again, a single definition does not exist. Huang et al. examined 987 women 55–75 years of age culled from a group health plan in Washington State, of whom 10 % had a PVR of 50–99 mL and 11 % had a PVR $\geq$ 100 mL at baseline [3]. In adjusted analyses, women with a PVR of $\geq$ 100 mL were more likely to report urinating more than eight times during the day and women with a PVR of $\geq$ 200 mL were more likely to report weekly urinary urgency incontinence (UUI) than those with a PVR $<$ 50 mL. High PVR was not associated with greater risk of stress urinary incontinence (SUI), nocturnal frequency, or urinary tract infection (UTI), indicating that many women with high PVR are asymptomatic. Similarly, the prevalence of elevated PVR ($\geq$ 100 mL) was 11 % in approximately 1,400 women with pelvic floor disorders undergoing evaluation at a large urogynecological referral center [4]. Symptoms alone did not predict which women had an elevated PVR, but the finding of prolapse at or beyond the hymen was associated with incomplete emptying. In another retrospective study, 15.9 % of 107 women with predominantly SUI and absence of previous pelvic surgery, advanced pelvic prolapse, and/or neurological deficit had a PVR $>$ 100 mL [5]. The prevalence of elevated PVR in the infirmed may be even higher. Tam et al. found that 22 % of 119 consecutive patients admitted into two convalescent wards were found to have a PVR $>$ 100 mL and in 9.2 % the PVR exceeded 400 mL [6]. There was an increased risk of UTI when the PVR exceeded 100 mL.

The definition of an elevated PVR in men is no clearer. Kolman et al. evaluated PVR in 477 randomly selected community-dwelling white men as part of a baseline urological evaluation and found that the distribution of PVR was highly skewed with a median of 9.5 mL and 25th and 75th percentiles equal to 2.5 mL and 35.4 mL, respectively [7]. There was a significant correlation of PVR with prostate volume and the odds of PVR $>$ 50 mL were 2.5 times greater for men with prostate volume greater than 30 mL than those with smaller prostates. In regression analyses PVR, did not appear to be associated with the AUA symptom index, age, or peak urinary flow rate. Men with enlarged prostate volume or PVR greater than 50 mL at baseline were about three times as likely to have subsequent acute urinary retention with catheterization during 3–4 years of follow-up.

Finally, the relationship between elevated PVR and urinary retention is likewise unclear [8]. In their review of MEDLINE literature, Kaplan et al. point out that the threshold for elevated PVR is often 100 mL, while the definitions of chronic urinary retention range widely in the literature (100–500 mL). Additionally, PVR does not seem to be a strong predictor of acute urinary retention. Furthermore, the authors conclude that there is no actual numerical value or relative increase in the volume of PVR that has been universally accepted or adopted into clinical practice. As such, the PVR measurement should act as a noninvasive screening test for evaluating voiding dysfunction. Taken with a good history, physical examination, and uroflowmetry, PVR measurement may aid in identifying patients in need of further evaluation and to evaluate treatment effect during follow-up.

Implications of Elevated PVR

Both an elevated PVR and urinary retention may be associated with some significant sequelae. Pelvic and suprapubic pain and pressure, as well as lower urinary tract symptoms (LUTS) such as urinary urgency and frequency may result from overdistention. Urinary stasis may result in UTIs and bladder calculi. Additionally, elevated intravesical pressure may result in hydroureteronephrosis, upper tract deterioration, and renal insufficiency. As mentioned previously, elevated PVRs may be caused by detrusor hypocontractility or acontractility, BOO, or, in rare cases, anatomic abnormalities such as large bladder diverticula. BOO can stem from an anatomic blockage (prostatic enlargement, urethral stricture, meatal stenosis) or a functional obstruction from poor sphincter relaxation (dyssynergia). Poor bladder contractility can result from neurogenic, myogenic, psychogenic, or pharmacologic causes.

Cases

Case 1: 61 years of man who presents with urinary retention

History: Patient voided small volumes with 2,200 mL PVR and subsequently placed on clean intermittent catheterization (CIC). He states he has always been a "slow voider" and denies urgency or UUI. He is otherwise healthy. DRE: >90 g benign prostate.

Course: Patient started on α-adrenergic antagonist (α-blocker) and 5-α reductase inhibitor (5-αRI) and CIC. He has been voiding on own with volumes 100–200 mL at a time. CIC volumes after volitional voiding are 100–150 mL.

Urodynamics (Fig. 18.1): Unable to perform pre-procedure UF; slightly decreased cystometric bladder capacity (~330 mL); no detrusor overactivity (DO); high

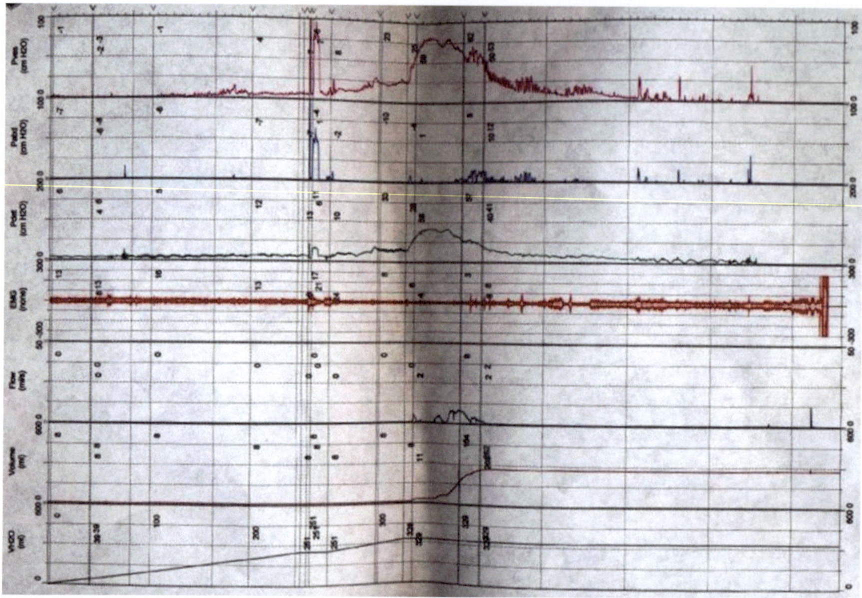

Fig. 18.1 CMG: slightly decreased cystometric bladder capacity (~330 mL); no DO; high compliance; no leak with valsalva maneuver; incomplete emptying on PFS with high-pressure, low-flow pattern ($P_{det}@Q_{max}=57$ cm H_2O); PVR$=115$ mL

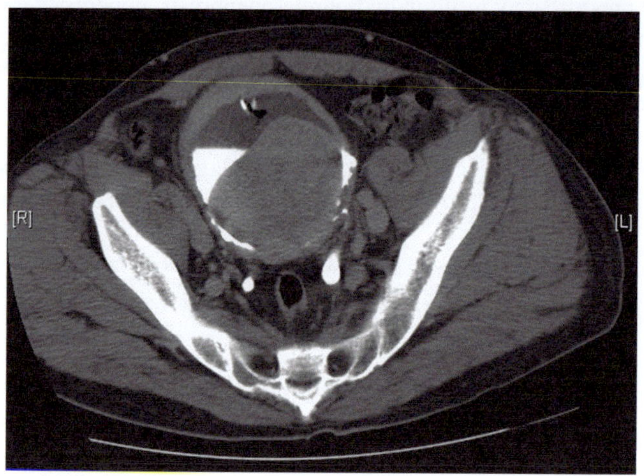

Fig. 18.2 CT: very large median lobe of the prostate

compliance; no leak with valsalva maneuver; incomplete emptying on PFS with high-pressure, low-flow pattern ($P_{det}@Q_{max}=57$ cm H_2O); PVR 115 mL.

Cystoscopy: Trilobar prostatic hypertrophy, very large median lobe, bladder trabeculations.

CT (for microscopic hematuria work-up): Very large median lobe (Fig. 18.2).

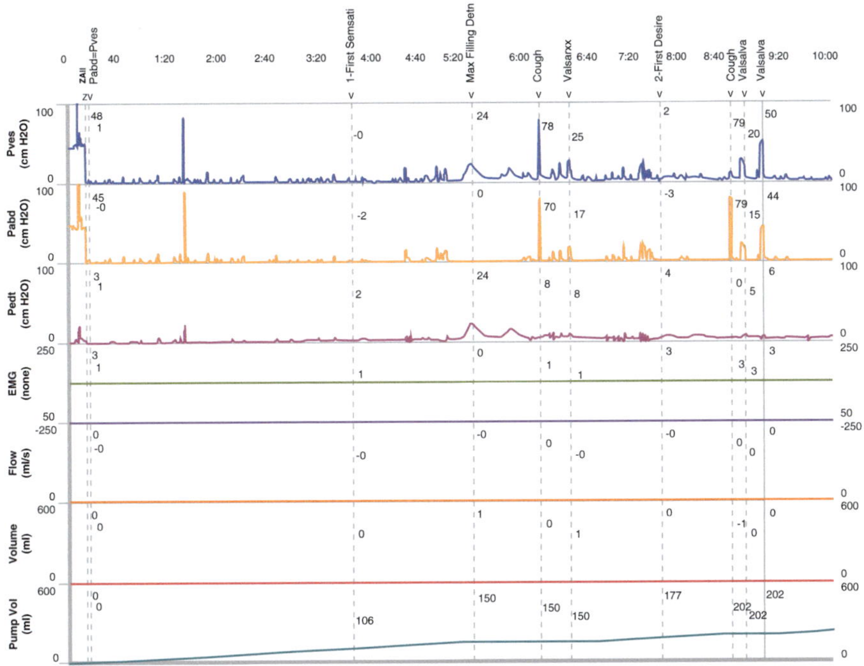

Fig. 18.3 CMG: first sensation at 106 mL; strong desire at 178 mL; cystometric bladder capacity at 247 mL; two episodes of DO at 150 mL of filling (pressures = 12–22 cm H_2O); both episodes associated with urgency but no leakage; high compliance; no leakage with cough or valsalva

Diagnosis: BOO due to benign prostatic obstruction (BPO).

Options: Continue α-blocker and 5-αRI, transurethral resection of prostate (TURP), suprapubic prostatectomy.

Commentary: This gentleman has clear evidence of BOO and options for relieving outlet resistance are effective in improving symptoms.

Case 2: 67 years of man presents for evaluation of UUI.

History: He complains of diurnal urgency, urinary frequency (10/day, 3/night), and UUI requiring 3–4 pads/24 h. He has subjective incomplete emptying. He denies weak stream or straining to urinate. DRE: 35 g benign prostate. The remainder of his history and exam are normal.

Course: Prostate specific antigen (PSA) is 0.45 ng/mL. Patient has been on dual therapy with α-blocker and 5-αRI for over a year and has also tried multiple muscarinic receptor antagonists (anticholinergics) in past without significant subjective improvement.

Urodynamics (Fig. 18.3): First sensation occurred at 106 mL, strong desire at 178 mL, and cystometric bladder capacity was 247 mL; Two episodes of DO at 150 mL of filling (pressures from 12 to 22 cm H_2O). Both were associated with urgency but no leakage; high compliance; no leakage with cough or valsalva; during PFS (Fig. 18.4), $P_{det}@Q_{max} = 65$ cm H_2O, $P_{detmax} = 84$ cm H_2O with a flow of 13.4 mL/s; Bladder Outlet Obstructive Index (BOOI) = 57.

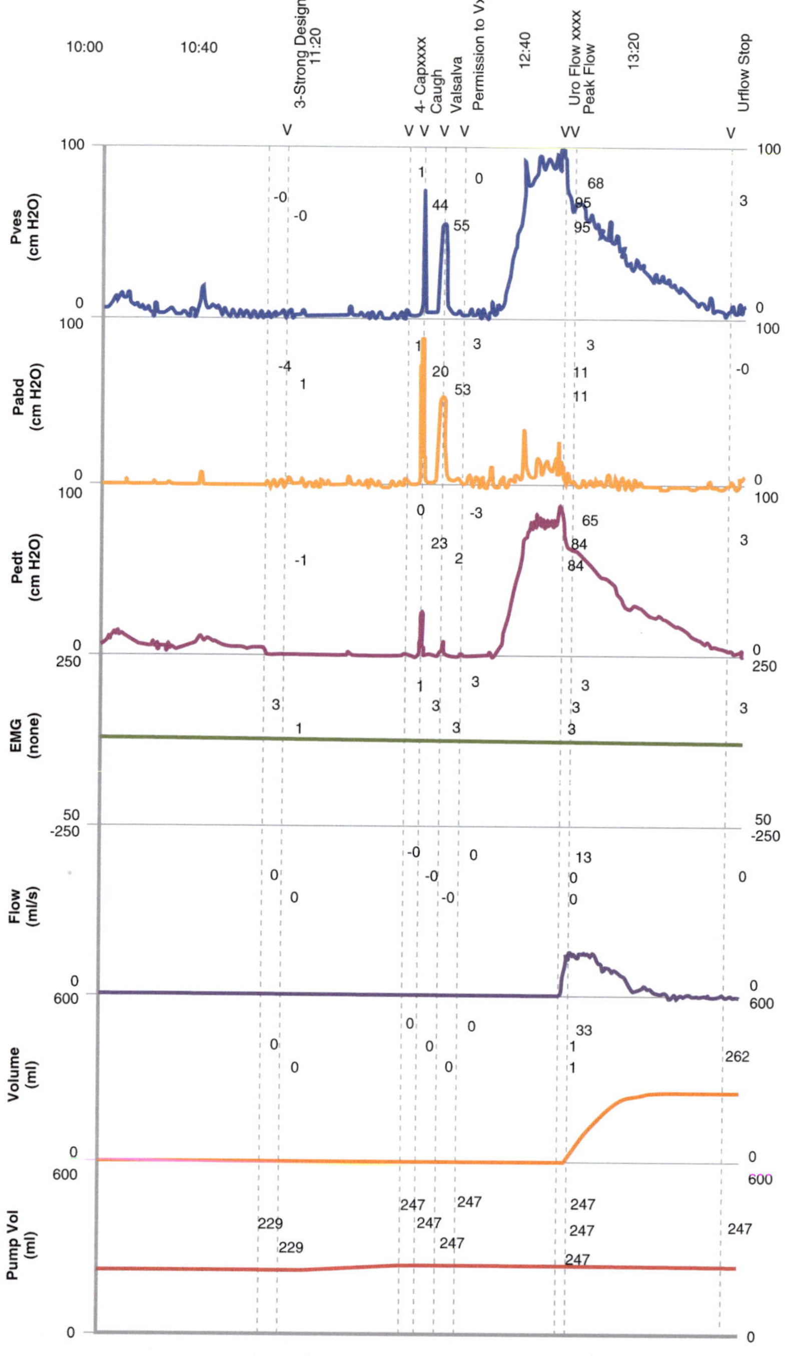

Fig. 18.4 PFS: P_{det} @ Q_{max} = 65 cm H$_2$O; P_{detmax} = 84 cm H$_2$O; flow = 13.4 mL/s; Bladder Outlet Obstructive Index (BOOI) = 57

Cystoscopy: Posterior urethra remarkable for high bladder neck with co-apting lateral lobes; moderate bladder trabeculations; small-bladder diverticulum.

Diagnosis: DO and BOO (due to BPO).

Options: Additional anticholinergics, β-3 adrenergic agonist, sacral neuromodulation, intravesical onabotulinumtoxinA injection, TURP.

Commentary: The $BOOI = P_{det}@Q_{max} - 2 \times Q_{max}$, with a value <20 representing no obstruction, 20–40 representing an equivocal result, and >40 representing obstruction. This gentleman has both a problem during bladder filling (DO) and voiding (BOO). As such, he may require more than one treatment to alleviate his symptoms. While TURP may improve his BPO, he may continue to have bothersome storage symptoms. Conversely, medical or surgical treatment of his DO is unlikely to improve, and, in some cases may negatively impact his voiding.

Case 3: 50 years of woman with progressively worsening emptying.

History: She urinates frequently during day (diary: 10–14 voids/day, 2 voids/night; volumes 100–200 mL) and strains to urinate; (+) incomplete emptying; denies SUI or UUI; (+) UTIs, 2–3/year; (+) lumbar back injury after MVA 7 years ago; no spinal or pelvic surgery; (+) constipation; no pelvic prolapse on examination.

Course: She has not tried any active therapy.

Urodynamics: Unable to perform pre-procedure UF (Fig. 18.5; catheterized PVR = 350 mL); delayed first desire (Fig. 18.6; 693 mL); large bladder capacity (>800 mL); no DO; high compliance; unable to generate coordinated detrusor contraction during PFS (Fig. 18.7); PVR at end of procedure >1,000 mL.

Diagnosis: Urinary retention due to detrusor acontractility.

Options: CIC, sacral neuromodulation.

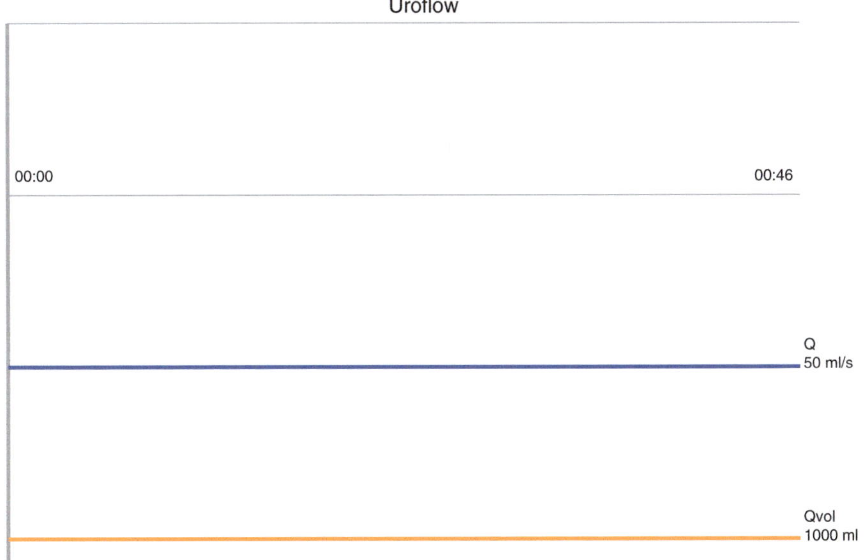

Fig. 18.5 Patient was unable to perform pre-procedure UF (catheterized PVR = 350 mL)

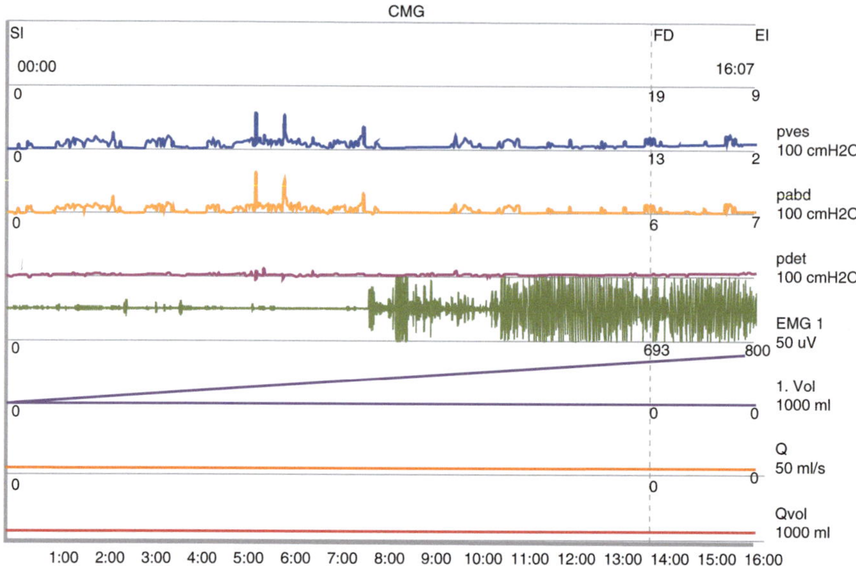

Fig. 18.6 CMG: delayed first desire (693 mL); large bladder capacity (>800 mL); no DO; high compliance

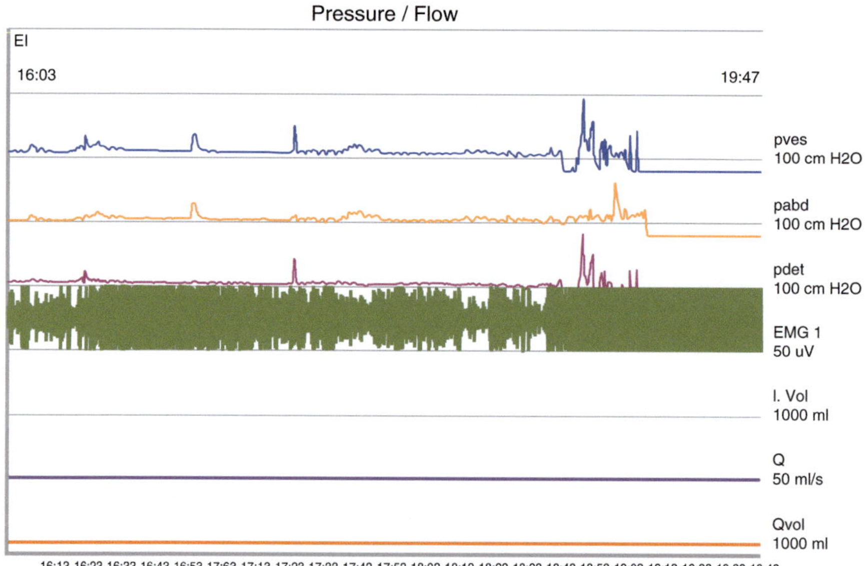

Fig. 18.7 PFS: patient unable to generate coordinated detrusor contraction; PVR at end of procedure > 1,000 mL

Commentary: This patient's symptoms stem from suboptimal emptying due to a lack of detrusor contractility. Her upper tracts are likely safe owing to high compliance and absence of DO. Her volitional voids during the day are most likely due to either valsalva voiding or overflow events.

Case 4: 55 years of man with overactive bladder symptoms.

History: He complains of urinary urgency and UUI 1–2 days/week. He voids 8/day and 2/night. Stream is "fair." He has tried two anticholinergics without significant benefit. He has had one recent culture-proven UTI (*E. coli*). Patient is otherwise healthy. DRE: 60 g benign prostate. He had a PVR of 198 and 187 mL on two consecutive visits.

Course: He had minimal improvement after a combination of an anticholinergic and α-blocker.

Urodynamics: Pre-CMG UF reveals Q_{max} 20 and continuous flow curve with adequate voided volume (277 mL; Fig. 18.8); PVR is high (375 mL); delayed first desire on CMG (463 mL; Fig. 18.9) and delayed normal desire (810 mL); no DO; high compliance; high-pressure, low-flow pattern on PFS (Fig. 18.10), small volume void, high PVR; low-flow and high PVR on post-PFS UF (Fig. 18.11).

Cystography: Large posterior bladder diverticulum (bladder is on the left) (Fig. 18.12); attempt to void (Fig. 18.13); post-void film showing empty bladder and full diverticulum (Fig. 18.14).

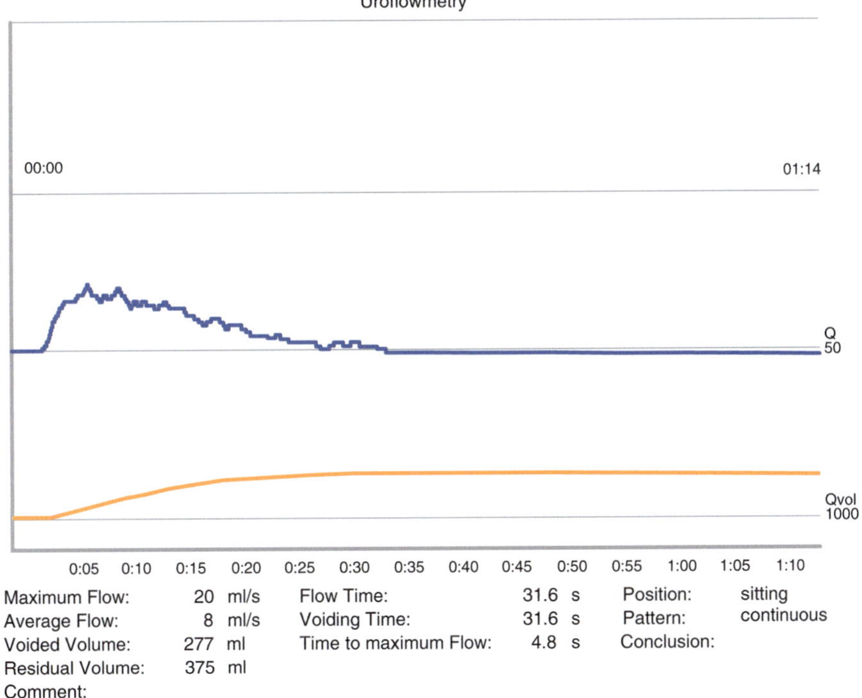

Fig. 18.8 Pre-CMG UF: $Q_{max} = 20$ mL/s with continuous flow curve with adequate voided volume (277 mL); PVR = 375 mL

Cystometry

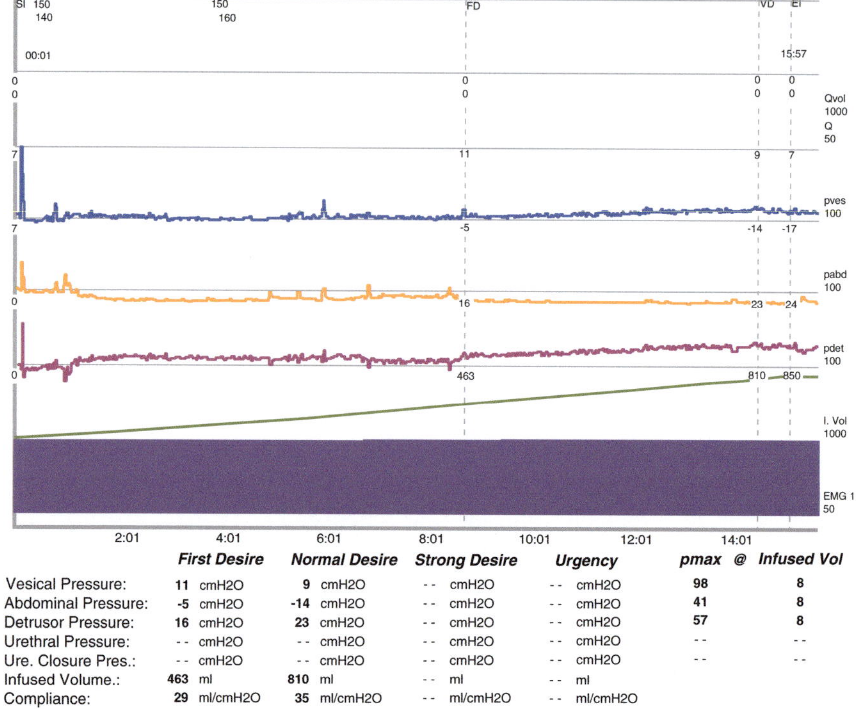

	First Desire	Normal Desire	Strong Desire	Urgency	pmax @	Infused Vol
Vesical Pressure:	11 cmH2O	9 cmH2O	-- cmH2O	-- cmH2O	98	8
Abdominal Pressure:	-5 cmH2O	-14 cmH2O	-- cmH2O	-- cmH2O	41	8
Detrusor Pressure:	16 cmH2O	23 cmH2O	-- cmH2O	-- cmH2O	57	8
Urethral Pressure:	-- cmH2O	-- cmH2O	-- cmH2O	-- cmH2O	--	--
Ure. Closure Pres.:	-- cmH2O	-- cmH2O	-- cmH2O	-- cmH2O	--	--
Infused Volume.:	463 ml	810 ml	-- ml	-- ml		
Compliance:	29 ml/cmH2O	35 ml/cmH2O	-- ml/cmH2O	-- ml/cmH2O		

Fig. 18.9 CMG: delayed first desire to void (463 mL); delayed normal desire (810 mL); no DO; high compliance

Pressure Flow

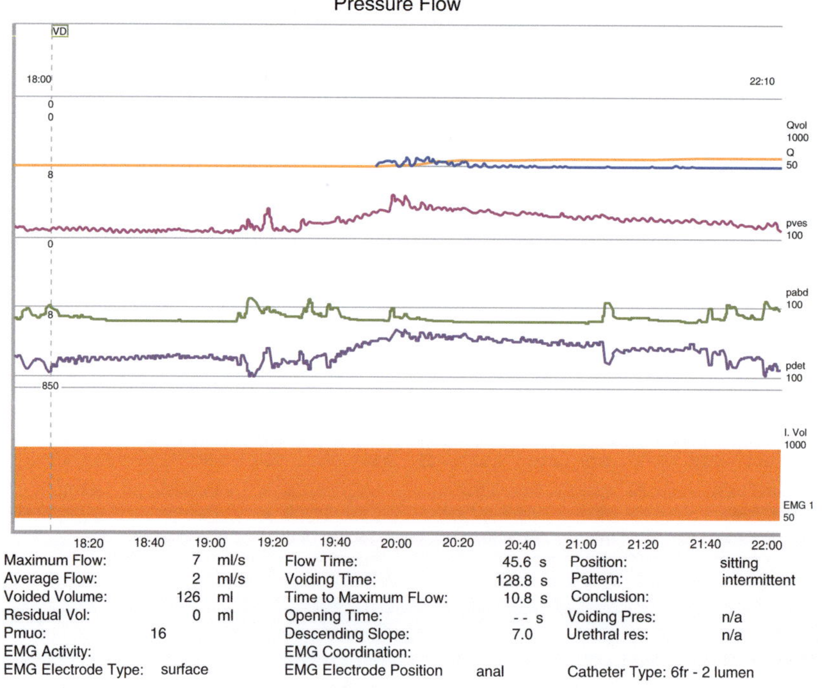

Maximum Flow:	7 ml/s	Flow Time:	45.6 s	Position:	sitting	
Average Flow:	2 ml/s	Voiding Time:	128.8 s	Pattern:	intermittent	
Voided Volume:	126 ml	Time to Maximum FLow:	10.8 s	Conclusion:		
Residual Vol:	0 ml	Opening Time:	-- s	Voiding Pres:	n/a	
Pmuo:	16	Descending Slope:	7.0	Urethral res:	n/a	
EMG Activity:		EMG Coordination:				
EMG Electrode Type:	surface	EMG Electrode Position	anal	Catheter Type: 6fr - 2 lumen		

Fig. 18.10 PFS: high-pressure, low-flow pattern; small-volume void; high PVR

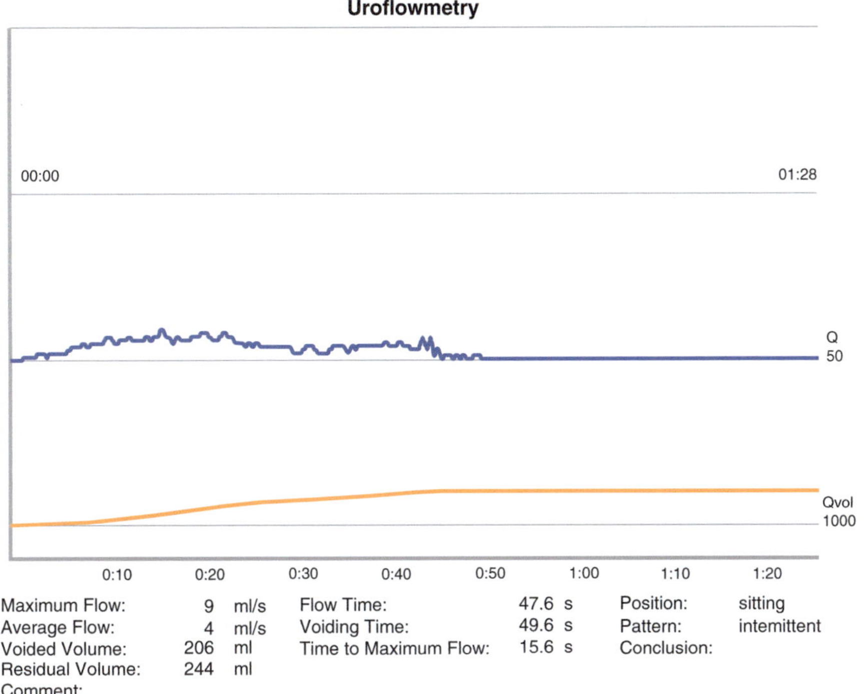

Maximum Flow:	9	ml/s	Flow Time:	47.6 s	Position:	sitting
Average Flow:	4	ml/s	Voiding Time:	49.6 s	Pattern:	intemittent
Voided Volume:	206	ml	Time to Maximum Flow:	15.6 s	Conclusion:	
Residual Volume:	244	ml				
Comment:						

Fig. 18.11 Post-PFS UF: low-flow; high PVR

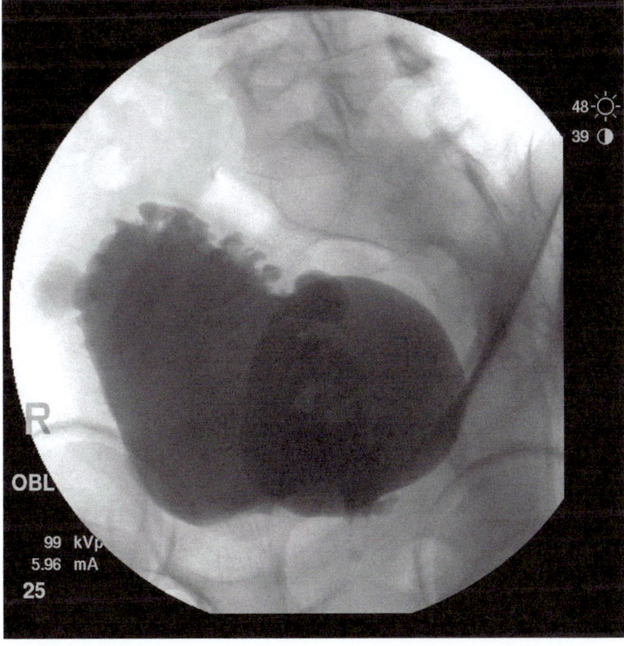

Fig. 18.12 Cystography: large posterior bladder diverticulum (bladder is on the *left*)

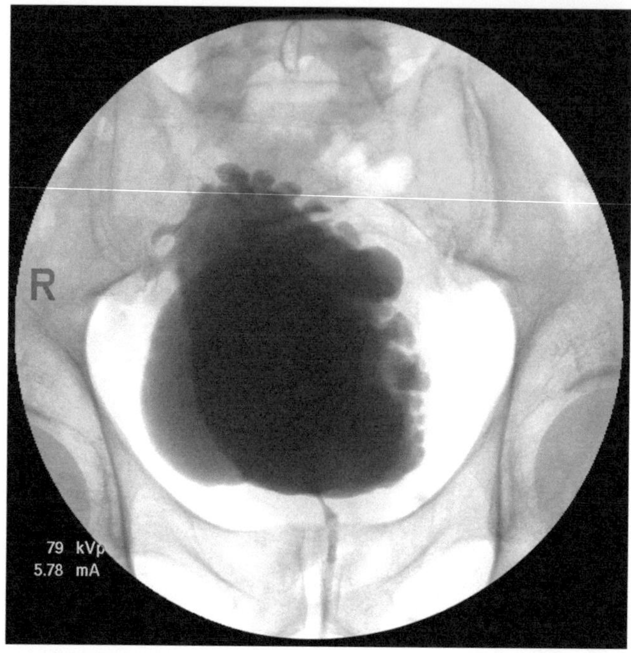

Fig. 18.13 Cystography during attempt to void

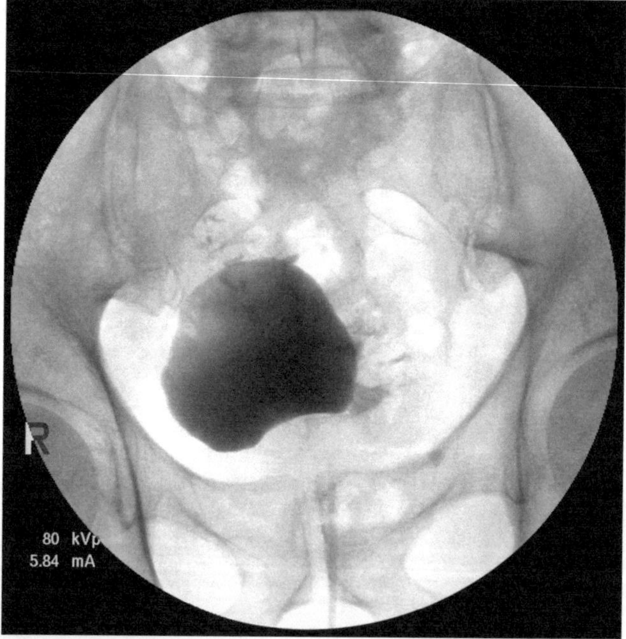

Fig. 18.14 Post-void cystography: empty bladder and full diverticulum

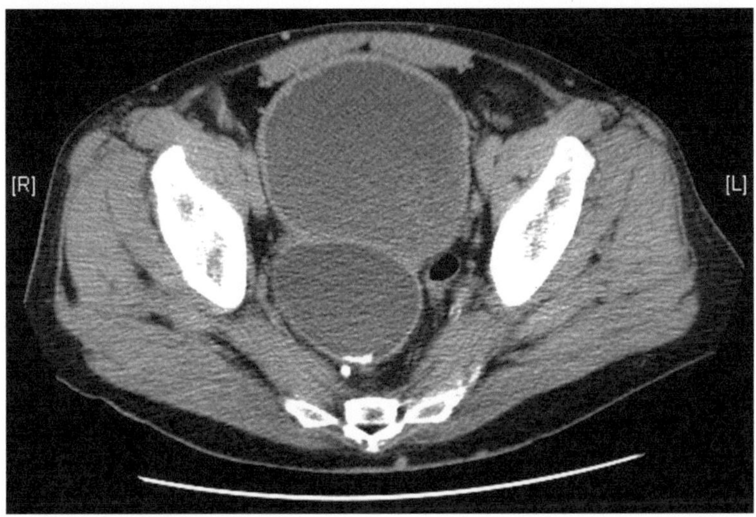

Fig. 18.15 CT: large bladder diverticulum

Cystoscopy: Mild trilobar prostatic enlargement, multiple trabeculations with small-bladder diverticula, and one large posterior bladder diverticulum with 24 F ostium.

CT (for work-up of microscopic hematuria): Large bladder diverticulum (Fig. 18.15).

Diagnosis: Stable bladder with evidence of BOO and large acquired bladder diverticulum.

Options: CIC, TURP, suprapubic prostatectomy ± bladder diverticulectomy, additional anticholinergics, β-3 adrenergic agonist.

Commentary: As with the man in *Case 2*, this gentleman has a problem with urinary storage and emptying, and thus may benefit from multiple treatments. Additionally, he has a large bladder diverticulum that is trapping urine and may be falsely elevating his PVR. Treating the outlet obstruction either first or concomitantly with the diverticulectomy is recommended.

Case 5: 62 years of man presents for evaluation of post-prostatectomy incontinence.

History: He has mild urinary urgency and frequency, mild incomplete emptying and mild weak stream. He does not strain to void. AUA SSI 7/35. He wears 1–2 pads/day for urinary incontinence that is worse with activity. His PSA is 0.0 ng/mL. He has a history of post-prostatectomy bladder neck contracture (BNC) and has undergone two previous BN incisions. The remainder of his history and physical examination are normal.

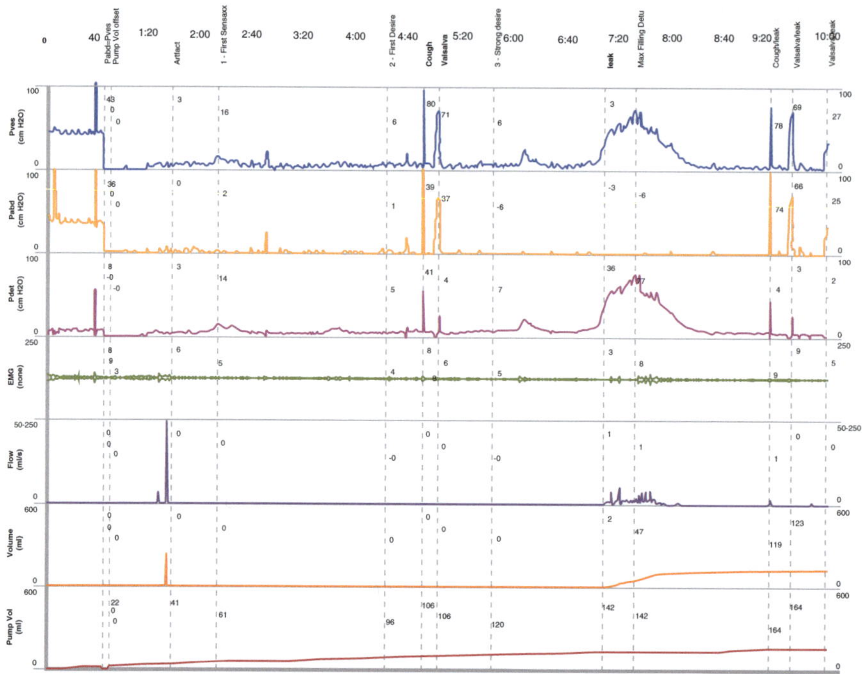

Fig. 18.16 CMG: First sensation (61 mL); strong desire (91 mL); bladder capacity (184 mL) after leakage volumes subtracted; high compliance; multiple episodes of DO starting at 65 mL, several with high-pressure (up to 70 cm H_2O) and leakage; SUI with VLPP=67–79 cm H_2O

Course: He has not improved on Kegel exercises and has tried one anticholinergic without significant benefit.

Urodynamics: (Figs. 18.16 and 18.17) First sensation, strong desire, and bladder capacity were 61, 91, and 184 mL (leakage volumes subtracted), respectively; compliance was high; multiple episodes of DO starting at 65 mL, several with high-pressure (up to 70 cm H_2O) and leakage; SUI with VLPP 67–79 cm H_2O; continuous leakage of urine at bladder capacity and patient was given permission to void (Fig. 18.18); $P_{detmax} \sim 62$ cm H_2O with a flow of 10 mL/s (BOOI=42).

Cystoscopy: Unable to pass scope through a ~12 F bladder neck contracture.

Diagnosis: BOO due to bladder neck contracture with SUI (ISD) and significant DO.

Options: Observation, BN incision, anticholinergics, urethral stent, artificial urinary sphincter (AUS), Cunningham clamp, and condom catheter.

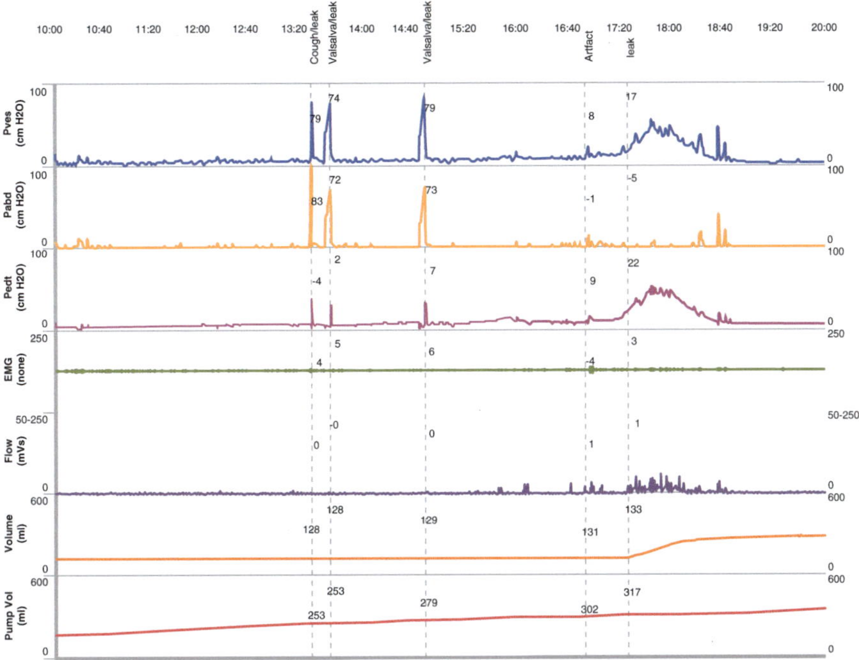

Fig. 18.17 Continuation of the tracing in 18.16. Additional episodes of DO and leakage following Valsalva maneuvers

Commentary: As with previous cases, this gentleman has complex urinary dysfunction that may require multiple therapeutic options to achieve symptom improvement. Regardless of the options chosen, BOO needs to be relieved in order to improve emptying, with subsequent pharmaceutical or surgical intervention to improve this gentleman's storage symptoms.

Case 6: 60 years of woman with SUI and mild emptying dysfunction

History: She has minimal diurnal urgency which is controlled with behavioral modification. She has some subjective incomplete emptying. She underwent one previous "bladder suspension" at time of abdominal hysterectomy 20 years ago. She has SUI with coughing, sneezing, and laughing, and requires 3 pads/day. No prolapse on exam (+). Urethral hypermobility.

Course: No improvement on behavioral modification, Kegel exercises. Patient did not want to pursue formal biofeedback and pelvic floor muscle training (PFMT).

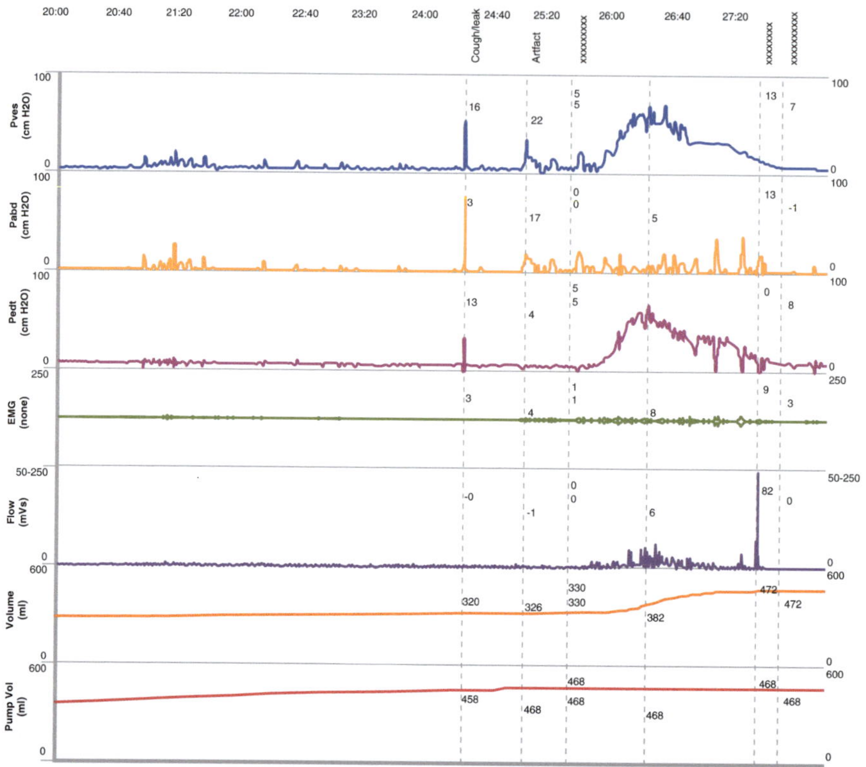

Fig. 18.18 CMG/PFS: continuous leakage of urine at bladder capacity; patient was given permission to void; $P_{\text{detmax}} \sim 62$ cm H_2O with flow $= 10$ mL/s (BOOI $= 42$)

Urodynamics: Adequate volume on pre-CMG UF with relatively low Q_{max}; PVR is low (Fig. 18.19); mildly decreased bladder capacity, one episode of DO (at 173 mL of filling) without leakage, and high compliance (Fig. 18.20); VLPP 92 and 126 cm H_2O; patient could not void on PFS despite detrusor contraction (Fig. 18.21); good post-procedure UF with $Q_{\text{max}} = 20$ mL/s, $Q_{\text{ave}} = 11$ mL/s, and continuous, bell-shaped flow curve (Fig. 18.22).

Diagnosis: SUI with high VLPP, DO, unobstructed emptying.

Options: Midurethral sling (MUS), pubovaginal sling (PVS), anticholinergics.

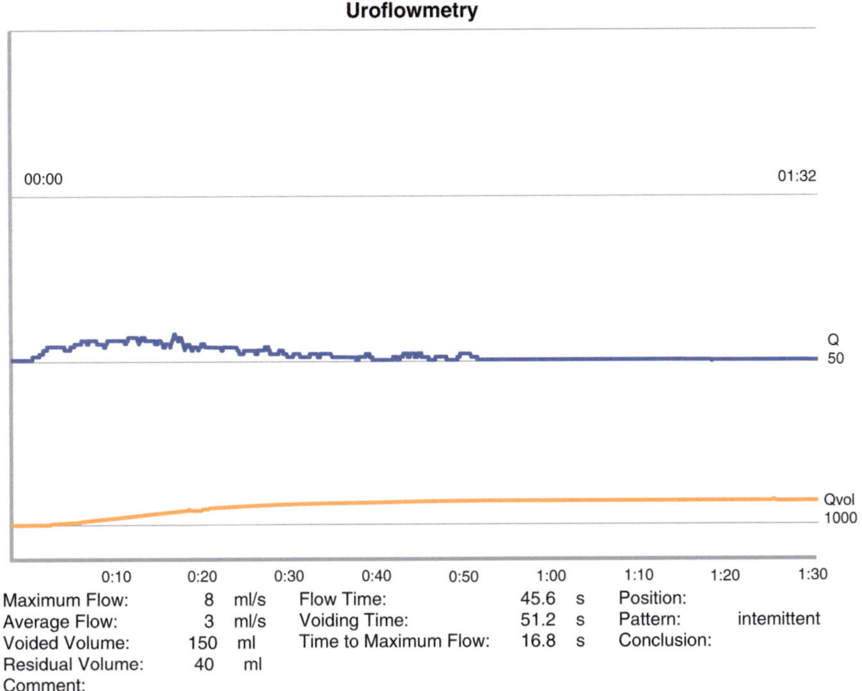

Fig. 18.19 Pre-CMG UF: adequate volume with low Q_{max}; PVR low

Commentary: This case represents a common scenario, where the whole is more than just the sum of the parts. If the initial uroflow and attempt at voiding on PFS are to be believed, then the patient may be thought to have some element of emptying dysfunction. However, the post-procedure uroflow (with a higher VV) provides some evidence to the contrary. The inability to void during a PFS may indicate some element of psychogenic inhibition (paruresis). Additionally, the patient appears to have tolerated a relatively modest amount of filling during the CMG indicating a potentially decreased bladder capacity. However, the VV on post-procedure uroflow was approximately twice the amount of infused volume, indicating that the patient may have produced a significant amount of urine during the study.

Case 7: 72 years of woman with Stage 2 cystocele and no overt SUI

History: (+) Positional emptying and often returning to commode 5 min later to complete voiding. No urinary incontinence. She underwent a previous hysterectomy without any concomitant procedures for incontinence or prolapse. There is no rectocele and minimal vault prolapse on pelvic exam (+). Urethral hypermobility. She is otherwise healthy.

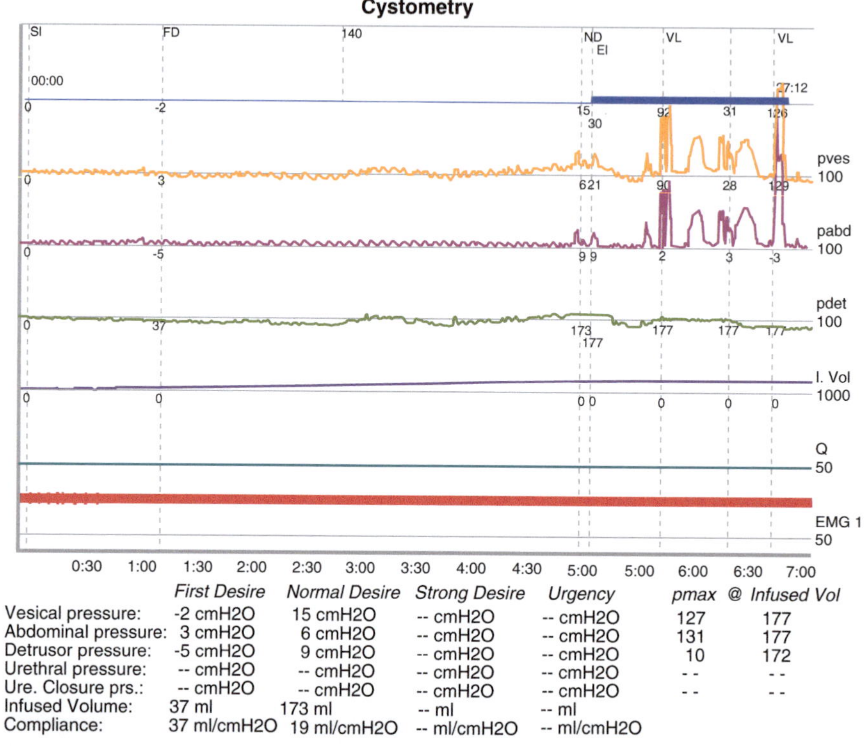

	First Desire	Normal Desire	Strong Desire	Urgency	pmax	@ Infused Vol
Vesical pressure:	-2 cmH2O	15 cmH2O	-- cmH2O	-- cmH2O	127	177
Abdominal pressure:	3 cmH2O	6 cmH2O	-- cmH2O	-- cmH2O	131	177
Detrusor pressure:	-5 cmH2O	9 cmH2O	-- cmH2O	-- cmH2O	10	172
Urethral pressure:	-- cmH2O	-- cmH2O	-- cmH2O	-- cmH2O	- -	- -
Ure. Closure prs.:	-- cmH2O	-- cmH2O	-- cmH2O	-- cmH2O	- -	- -
Infused Volume:	37 ml	173 ml	-- ml	-- ml		
Compliance:	37 ml/cmH2O	19 ml/cmH2O	-- ml/cmH2O	-- ml/cmH2O		

Fig. 18.20 CMG: mildly decreased bladder capacity; one episode of DO (173 mL of filling) without leakage; high compliance

Course: Voiding symptoms improved after pessary, but patient now complains of SUI. She had difficulty removing and reinserting several different pessaries and was interested in surgical intervention.

Urodynamics: Patient unable to perform pre-CMG UF, but PVR was low (30 mL) (Fig. 18.23); no DO, high compliance, and VLPP (with prolapse reduction) was 86 and 93 cm H_2O at 306 mL of filling (Fig. 18.24); she had a small-volume void on PFS (92 mL) with a combination of detrusor contraction and valsalva (Fig. 18.25); good post-procedure UF with $Q_{max} = 20$ mL/s, $Q_{ave} = 10$ mL/s, and continuous, bell-shaped flow curve (Fig. 18.26).

Diagnosis: Cystocele with occult SUI.

Options: Pessary with anti-incontinence knob, PFMT, anterior colporrhaphy with MUS / PVS / bulking therapy.

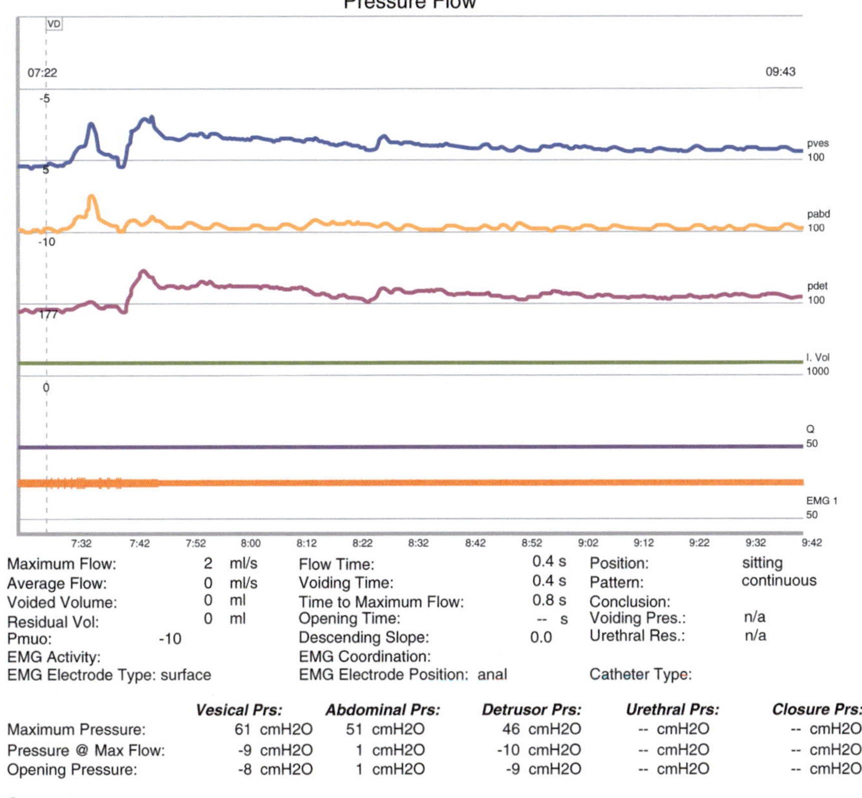

Maximum Flow:	2 ml/s	Flow Time:	0.4 s	Position:	sitting
Average Flow:	0 ml/s	Voiding Time:	0.4 s	Pattern:	continuous
Voided Volume:	0 ml	Time to Maximum Flow:	0.8 s	Conclusion:	
Residual Vol:	0 ml	Opening Time:	-- s	Voiding Pres.:	n/a
Pmuo:	-10	Descending Slope:	0.0	Urethral Res.:	n/a
EMG Activity:		EMG Coordination:			
EMG Electrode Type: surface		EMG Electrode Position: anal		Catheter Type:	

	Vesical Prs:	Abdominal Prs:	Detrusor Prs:	Urethral Prs:	Closure Prs:
Maximum Pressure:	61 cmH2O	51 cmH2O	46 cmH2O	-- cmH2O	-- cmH2O
Pressure @ Max Flow:	-9 cmH2O	1 cmH2O	-10 cmH2O	-- cmH2O	-- cmH2O
Opening Pressure:	-8 cmH2O	1 cmH2O	-9 cmH2O	-- cmH2O	-- cmH2O

Comment:
   Pt unable to void from urochair:

Fig. 18.21 CMG: VLPP = 92 and 126 cm H_2O; patient could not void on PFS despite generating detrusor contraction

Commentary: This is similar to *Case 5* in that the voiding pattern becomes clearer on a post-procedure uroflow when there is a sufficient amount of urine in the bladder. The significant straining during PFS may be a response to the urethral catheter. Once again, the VV after PFS and uroflow significantly exceeds the filling volume.

Case 8: 30 years of woman with C7 spinal cord injury (SCI).

History: S/p automobile accident 1 year ago. Performs CIC every 4 h and leaks in between. She has an effective bowel protocol. On exam, there is skeletal spasticity, hyperreflexic deep tendon reflexes, and abnormal plantar response.

Course: She is currently on oxybutynin 15 mg twice/daily without significant benefit.

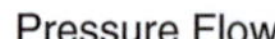

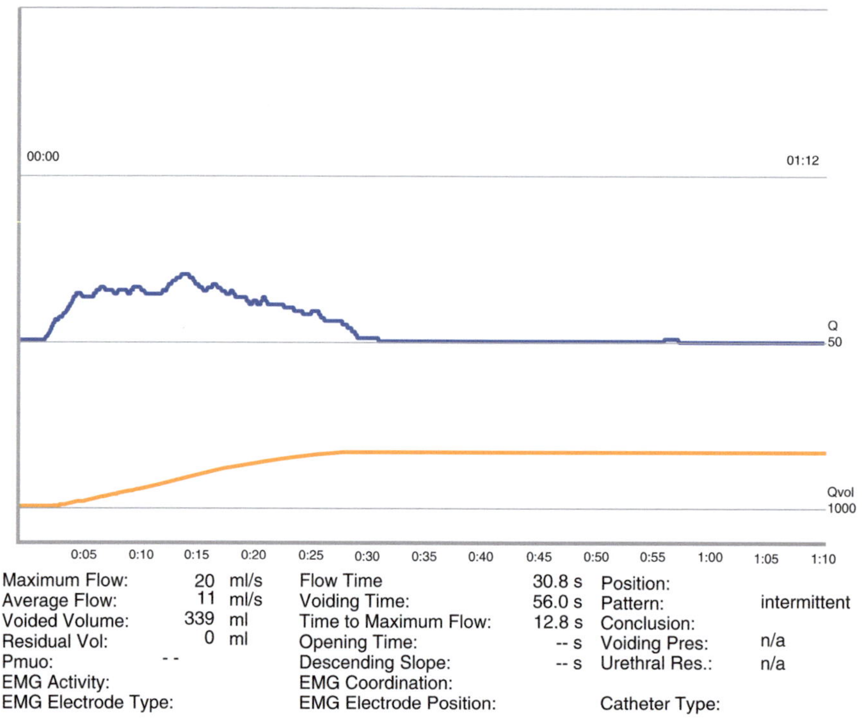

Maximum Flow:	20 ml/s	Flow Time	30.8 s	Position:	
Average Flow:	11 ml/s	Voiding Time:	56.0 s	Pattern:	intermittent
Voided Volume:	339 ml	Time to Maximum Flow:	12.8 s	Conclusion:	
Residual Vol:	0 ml	Opening Time:	-- s	Voiding Pres:	n/a
Pmuo:	- -	Descending Slope:	-- s	Urethral Res.:	n/a
EMG Activity:		EMG Coordination:			
EMG Electrode Type:		EMG Electrode Position:		Catheter Type:	

Fig. 18.22 Post-CMG UF: good (Q_{max} = 20 mL/s, Q_{ave} = 11 mL/s) with continuous, *bell-shaped flow curve*

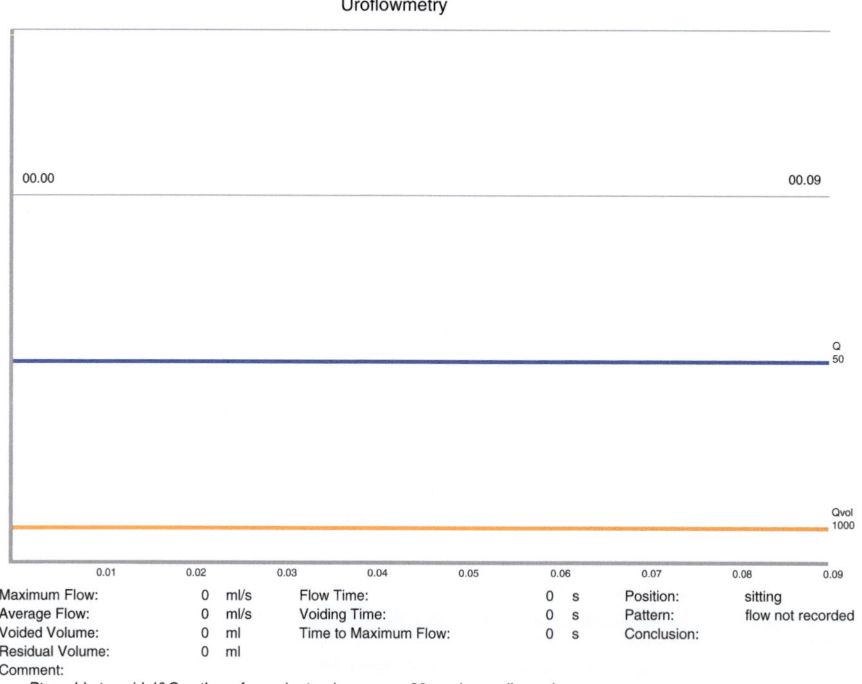

Maximum Flow:	0 ml/s	Flow Time:	0 s	Position:	sitting
Average Flow:	0 ml/s	Voiding Time:	0 s	Pattern:	flow not recorded
Voided Volume:	0 ml	Time to Maximum Flow:	0 s	Conclusion:	
Residual Volume:	0 ml				

Comment:
  Pt unable to void. I&O cath performed returning approx 30 cc clear yellow urine.

Fig. 18.23 Pre-CMG UF: patient unable to perform; PVR low (30 mL)

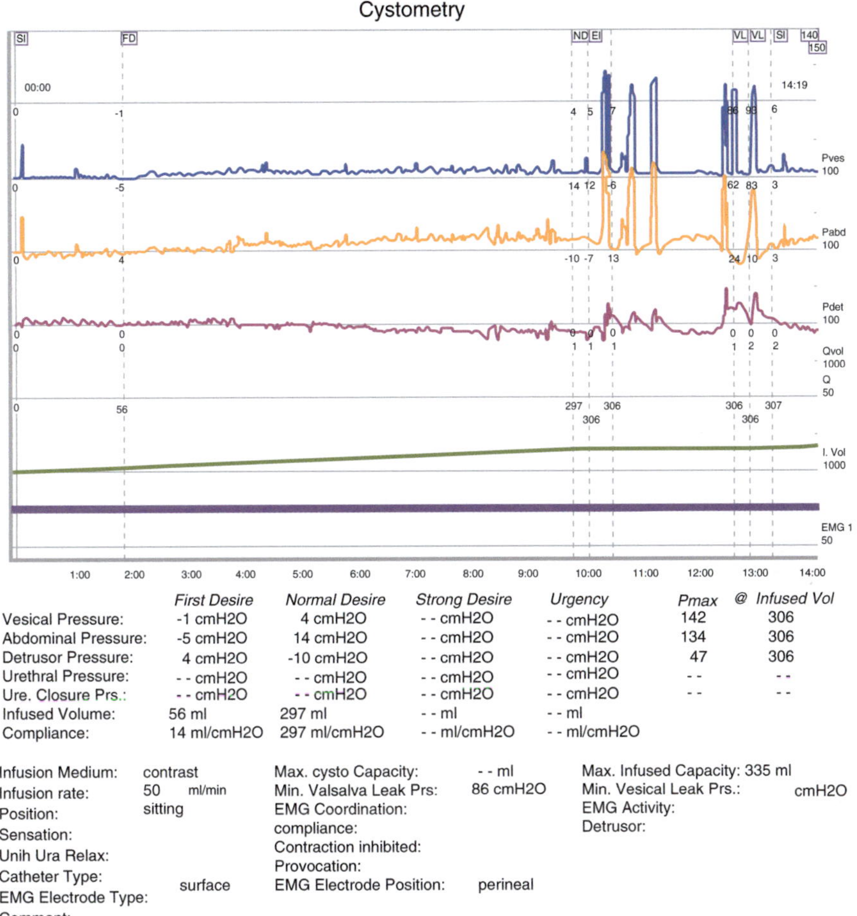

Fig. 18.24 CMG: no DO; high compliance; VLPP (with prolapse reduction) = 86 and 93 cm H_2O at 306 mL of filling

Urodynamics (Fig. 18.27): Stable detrusor until ~150 mL of filling; DO demonstrated with a peak detrusor pressure of 55 cm H_2O; increased EMG activity at time of DO.

Cystography (Fig. 18.28): Narrowing at external sphincter at the time of unstable detrusor contraction.

Diagnosis: Small-bladder capacity, detrusor-external sphincter dyssynergia (DESD).

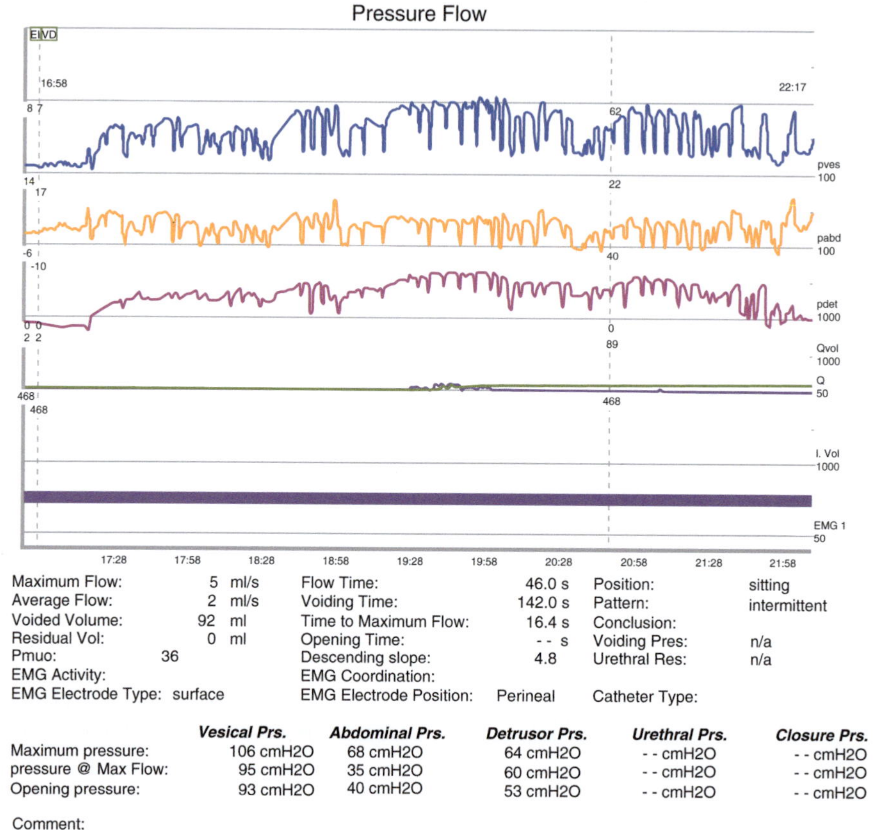

Maximum Flow:	5 ml/s	Flow Time:	46.0 s	Position:	sitting
Average Flow:	2 ml/s	Voiding Time:	142.0 s	Pattern:	intermittent
Voided Volume:	92 ml	Time to Maximum Flow:	16.4 s	Conclusion:	
Residual Vol:	0 ml	Opening Time:	- - s	Voiding Pres:	n/a
Pmuo:	36	Descending slope:	4.8	Urethral Res:	n/a
EMG Activity:		EMG Coordination:			
EMG Electrode Type:	surface	EMG Electrode Position:	Perineal	Catheter Type:	

	Vesical Prs.	Abdominal Prs.	Detrusor Prs.	Urethral Prs.	Closure Prs.
Maximum pressure:	106 cmH2O	68 cmH2O	64 cmH2O	- - cmH2O	- - cmH2O
pressure @ Max Flow:	95 cmH2O	35 cmH2O	60 cmH2O	- - cmH2O	- - cmH2O
Opening pressure:	93 cmH2O	40 cmH2O	53 cmH2O	- - cmH2O	- - cmH2O

Comment:
  pt unable to empty to completion from urochair.

Fig. 18.25 PFS: small-volume void (92 mL) with a combination of detrusor contraction and valsalva maneuver

Options: Additional anticholinergics, intravesical onabotulinumtoxinA injection, bladder augmentation (with or without catheterizable channel), urinary diversion.

Commentary: DESD is caused when the coordinated voiding reflex between the bladder and external sphincter is disrupted. This finding is typically seen in patients with SCI or multiple sclerosis, but can also be seen in any lesion between the brainstem and sacral spinal cord (e.g., myelodysplasia or transverse myelitis). Symptomatically, people with DESD experience diurnal incontinence, urinary retention, and often have a history of UTIs. A build-up of pressures in the bladder can result in vesicoureteral reflux, UTIs, hydronephrosis, urinary tract calculi, and renal insufficiency. The goal of therapy for DESD is to

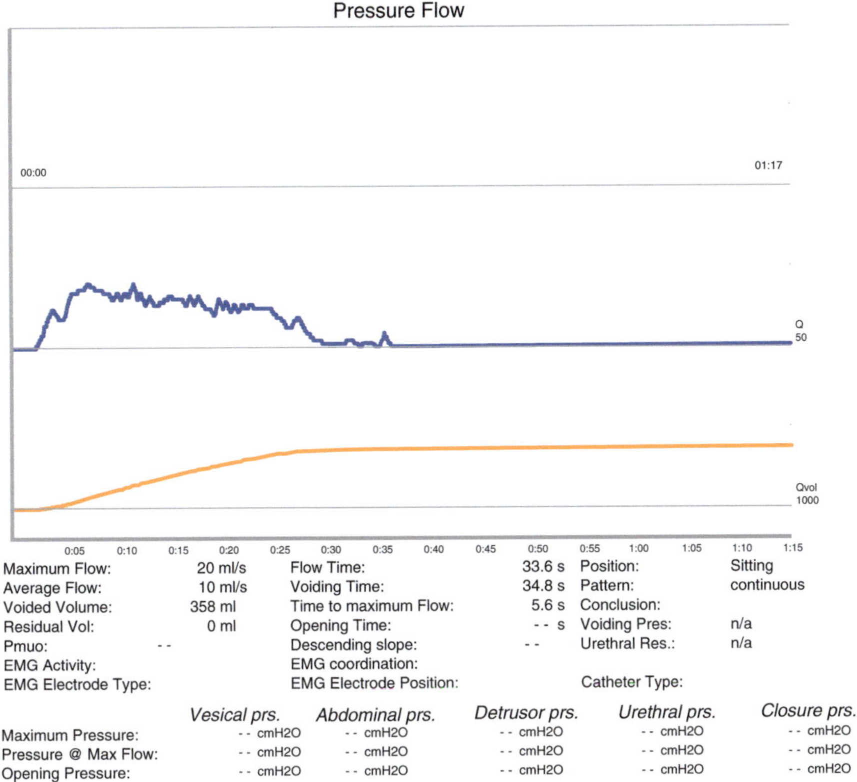

Maximum Flow:	20 ml/s	Flow Time:	33.6 s	Position:	Sitting
Average Flow:	10 ml/s	Voiding Time:	34.8 s	Pattern:	continuous
Voided Volume:	358 ml	Time to maximum Flow:	5.6 s	Conclusion:	
Residual Vol:	0 ml	Opening Time:	- - s	Voiding Pres:	n/a
Pmuo:	- -	Descending slope:	- -	Urethral Res.:	n/a
EMG Activity:		EMG coordination:			
EMG Electrode Type:		EMG Electrode Position:		Catheter Type:	

	Vesical prs.	Abdominal prs.	Detrusor prs.	Urethral prs.	Closure prs.
Maximum Pressure:	- - cmH2O	- - cmH2O	- - cmH2O	- - cmH2O	- - cmH2O
Pressure @ Max Flow:	- - cmH2O	- - cmH2O	- - cmH2O	- - cmH2O	- - cmH2O
Opening Pressure:	- - cmH2O	- - cmH2O	- - cmH2O	- - cmH2O	- - cmH2O

Fig. 18.26 Post-procedure UF: good (Q_{max} = 20 mL/s, Q_{ave} = 10 mL/s) with continuous, *bell-shaped flow curve*

decrease bladder storage pressures and facilitate bladder emptying. Since this patient is already performing CIC, the remaining goal is to eliminate DO to re-establish continence and potentially increase the interval between catheterizations. The bladder may be paralyzed pharmacologically or may be surgically converted to a low-pressure urinary reservoir by augmentation cystoplasty. Urinary diversion is typically reserved for patients failing less-complex measures and/or those unable to perform CIC. In men, additional options include an external sphincterotomy or urethral stent and an external urinary appliance (condom catheter). Without proper treatment over 50 % men with DESD develop serious urological complications within 5 years, while in women the complications are less common [9].

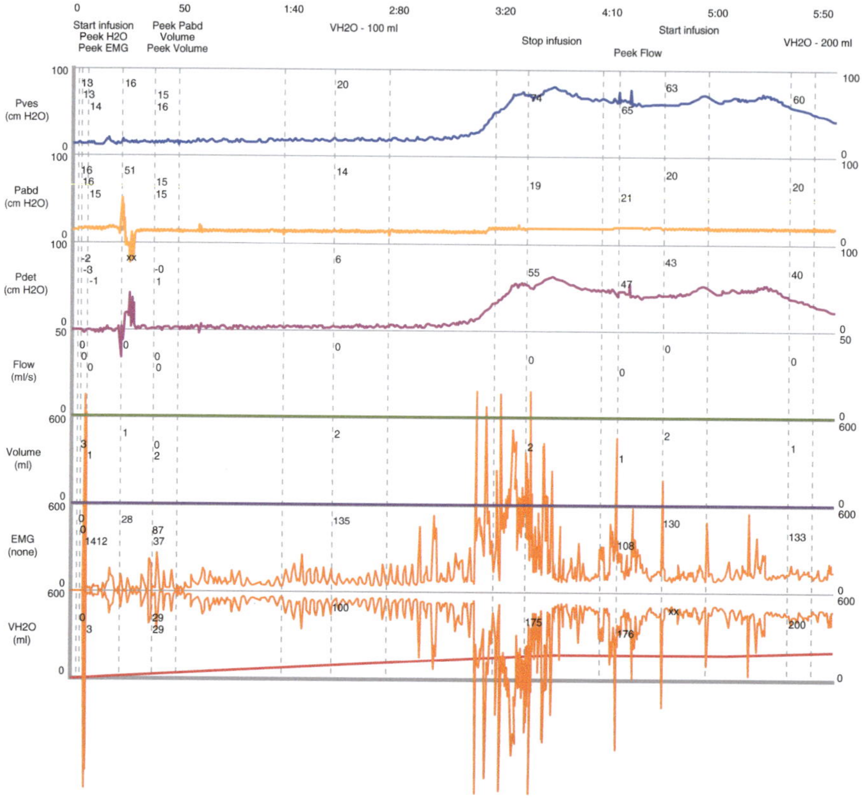

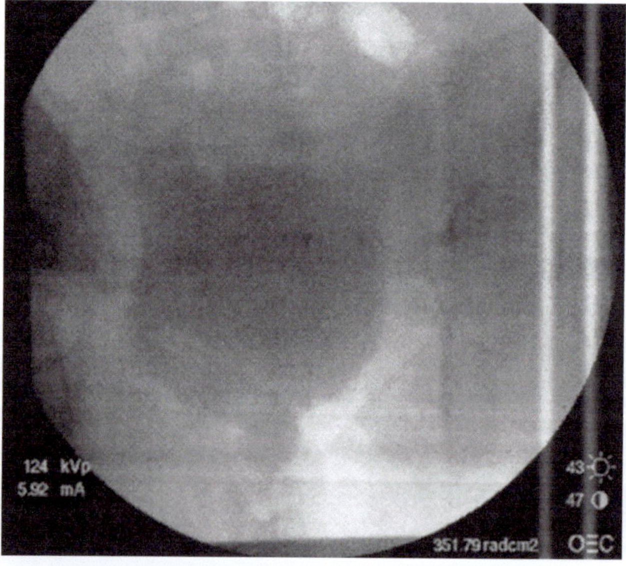

Fig. 18.27 CMG: stable detrusor until ~150 mL of filling; DO with a peak $P_{det}=55$ cm H_2O; increased EMG activity at time of DO

Fig. 18.28 Cystography: narrowing at external sphincter at the time of DO

References

1. Bates CP, Whiteside CG, Turner WR. Synchronous urine pressure flow cystourethrography with special reference to stress and urge incontinence. Br J Urol. 1970;42:714–23.
2. Abrams P, Cardozo L, Fall M, Griffiths D, Rosier P, Ulmsten U, van Kerrebroeck P, Victor A, Wein A. Standardisation of terminology of lower urinary tract function: report from the standardisation sub-committee of the International Continence Society. Neurourol Urodyn. 2002;21:167–78.
3. Huang AJ, Brown JS, Boyko EJ, Moore EE, Scholes D, Walter LC, Lin F, Vittinghoff E, Fihn SD. Clinical significance of postvoid residual volume in older ambulatory women. J Am Geriatr Soc. 2011;59:1452–8.
4. Lukacz ES, DuHamel E, Menefee SA, Luber KM. Elevated postvoid residual in women with pelvic floor disorders: prevalence and associated risk factors. Int Urogynecol J Pelvic Floor Dysfunct. 2007;18:397–400.
5. Tseng LH, Liang CC, Chang YL, Lee SJ, Lloyd LK, Chen CK. Postvoid residual urine in women with stress incontinence. Neurourol Urodyn. 2008;27:48–51.
6. Tam CK, Wong KK, Yip WM. Prevalence of incomplete bladder emptying among elderly in convalescent wards: a pilot study. Asian J Gerontol Geriatr. 2006;1:66–71.
7. Kolman C, Girman CJ, Jacobsen SJ, Lieber MM. Distribution of post-void residual urine volume in randomly selected men. J Urol. 1999;161:122–7.
8. Kaplan SA, Wein AJ, Staskin DR, Roehrborn CG, Steers WD. Urinary retention and post-void residual urine in men: separating truth from tradition. J Urol. 2008;180:47–54.
9. Chancellor MB, Kaplan SA, Blaivas JG. Detrusor-external sphincter dyssynergia. Ciba Found Symp. 1990;151:195–206.

Chapter 19
Bladder Emptying: Clinical Bladder Outlet Obstruction

Michael E. Albo

Introduction

Patients with bladder outlet obstruction (BOO) commonly present with bothersome lower urinary tract symptoms (LUTS) unfortunately, the symptoms are non-specific to BOO and do not correlate with the outcomes following treatment of obstruction [1]. BOO can also present without symptoms or with secondary conditions such as urinary tract infections, bladder diverticuli, bladder stones, or renal failure. During the evaluation of LUTS, the clinician must distinguish BOO from other conditions that may be the cause of the patient's symptoms through a combination of a focused history, physical exam findings, laboratory tests, and more invasive testing when necessary. The goal of the evaluation is to identify patients who are more likely to deteriorate from untreated LUTS, to identify patients who will respond to a particular therapy, and to identify additional lower urinary tract pathology that can either be a contributing factor to the symptoms or could be a poor prognosticator after treatment of the obstruction. This chapter will review a number of urodynamic tracings obtained during the course of evaluating patients with symptoms of clinical BOO.

Simultaneous measurement of detrusor pressure and urinary flow rate during voluntary voiding in a pressure flow study (PFS) is the best method currently available to diagnose BOO [2]. The International Continence Society in fact defines BOO as "an **urodynamic** observation characterized by increased detrusor pressure and reduced urinary flow rate during voiding" [3]. The AUA Guidelines on Urodynamics in Adults state that "PFS remains the only means of definitely establishing or ruling out the presence of BOO in men" [4]. Although there is no urodynamic standard for obstruction in women, the AUA Guidelines state "the finding of

M.E. Albo, MD (⊠)
Department of Urology, UC San Diego Health Systems,
200 West Arbor Drive, San Diego, CA 92103-8897, USA
e-mail: malbo@ucsd.edu

© Springer Science+Business Media New York 2015
E.S. Rovner, M.E. Koski (eds.), *Rapid and Practical Interpretation of Urodynamics*, DOI 10.1007/978-1-4939-1764-8_19

an elevated detrusor voiding pressure in association with low flow may suggest obstruction, particularly in the presence of new onset filling, storage or emptying symptoms after surgery" [4].

Non-invasive diagnostic methods including non-invasive uroflowetry (NIF), surface electromyography (EMG), and fluoroscopy are commonly used in the evaluation of BOO but do not have the diagnostic accuracy of the PFS. The primary limitation of non-invasive uroflowmetry is that it provides no information about the pressure required to generate a given flow rate and consequently cannot distinguish obstruction from impaired detrusor contractility as a cause of reduced flow. Similarly, it cannot distinguish between a normal flow rate that is produced by an obstructed bladder capable of generating high pressures. Studies have shown variability in the diagnostic accuracy of non-invasive uroflowmetry in detecting BOO in men that range from moderately high to low [5]. Surface electrode EMG testing can be utilized to evaluate urethral sphincter and pelvic muscle function during voiding, however it is technically challenging to perform with accuracy, artifacts are common, and the EMG diagnosis must be taken in context with bladder pressure, urinary flow, and anatomic imaging to obtain the most useful information [6]. Retrograde and antegrade fluoroscopy can define lower urinary tract anatomy and potentially identify the location of obstruction, but cannot diagnose obstruction without also measuring bladder pressure. Efforts to identify less invasive or non-urodynamic techniques are ongoing and include ultrasound assessment of bladder or detrusor wall thickness, ultrasound estimation of bladder weight, and infrared spectroscopy to assess bladder oxygenation. None of these has yet replaced the PFS as the gold standard diagnostic test for BOO [7].

A variety of nomograms based on the pressure flow relationship have been developed to standardize the analysis of pressure flow studies and to assist the clinician in the diagnosis of lower urinary tract dysfunction in men. They have been discussed in detail in earlier chapters. In 1997 the ICS attempted to standardize the urodynamic diagnosis of outlet obstruction using the ICS provisional nomogram, which divides patients into 3 classes: unobstructed, equivocal, and obstructed, based on the Bladder Outlet Obstruction Index (BOOI) [8]. Using this nomogram, the sensitivity and specificity of the PFS in diagnosing obstruction are 81 and 83 %, respectively, when the unobstructed and equivocal classes on the ICS nomogram are amalgamated with an overall accuracy of 82 %, a figure that has been reproduced by other studies [9].

While the nomograms have been helpful in the diagnosis of BOO in men, the evidence supporting the use of UDS in the evaluation of BOO in women is much less developed and the applicability of nomograms in assessing BOO in women remains controversial. A variety of definitions of BOO, incompletely defined normative PFS parameters, and a lack of literature that correlates PFS findings with outcomes all contribute to this lack of evidence [10]. Additionally the differences between male and female voiding both in regard to the normal voiding mechanism as well as the pathophysiology leading to voiding abnormalities makes it unlikely that the same nomograms will be sufficient. Many women are able to void by relaxing the pelvic floor muscles in the face of low detrusor pressures or by increasing intra-abdominal pressures. Multiple investigators have attempted to define BOO in women using urodynamic parameters including Q_{max}, $P_{det}@Q_{max}$, fluoroscopic imaging, or some combination of values with the intent of defining parameters for construction of the nomograms [11–15]. At this time, most organizations support the use of PFS in the evaluation of BOO in women when potentially morbid therapy is being considered [4].

While there is little argument that pressure flow studies are the gold standard for the diagnosis of BOO, whether they are necessary to confirm urodynamic obstruction before proceeding with invasive therapy remains controversial. Systematic reviews have identified only low quality evidence or expert opinion on the subject [16]. There is morbidity associated with PFS with 19 % of men having experienced hematuria, UTI, sepsis, or urinary retention following PFS [17]. The AUA Guidelines state that "clinicians should perform PFS in men when it is important to determine if urodynamic obstruction is present in men with LUTS, particularly when invasive, potentially morbid, or irreversible treatments are considered" (Standard; Evidence Strength: Grade B). They go on to say "However, patients should also be made aware of the risks of PFS as well as some of the diagnostic pitfalls of the studies" [4]. The European Association of Urology Guidelines on the Assessment of BPH recommend PFSs in "men with LUTS who voided a volume of less than 150 mL or a maximum urinary flow greater than 15 mL/s prior to surgery, very young (<50 years) or old patients (>80 years), post-void residual urinary volumes greater than 300 mL, suspicion of neurogenic bladder dysfunction, post radical pelvic surgery, or previous unsuccessful invasive treatment of BPH" [18].

The diagnostic utility of PFS is perhaps most helpful in the neurogenic population because the underlying neurologic disease can affect or obscure patient symptomology. Neurogenic patients with LUTS are particularly difficult to diagnose given the multifactorial nature of their lower urinary tract dysfunction. The AUA Guidelines state "Clinicians should perform pressure flow analysis in patients with relevant neurologic disease with or without symptoms or in patients with other neurologic disease and elevated PVR or urinary symptoms" [4].

Once the decision has been made to utilize urodynamics as a diagnostic test, in order to maximize their value, it is imperative that the performance and interpretation of those studies meet the standards established by the international community [19]. Quality control techniques, such as having the patient cough before, during, and after the study check concordance of the pressure lines and help identify potential artifact in order to adequately differentiate voluntary events from involuntary events. Most importantly, the urodynamic study requires interaction with the patient. The intent of the study is to apply pressure flow values to a patient's typical voiding experience. Asking the patient whether their void during the urodynamic study was typical of how they normally void helps assure that the urodynamic values obtained are truly measuring the voiding parameters of that patient. If the patient states that the void was not typical for them, the values must be suspect and the study should be repeated.

There are a number of factors the clinician must take into consideration when applying urodynamic results to a given patient. Not every instance of high pressure/ low flow voiding during a PFS is due to pathologic obstruction. Pressure flow parameters vary with the volume of urine voided, whether the catheter is causing anatomic or functional obstruction, as well as the patient's ability to relax the urethral sphincter and/or pelvic muscles during the void. At times the catheter can slip into the prostatic urethra measuring urethral pressure as opposed to detrusor pressure during the void, resulting in artificially elevated pressure. To avoid these pitfalls, it is important to compare the pressure flow parameters with the non-invasive flow parameters. If the non-invasive uroflow demonstrates a normal flow rate and pattern, then the PFS is less likely an accurate representation of the patients voiding dynamics. Finally, PFS may not be able to identify the presence of obstruction in two situations, first if the patient doesn't void and secondly if the patient has detrusor underactivity which will result in a low flow regardless of the urethral resistance.

The eight urodynamic studies presented in this chapter are tracings obtained during the work-up of patients presenting with LUTS. They represent a wide variety of pathophysiology from both male and female patients. The urodynamic findings highlight the issues discussed above. The format includes a brief, pertinent history and physical exam findings with the bulk of the discussion centering on the tracing itself. Each tracing is interpreted by first assessing whether the study meets minimum requirements for validity and recognizing potential areas of artifact. Those validity requirements include active and concordant pressure lines at the beginning, during, and at the conclusion of the study, baseline pressure values within the normal range, adequate annotation of events, and delineation of storage and voiding phases. Once it has been determined that the minimal criteria for validity are present, most of the focus is on the pressure flow portion of the study. When artifacts are present they are noted and taken into consideration when interpreting the study.

Case 1

Sixty-five-year-old male presents with symptoms of hesitancy, slow stream, and urgency. In addition he is getting up twice a night to urinate. IPSS 20 with QoL score of 4. His primary care physician placed him on an alpha-blocker 6 months ago and he thought it initially helped. He is otherwise healthy. On physical exam he has a normal penis and testes, 60 g prostate, smooth and symmetrical, normal anal sphincter tone, grossly normal neurologic exam. Urinalysis normal and PVR 25 mL. Patient was unable to void for a non-invasive uroflow at time of his initial evaluation. He was scheduled for urodynamic evaluation.

Non-invasive uroflow metry (NIF): In spite of being instructed to come with a full bladder, the patient had urinated immediately prior to leaving home and could not void for a non-invasive uroflow. This is a common occurrence and one should consider refilling the bladder at the conclusion of the PFS, remove the vesical catheter and other tubing, and allow the patient to void in the uroflow for a non-invasive study.

Cystometrogram/Pressure Flow Study (CMG/PFS) (Fig. 19.1a). We will first assess the tracing for validity. Both the vesical and abdominal pressure lines are live, baseline pressures are within the normal range for a patient standing, P_{ves} 36, P_{abd} 29, and P_{det} 8 cm/H_2O (a) and they correlate with one another as is demonstrated by similar amplitude cough spikes. (b) The study clearly demarcates the transition between filling and emptying phases with the annotation of maximum cystometric capacity and permission to void (c) and reestablishes baseline pressures and concordance between P_{ves} and P_{abd} prior to the void (d). The patient was able to initiate a voluntary void (e). There is evidence that both P_{ves} and P_{abd} remain active and concordant at the conclusion of the void (f). The storage phase demonstrates no

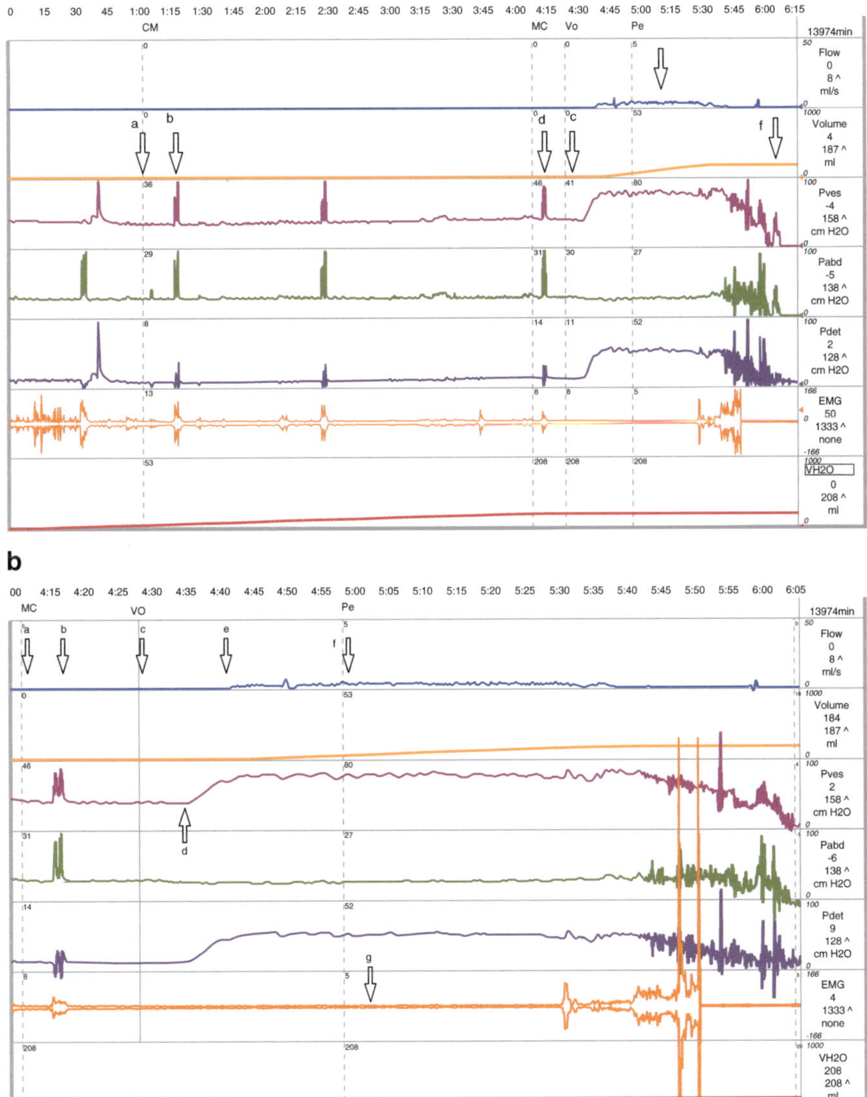

Fig. 19.1 (**a**) CMG and PFS, (**b**) expanded PFS segment, (**c**) pressure flow nomogram, (**d**) post-PFS non-invasive uroflow

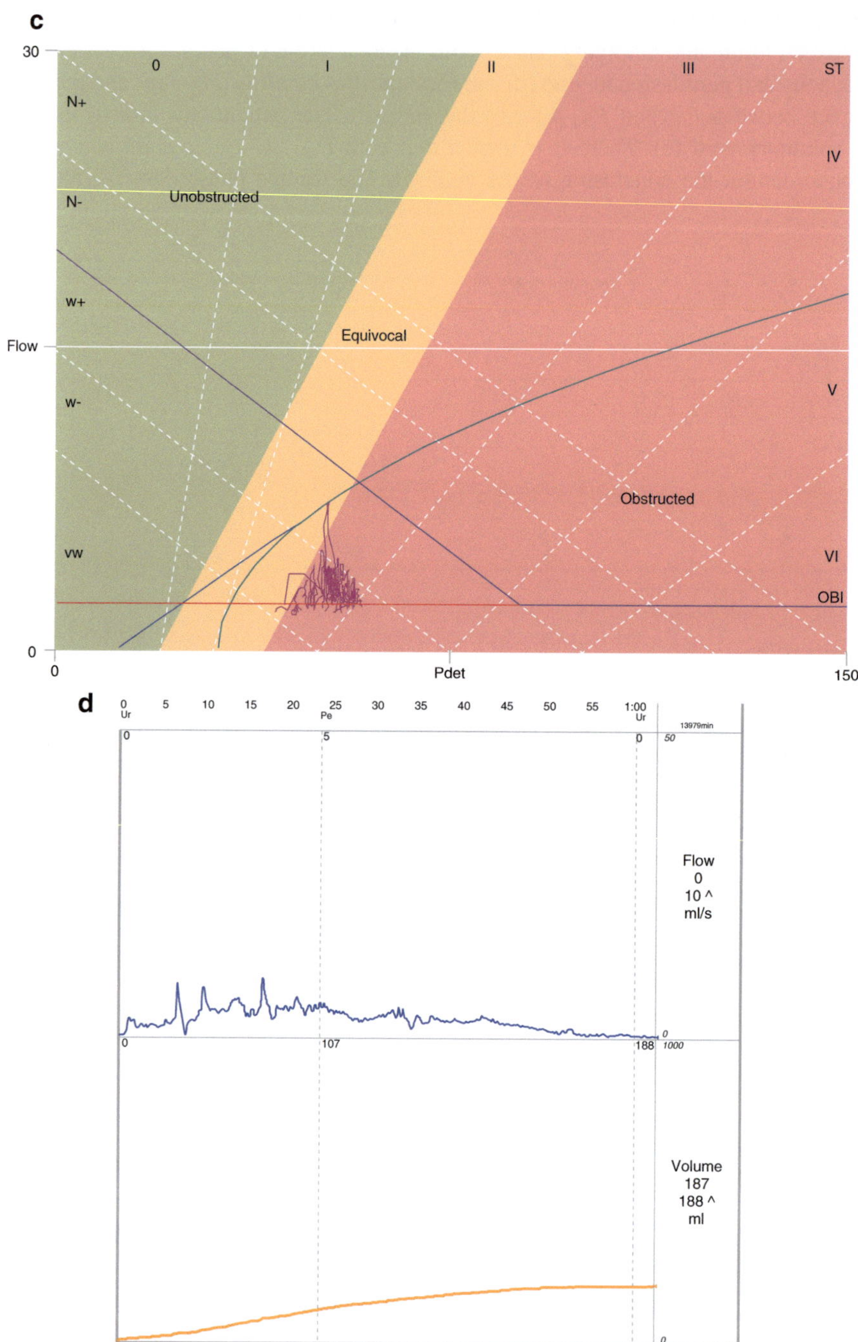

Fig. 19.1 (continued)

evidence of involuntary detrusor activity and normal compliance. The pressure flow segment of the study is expanded in Fig. 19.1b.

Expanded PFS Segment (Fig. 19.1b). This segment of the tracing begins at the end of the storage phase labeled as MCC. (a) Prior to voiding the patient is asked to cough to assess accuracy of pressure lines. (b) The patient is then given permission to void. (c) The P_{ves} rises rapidly without concomitant change in P_{abd} confirming that the intravesical pressure change is due to a detrusor contraction. (d) Flow is initiated (e) and he voids 184 mL with a post-void residual of 21 mL. The Q_{max} is 5 mL/s and the $P_{det}@Q_{max}$ is 52 cm/H_2O (f) and the flow pattern is continuous with a prolonged plateau phase. EMG activity has decreased throughout the voiding portion of the study. (g) Based on what we have interpreted as accurate pressure flow measurements the nomogram can be considered accurate and with a curve pressure/flow curve wholly contained in the obstructed zone (Fig. 19.1c).

The patient underwent refilling and the catheters were removed. He was asked to void in the uroflowmeter for a non-invasive uroflow (Fig. 19.1d).

This case demonstrates a classical presentation of outlet obstruction. The patient presents with obstructive type LUTS not well controlled with pharmacologic therapy and has urodynamic findings consistent with low flow/high pressure that meets the urodynamic definition of outlet obstruction. What the study does not do is identify the anatomic location of the obstruction. The differential diagnosis in this patient includes outlet obstruction from bladder neck dysfunction, BPH, or voiding dysfunction not identified by EMG. A urethral stricture is less likely but possible. Finally, if the non-invasive uroflow and PFS flow parameters were markedly different one would have had to consider that the PFS findings were secondary to artifact.

Case 2

Seventy-five-year-old male presents with symptoms of urgency, frequency, urge incontinence, and nocturia ×5. He has not been on any medication. He also has a history of Parkinson's disease, which has been stable for the past 5 years. He denies any problems with urinary tract infection, hematuria, or previous pelvic surgery. Urinalysis negative. Non-invasive uroflow was attempted (Fig. 19.2a) but the patient only voided 90 mL with a PVR 10 mL. This is an insufficient volume to assess uroflow parameters. Urodynamic studies were ordered and depicted in Fig. 19.2b–d.

CMG/PFS (Fig. 19.2b). Assessment of study validity demonstrates baseline pressures within normal range for standing patient and good concordance of the P_{ves} and P_{abd} at onset of studies. During the storage segment there is evidence of detrusor overactivity beginning at volume of 70 mL (a) and continuing with increasing amplitude until capacity at which time the patient could no longer hold back the flow. (b) The pressure lines are concordant after voiding is complete. Expanded PFS segment of the tracing is shown in Fig. 19.2c.

Expanded PFS (Fig. 19.2c). The initial event depicted in this tracing is a sudden rise in P_{ves} that is not associated with a rise in P_{abd} indicating that this is an

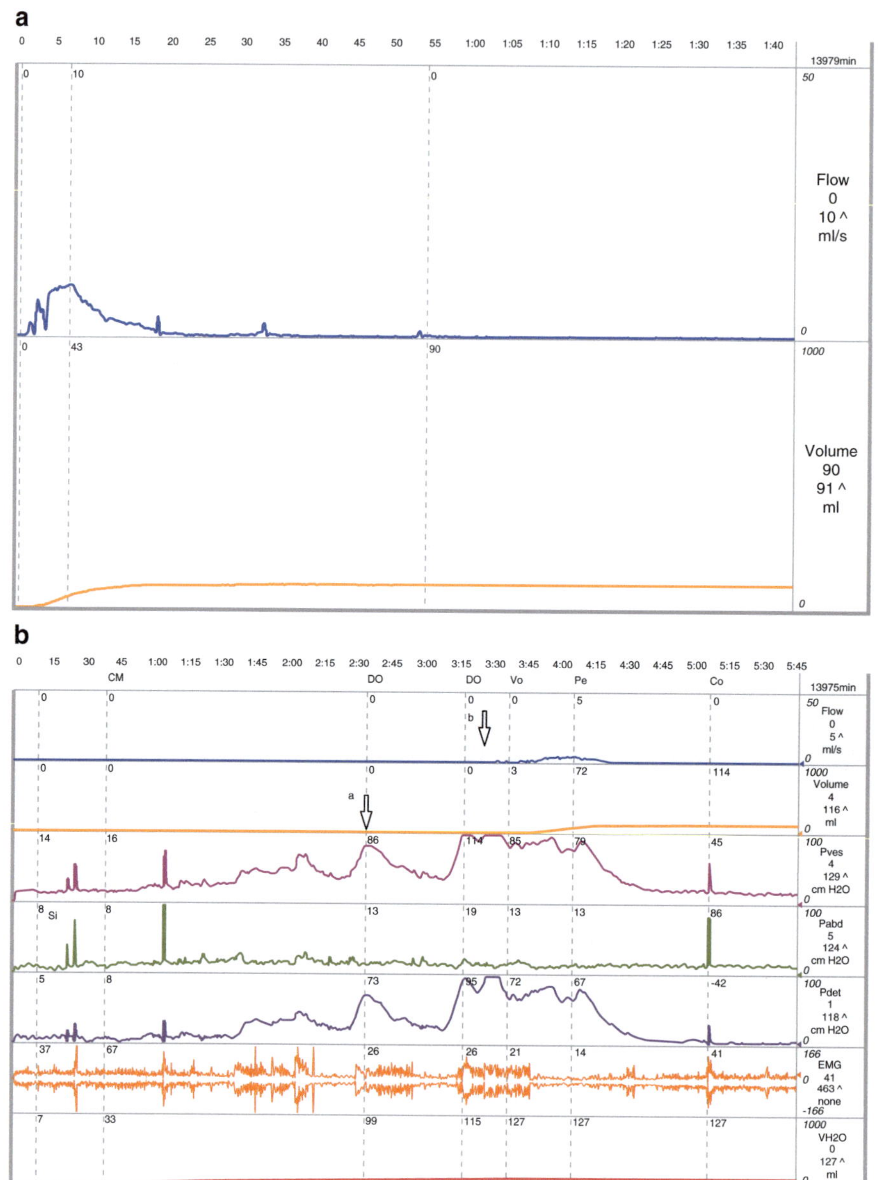

Fig. 19.2 (**a**) Non-invasive uroflow, (**b**) CMG and PFS, (**c**) expanded PFS, (**d**) nomogram

involuntary detrusor contraction. (a) It is accompanied by a voluntary increase in EMG activity (b) and eventually a small amount of flow (c), representing an involuntary detrusor contraction associated with incontinence. As the patient begins to leak, the P_{det} decreases slightly (d). The patient indicates he could no longer resist

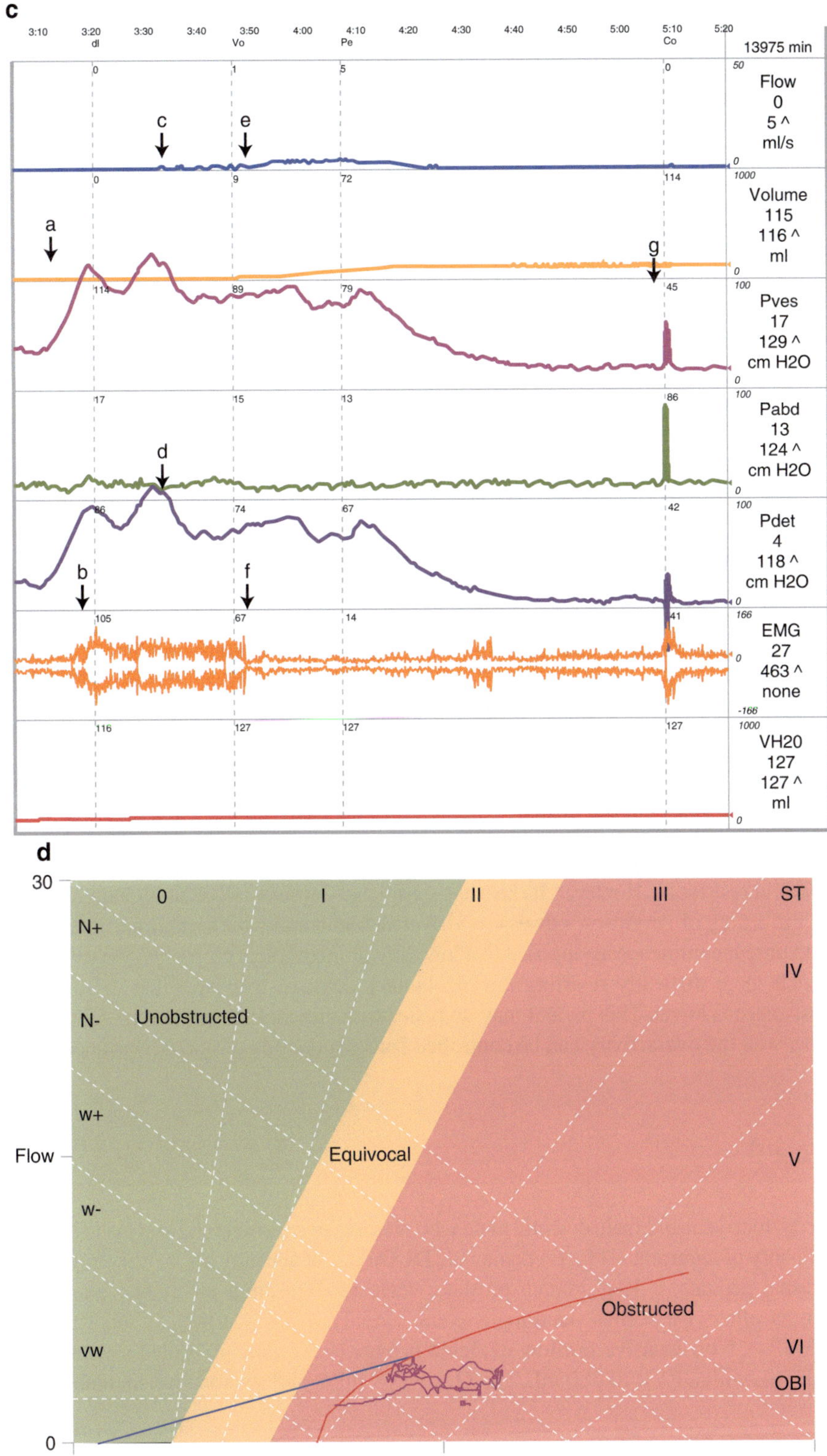

Fig. 19.2 (continued)

the urge and is given permission to void (e). As he begins to void, the flow rate rises, the EMG activity decreases (f), and the P_{det} remains constant throughout the void. The Q_{max} is 5 mL/s, the $P_{det}@Q_{max}$ is 67 cm/H_2O, and the flow pattern is continuous with a prolonged plateau. The patient voids 116 mL with a PVR of 11 mL. At the conclusion of the study, both P_{ves} and P_{abd} remain active and concordant during cough spike. (g) The entire pressure flow relationship is in the obstructed zone of the nomogram (Fig. 19.2d). The non-invasive uroflow and pressure flow tracings are consistent with one another suggesting this is not due to artifact from the study.

The study highlights a number of interesting findings in addition to the obstructed voiding parameters that may affect the selection of treatment. First, the patient has a small capacity bladder of 127 mL and high amplitude detrusor overactivity with incontinence. These findings are consistent with the patient's symptoms of urgency, frequency, and urge incontinence.

The combination of a detrusor contraction and a concomitant increase in EMG activity displayed in this tracing are similar to the urodynamic findings one sees with detrusor external sphincter dyssynergia (DESD). What separates this tracing from DESD is the fact that the patient is voluntarily increasing the EMG activity in an effort to resist the urge to urinate whereas DSD occurs as an involuntary reflex. Without being present during the study or having proper annotation, there would be no way to distinguish by looking at the tracing alone. Another consideration in a patient with Parkinson's Disease is pseudodyssynergia secondary to abnormal sphincter and pelvic floor relaxation during voiding, referred to as sphincter bradykinesia [20]. Since the EMG activity decreased the moment the patient was allowed to void, it is likely that the EMG activity in this study is mostly voluntary.

The patient clearly meets the definition for outlet obstruction secondary to BPH with high pressure/low flow that would likely respond to treatments aimed at reducing urethral resistance. However, he also has significant detrusor overactivity incontinence in the setting of Parkinson's disease and is most bothered by the symptoms of urgency and urge incontinence as opposed to a low flow or incomplete emptying. He will have much more difficulty resisting the involuntary detrusor activity when the urethral resistance is lower. This patient may do better with anticholinergic therapy first to see how well the overactivity can be controlled before reduction of outlet resistance.

Case 3

Sixty-four-year-old male diabetic male who presents in consultation from his PCP with a history of recurrent UTIs. He denies LUTS. On physical exam, his is overweight, has normal genitals, a 40-g smooth prostate, decreased sensation in his feet bilaterally but an otherwise normal neurologic exam. Urinalysis positive for LE and Ketones. PSA 1.4. Non-invasive uroflow depicted in Fig. 19.3a. Patient voided a volume of 103 mL with a PVR of 380 mL. His Q_{max} was 9 mL/s and a somewhat flattened flow pattern. He stated that was a normal void and he could not empty any more urine on a second try. CMG and PFS depicted in Fig. 19.3b.

Baseline pressures are within normal range and pressure lines are concordant during cough spikes (a). No evidence of detrusor overactivity during storage and normal compliance at MCC of 619 mL. (b) Voiding phase demarcated (c) and patient

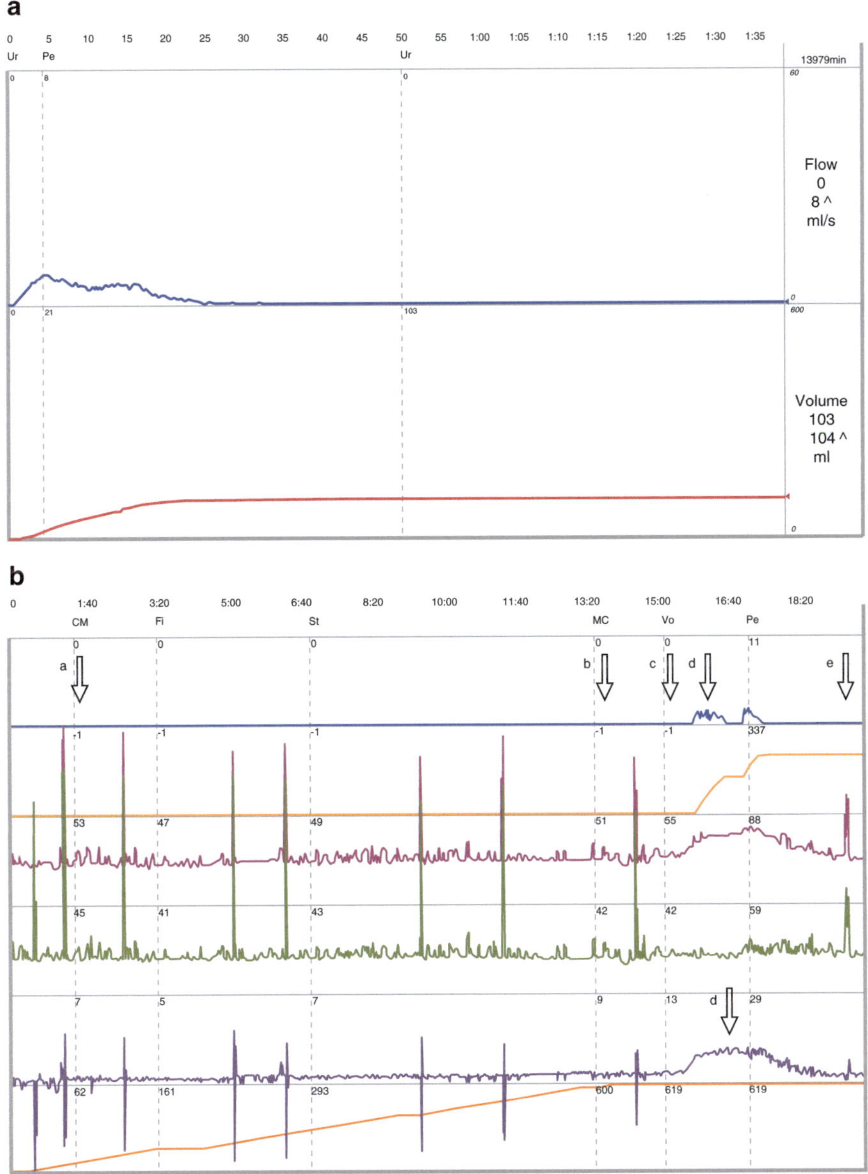

Fig. 19.3 (**a**) Non-invasive uroflow, (**b**) CMG and PFS, (**c**) nomogram

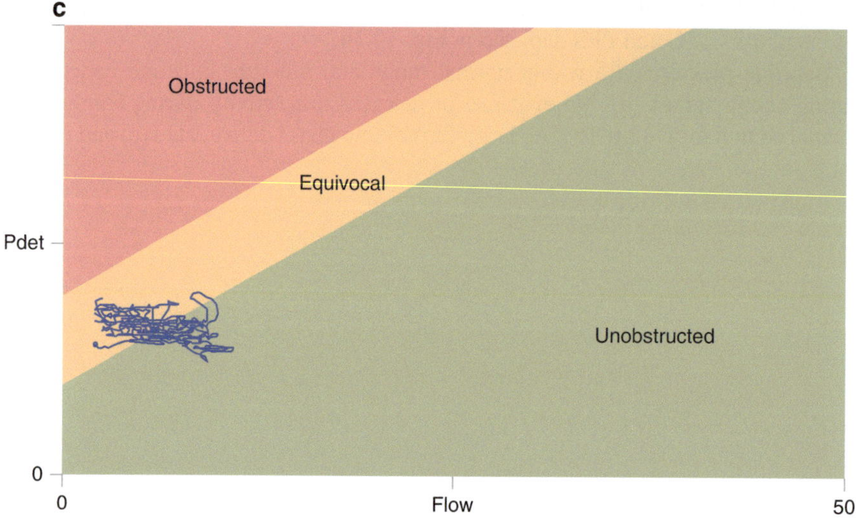

Fig. 19.3 (continued)

initiated voided with a detrusor contraction (d) and an intermittent flow pattern (d). The second portion appears to be associated with valsalva. At the conclusion of the void there is concordance between P_{ves} and P_{abd} during cough spikes (g). Q_{max} is 11 mL/s and $P_{det}@Q_{max}$ is 29 cm/H_2O. He voided a volume of 313 mL with a PVR 303 mL. The nomogram places him in the equivocal range for obstruction (Fig. 19.3c).

This patient has no clinical symptoms of obstruction but has an elevated post-void residual. The question is whether the poor bladder emptying is from obstruction or detrusor underactivity. The non-invasive flow is not helpful. While the flow rate is low, the pattern is continuous. The PFS demonstrates a large capacity bladder with delayed sensation. While he does void with a sustained detrusor contraction, the P_{det} max is only 30 cm/H_2O. The likely diagnosis for this patient is detrusor under activity, possibly related to his diabetes. However, he also likely has a relative outlet obstruction meaning that the relationship between the amount of pressure his bladder can generate and urethral resistance is unfavorable for him emptying efficiently. We would treat this patient as if he were obstructed, since by reducing urethral resistance the bladder pressure that he does generate may be sufficient to empty his bladder more completely.

Case 4

Forty-year-old male with frequency, urgency, decreased flow, and recurrent UTIs. He was found to have high PVRs by bladder ultrasound of over 800 mL. He was placed on CIC but found that the PVRs were very inconsistent in volume. He reported having many catheter volumes of 10–30 mL but then having to urinate again within a short time. He continued to have frequency that he could not explain by bladder volume and continued to have culture proven UTIs. He was scheduled for a videourodynamic study. The non-invasive uroflow is depicted in Fig. 19.4a. He voided 61 mL with an intermittent flow pattern, a Q_{max} of 8 mL/s and a PVR of 400 mL.

CMG and PFS depicted in Fig. 19.4b. Patient is standing, baseline pressures are within normal range, P_{ves} 29 cm/H$_2$O, P_{abd} 26 cm/H$_2$O (a) and both respond to cough with concordant spikes (b). In the middle of the tracing there is a sudden drop in both P_{abd} and P_{ves} and they remain concordant (c). This represents a point during the study that the patient became dizzy and was placed in the supine position. When he resumed the standing position, the pressures returned to their previous values and were again concordant during cough (d). The patient reached maximum capacity of 500 mL and was given permission to void (e).

The PFS portion of the study has been expanded in Fig. 19.4c starting at the point that the patient was given permission to void. (a) After a minute delay the P_{det} begins to rise and he voids 25 mL before the P_{det} returns to zero. Q_{max} is 5 mL/s and $P_{det}@Q_{max}$ is 67 cm/H$_2$O and PVR of 475 mL. Filling resumed slowly over a 4-min period (c) until he developed a second urge and again he attempted to void.

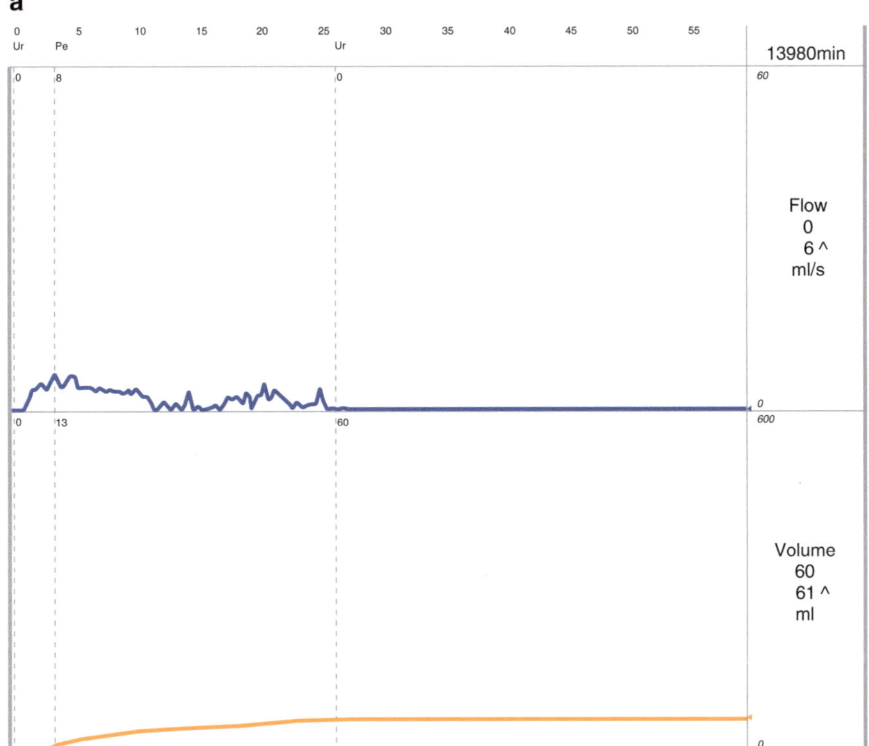

Fig. 19.4 (**a**) Non-invasive Uroflow, (**b**) CMG and PFS, (**c**) expanded PFS, (**d**) nomogram, (**e**) fluoroscopic image—capacity, (**f**) fluoroscopic image—void, (**g**) fluoroscopic image—filling

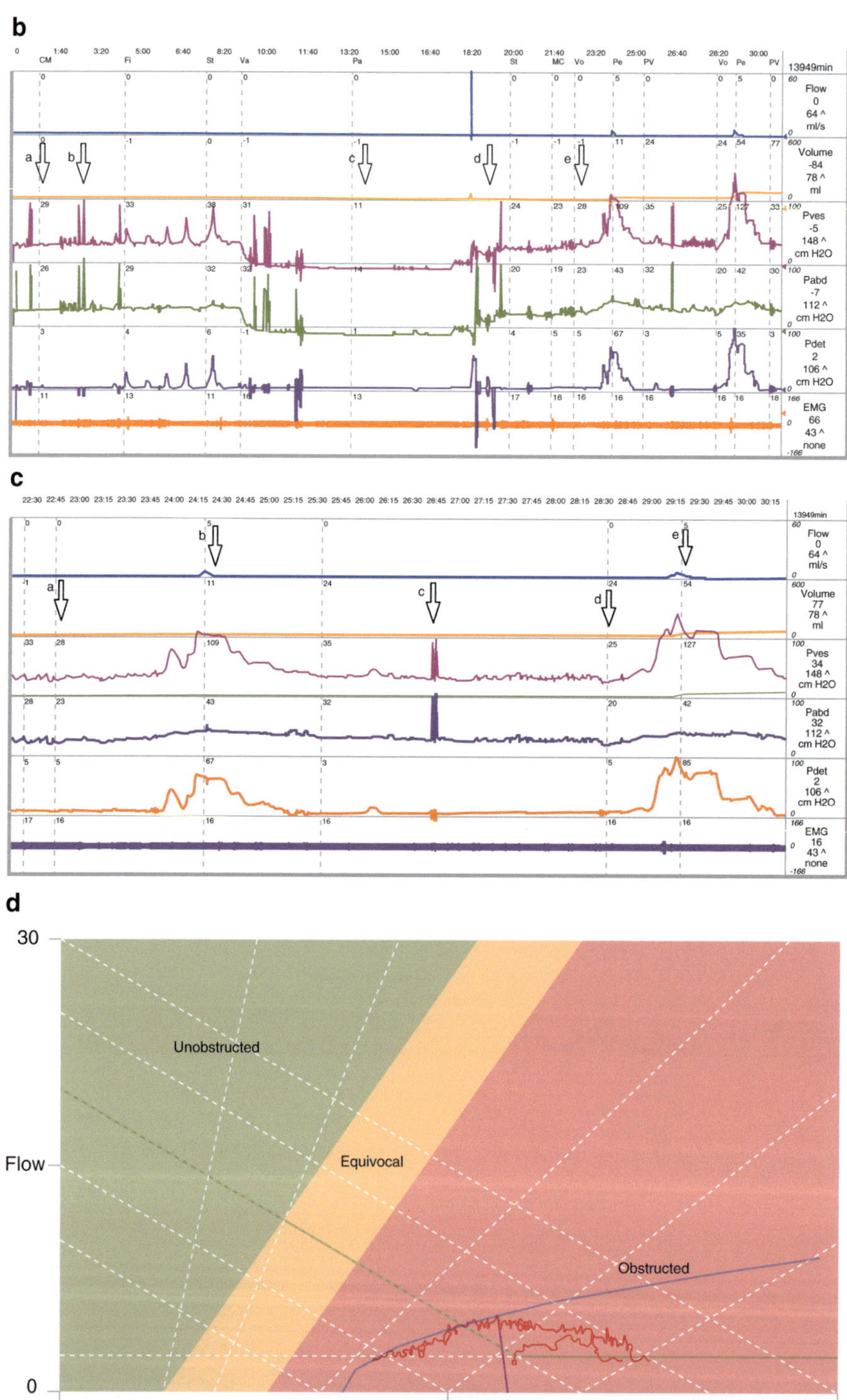

Fig. 19.4 (continued)

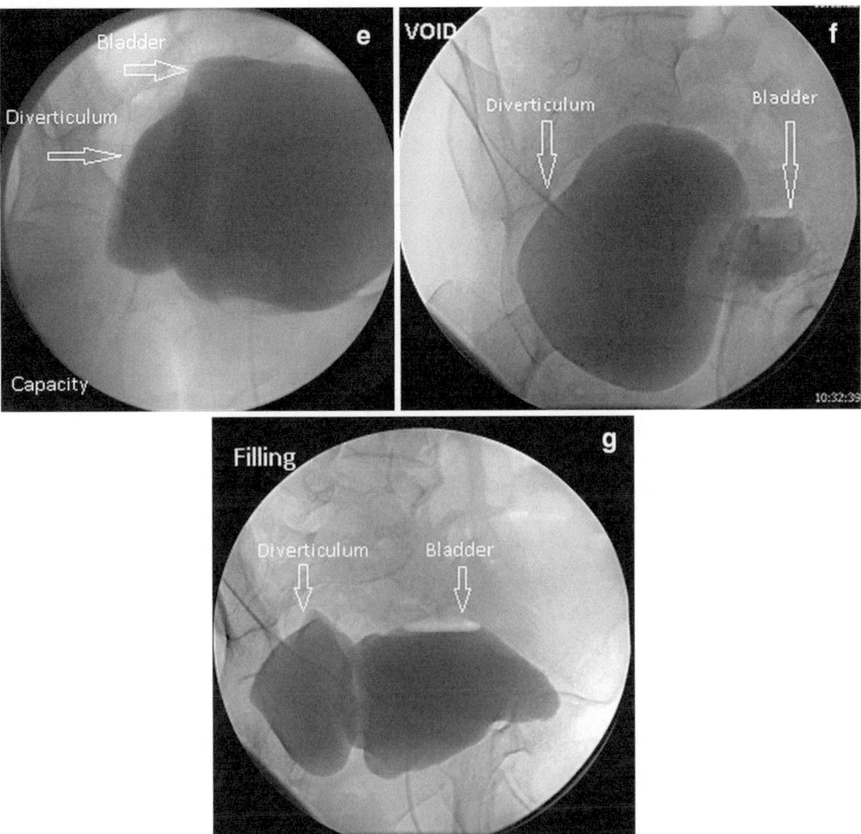

Fig. 19.4 (continued)

The second attempt to void (d) resulted in voided volume of 52 mL, a Q_{max} of 5 mL/s, a $P_{det}@Q_{max}$ of 85 cm/H$_2$O, and PVR of 450 mL (e). The nomogram suggests obstruction (Fig. 19.4d).

Fluoroscopy during urodynamics is termed videourodynamics and allows for evaluation of lower urinary tract anatomy and bladder pressure simultaneously. In this case, (Fig. 19.4e–g) we see that the patient has a large bladder diverticulum that fills during voiding and then empties back into the bladder during rest. Figure 19.4e corresponds to point (a) on the tracing in Fig. 19.4c when the patient reached capacity with a low P_{det} and the bladder diverticulum is small in comparison to the bladder. Figure 19.4f corresponds to point (b) on the tracing in Fig. 19.4c taken during voiding. It shows an enlarging bladder diverticulum, a poorly funneling bladder neck, and poorly filled prostatic urethra in spite of the rising intravesical pressure. This suggests that there is a more resistance at the level of the bladder outlet than there is at the diverticular opening resulting in flow in the direction of the diverticulum. The patient feels that the bladder is empty when the flow stops and if he were to catheterize at this point he would have indeed have a very small PVR. Figure 19.4g is taken during the period of refilling corresponding to point (c) on the tracing in Fig. 19.4c The P_{det} is again low and urine flows from the diverticulum back into the native bladder.

The patient has outlet obstruction associated with a bladder diverticulum. The videourodynamic findings correlate with the patient's symptoms and also help us understand why the patient did not have relief after beginning self-catheterization. He was catheterizing immediately after voiding when the bladder was still empty, prior to refilling from the diverticulum. When the patient began performing CIC without trying to void and allowed the catheter to remain in until the flow stopped, he emptied completely. This took care of the urgency and frequency. In order to resolve his symptoms he will need to address both the obstruction and the bladder diverticulum. By simply addressing outlet obstruction, he will likely continue to fill the diverticulum continuing to have high PVRs and have unresolved symptoms. Removing the diverticulum without addressing the obstruction will leave him at a high risk for recurrence of the diverticulum.

Case 5

Seventy-year-old male presents 3 years after radical retropubic prostatectomy for prostate cancer, with a history of post-prostatectomy incontinence previously treated with a male sling 5 years earlier. Recently developed urinary retention and underwent a procedure for a "scar at the bladder neck." Now he is experiencing incontinence during the daytime that is worse when he is active. The patient underwent urodynamics and a voiding cystourethrogram (VCUG) to evaluate both the function and anatomy of the lower urinary tract (Fig. 19.5a).

Baseline P_{ves}, and P_{abd} pressures are in the normal range for standing. (a) P_{abd} and P_{ves} lines are active and concordant in measurement as demonstrated by the cough pressure spikes. Due to the slightly higher P_{abd} at the beginning of the study the P_{det} starts out with a non-physiologic value of negative 5 cm/H_2O. (b) Attempts to correct this should be made prior to starting the study by adjusting the abdominal catheter or the fluid in the balloon. During the storage phase, detrusor overactivity occurs at a volume of 154 mL. (c) Once the detrusor contraction ends, the patient is asked to cough and perform valsalva maneuvers, but no urodynamic stress incontinence is identified. (d). When he reaches capacity he is given permission to void. (e) Patient is unable to void in spite of a detrusor contraction of over 100 cm/H_2O. (f) He subsequently attempts to augment the detrusor contraction with a valsalva maneuver (g) and is still unable to produce flow. The vesical catheter is then removed as illustrated by the sudden drop in P_{ves} (h) and he is asked to cough and valsalva without the vesical catheter and urodynamic stress incontinence is and noted (i).

At rest, in the right anterior oblique position, fluoroscopy demonstrates bilateral vesicoureteral reflux left>right and a closed bladder neck (Fig. 19.5b). Voiding image in left anterior oblique position demonstrates the catheter in the urethra, partially open bladder neck, contrast narrowing at the level of the external sphincter and bone anchors bilaterally in the inferior rami of pubis (Fig. 19.5c).

This patient has a clinical presentation of urinary incontinence secondary to urethral dysfunction and BOO from a post-prostatectomy bladder neck contracture.

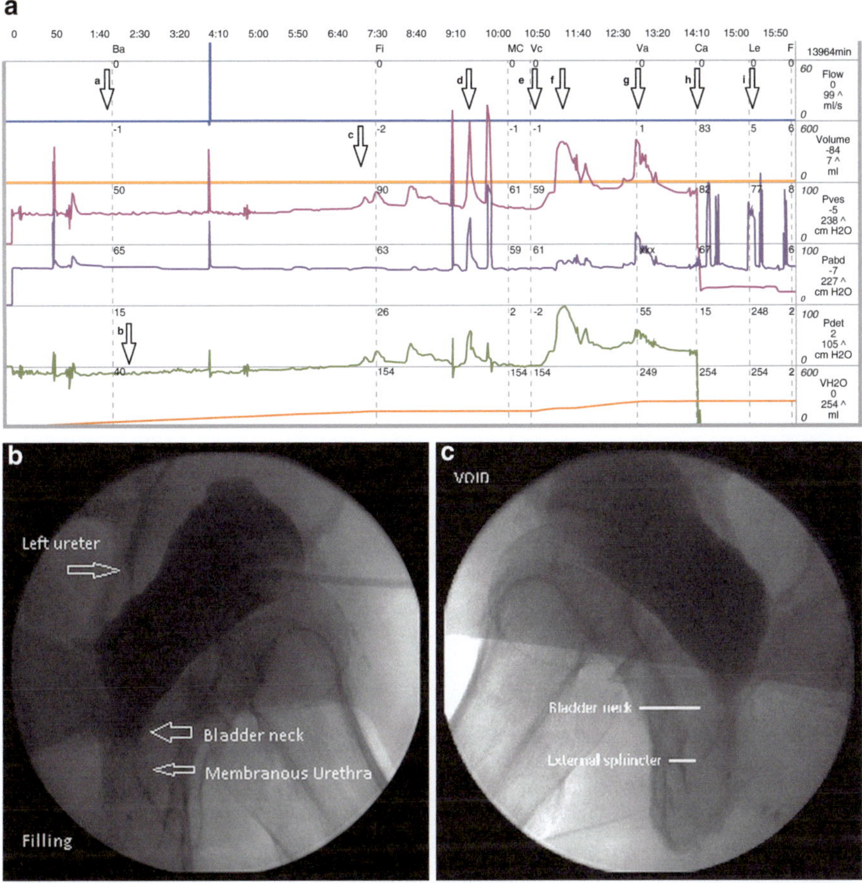

Fig. 19.5 (**a**) CMG and PFS, (**b**) fluoroscopic image—resting cystogram, (**c**) fluoroscopic image voiding cystourethrogram

The urodynamic study demonstrates obstructive parameters and fluoroscopy identifies anatomic evidence that the obstruction is at the level of the bladder neck. It also demonstrates bilateral vesicoureteral reflux. Subsequent cystoscopy confirmed a bladder neck contracture.

Case 6: Relative Outlet Obstruction After Sling

Sixty-five-year-old woman, 6 months status post a midurethral sling, presents with slow, intermittent flow and incomplete emptying. No urinary incontinence symptoms. The physical exam was normal; specifically there was no evidence of mesh exposure on vaginal exam. The sling could be palpated at the proximal urethra. Urinalysis negative. Non-invasive uroflow depicted in Fig. 19.6a. The initial spike (a) should be

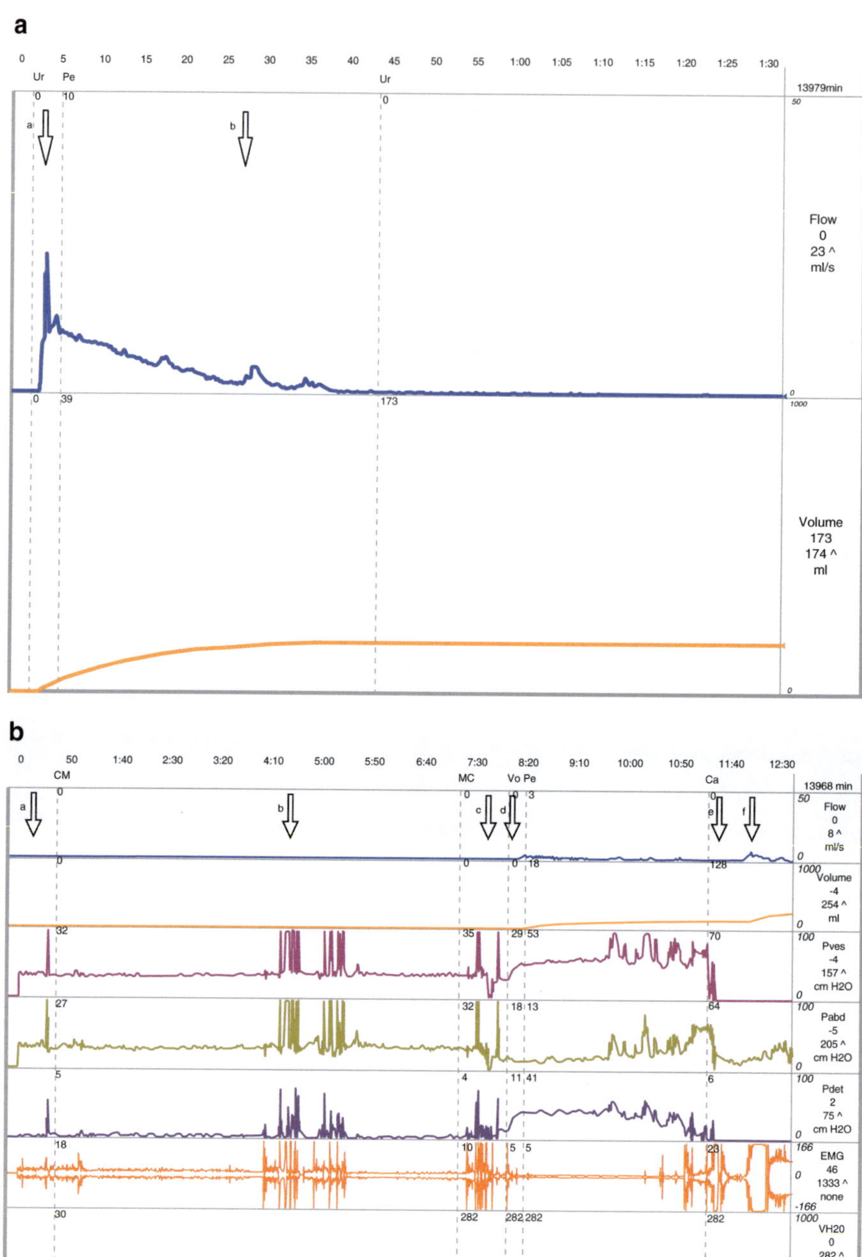

Fig. 19.6 (**a**) Non-invasive uroflow, (**b**) CMG and PFS, (**c**) PFS expanded

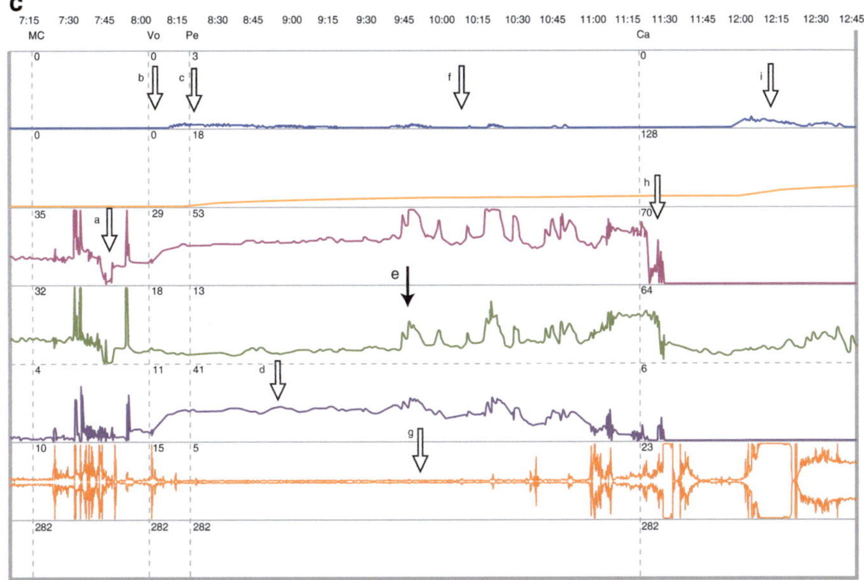

Fig. 19.6 (continued)

disregarded as artifact since it lasts less than 2 s. Taking that into consideration the Q_{max} is 12 cc/s and the curve has a prolonged terminal portion as opposed to being bell-shaped (b).

CMG and PFS (Fig. 19.6b) Baseline pressures are within the normal range and concordant with one another (a). Multiple cough and valsalva maneuvers performed to assess for urinary incontinence (b). Storage phase demonstrates no evidence of urodynamic incontinence and normal compliance. Patient moved from a standing to a sitting position between storage and emptying with adjustment of transducers (c) and reestablishment of PFS baseline and concordance. Patient was given permission to void and did so with a combination of detrusor contraction and Valsalva (d). At the conclusion of the study the vesical catheter was removed (e) and she completed her void (f). The PFS is expanded in Fig. 19.6c for closer examination.

Expanded PFS section (Fig. 19.6c). The patient's position adjusted (a) and baseline pressures and concordance are reestablished. After she is given permission to void (b), she initiates flow and rapidly reaches her Q_{max} of 8 mL/s with a $P_{det}@Q_{max}$ of 41 cm/H_2O (c). The flow is intermittent. (f) During the initial phase of voiding, she voids only 28 mL with a sustained detrusor contraction that lasts the duration of the void (d). Halfway through this portion of the voiding phase she begins to augment the void with valsalva (e). EMG activity decreases during void (g). The vesical catheter is removed and she is able to void another 200 mL (h). The flow pattern is similar in shape to the pattern on her NIF.

This study is suggestive of a relative obstruction.

Case 7: Post Sling Obstruction

Fifty-four year-old female presents 6 months following placement of a midurethral sling for stress urinary incontinence. Her stress incontinence has improved but she now is bothered by urge incontinence. She reports being in urinary retention following her sling for the first 2 weeks during which time she used an indwelling catheter. She is currently on anticholinergic medication that has helped somewhat, but remains bothered. A non-invasive flow was obtained (Fig. 19.7a), during which she voided 307 mL with a Q_{max} of 8 mLs/s, a prolonged flow pattern and a PVR of 30 mL.

CMG and PFS (Fig. 19.7b) Baseline pressures are within normal range for a patient standing and are concordant during a cough spike (a). There is significant activity in the abdominal pressure line throughout study that is not associated with patient moving around and which creates artifact in the P_{det} tracing. However, there is definitive evidence of detrusor overactivity beginning at a volume of 116 mL associated with strong urge to urinate (b) and then continuing episodically throughout the duration of the study (c–e). No evidence of urodynamic stress incontinence with cough or valsalva. The maximum capacity is 266 mL. After changing positions and reestablishing baseline pressures by adjusting the transducers to the height of the symphysis (f), she is given permission to void (g). She voids with a detrusor contraction (h) and continuous flow pattern (i). Transducers are active at end of study during cough spike (j). The expanded PFS study is displayed in Fig. 19.7c.

Expanded PFS (Fig. 19.7c) This tracing begins at the time of her last involuntary detrusor contraction (a). After she reached capacity she is moved from standing to sitting position, the transducers are adjusted, and a new baseline is established (b). Her voiding attempt is initiated with both a detrusor contraction and valsalva (c), followed by cessation of EMG activity (d) and a persistent detrusor contraction (e). She voids a total of 228 mL with a Q_{max} of 5 mL/s, $P_{det}@Q_{max}$ of 51 cm H_2O, and a prolonged pattern, consistent with obstruction. Fluoroscopy revealed an open bladder neck with narrowing at proximal urethral and slight indentation in the area of the previous sling (Fig. 19.7d).

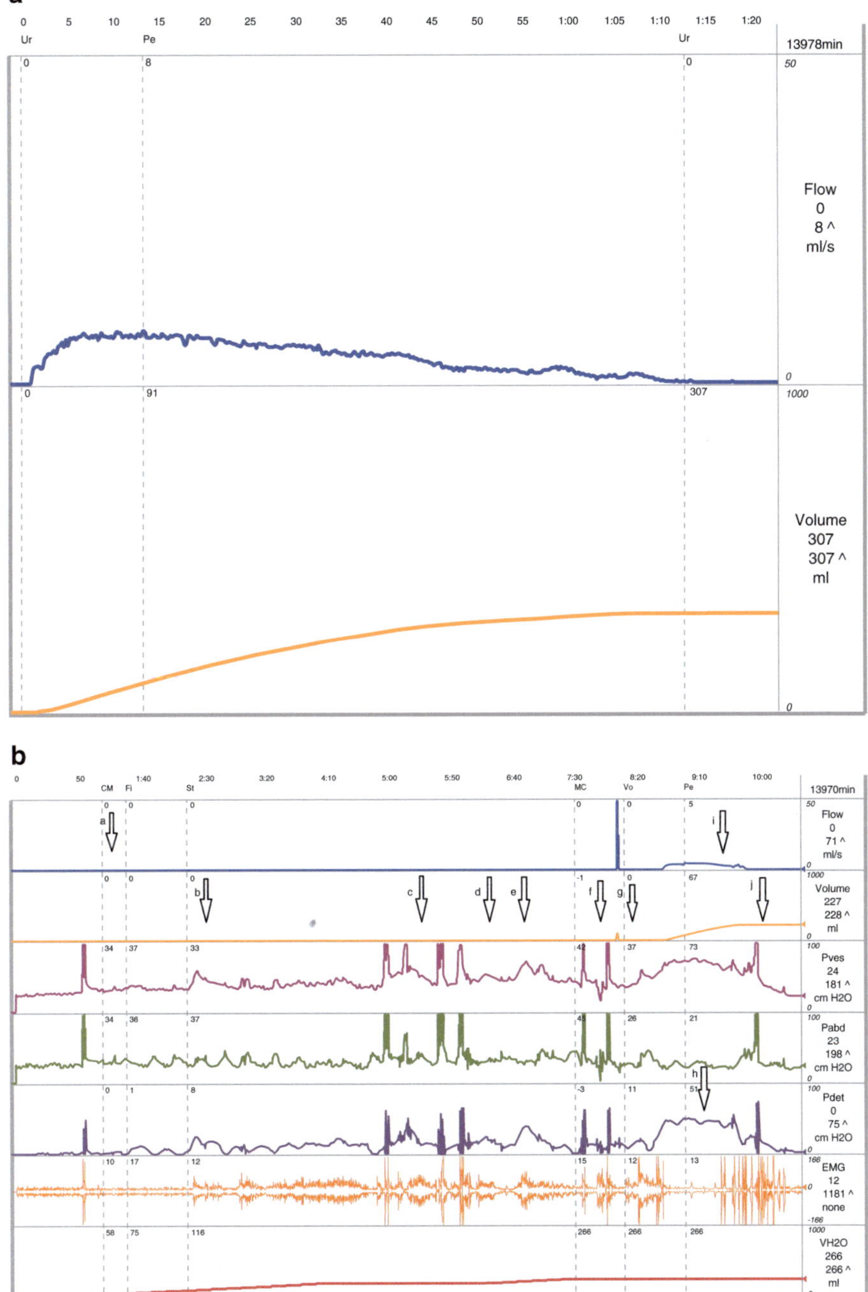

Fig. 19.7 (**a**) Non-invasive uroflow, (**b**) CMG and PFS, (**c**) expanded PFS, (**d**) fluoroscopic image—voiding cystourethrogram corresponding to (**c**)

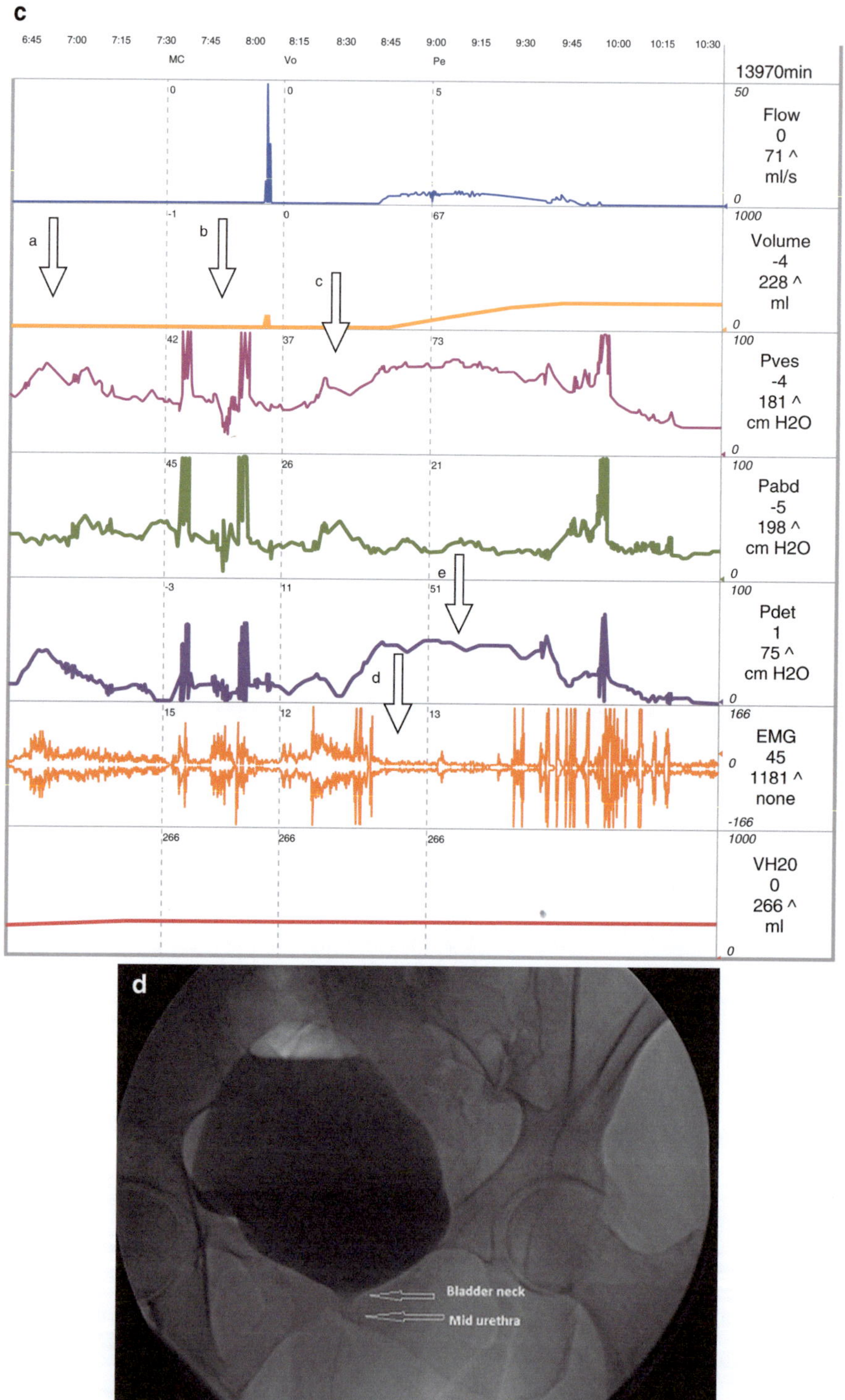

Fig. 19.7 (continued)

Case 8

Sixty-four year-old patient who presents with a history of stress urinary incontinence symptoms for many years. She denies urgency or urge incontinence. Denies previous therapy or history of urinary tract infection. Does state that she strains to urinate. No evidence of prolapse on physical exam. Non-invasive uroflow demonstrates a voided volume of 284 mL with a Q_{max} of 29 mL/s, (after smoothing the curve) and an intermittent flow pattern. PVR of 30 mL (Fig. 19.8a).

CMG and PFS (Fig. 19.8b) Baseline pressures within normal range for standing patient P_{ves} 27, P_{abd} 21, and P_{det} of 6 cm/H$_2$O. (a) Good concordance of both lines during cough spikes (b) No evidence of detrusor overactivity. Urodynamic stress incontinence is identified during valsalva maneuvers performed at a volume of 207 mL with VLPPs of 67 and 71 cm/H$_2$O. Patient is moved from standing to sitting position, transducers are adjusted, and new baseline pressures are established prior to voiding (d). Patient voids with a sustained valsalva maneuver for the initial 100 mL of the void (e) and then with intermittent valsalva during the remaining 200 mL (f) with flow patterns that reflected that voiding mechanism. The EMG is increasingly active during this period, (g) demonstrating how difficult it is to assess pelvic relaxation with surface electrodes when the patient is straining.

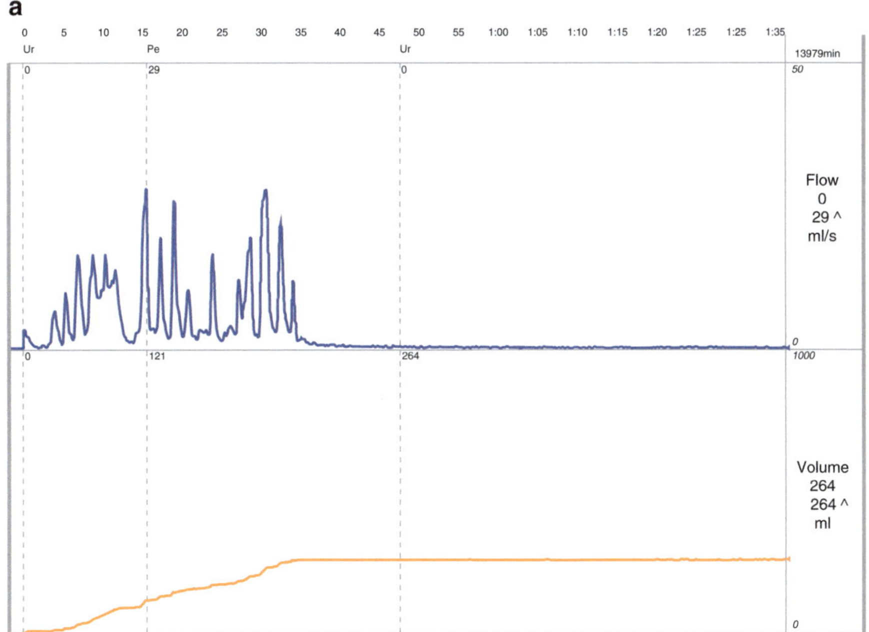

Fig. 19.8 (a) Non-invasive uroflow, (b) CMG and PFS, (c) expanded PFS

b

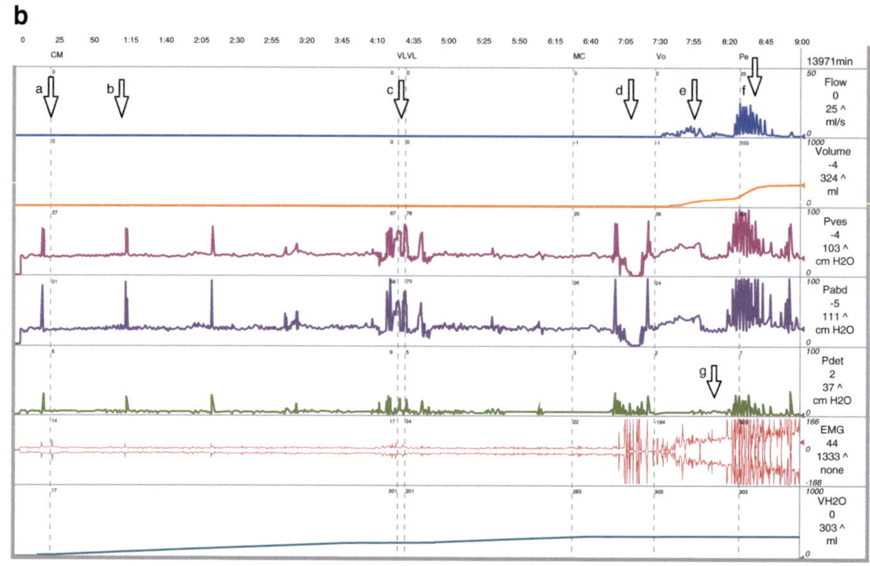

c

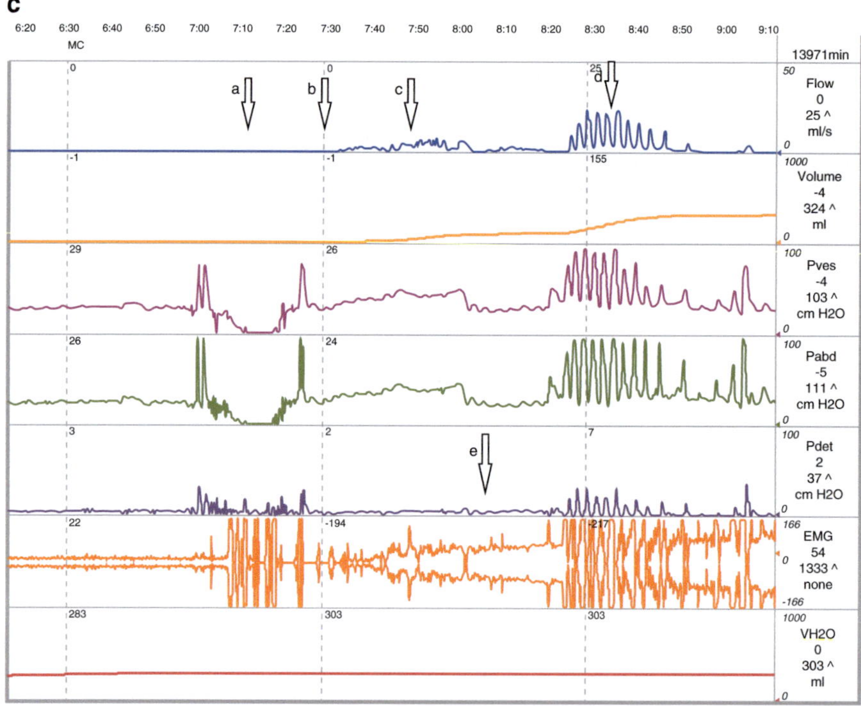

Fig. 19.8 (continued)

Expanded PFS (Fig. 19.8c) This section demonstrates a position change with readjustment of transducers (a). Permission to void. (b) Flow pattern that is initially continuous and low in amplitude (c). Flow pattern that becomes more intermittent with higher amplitude spikes (d). This flow pattern is mirrored by both the P_{ves} and P_{abd} tracings suggesting a valsalva voiding mechanism. The subtracted P_{det} suggests there is minimal if any detrusor functions (e). This study confirms the suspicion from the non-invasive uroflow that the patient is a valsalva voider. This may have implications for the type of anti-incontinence procedure the patient is offered.

Conclusion

BOO can be associated with LUTS or can remain "silent" leading to secondary conditions such as urinary tract infections, bladder diverticulum, bladder stones, or renal failure. Categorizing and understanding these entities is crucial when evaluating a patient with potential BOO. Urodynamic evaluation, specifically the PFS, is currently the gold standard diagnostic tool. Professional medical societies recommend a focused use of urodynamics in the evaluation of patients at risk for BOO. While it is not necessary to perform pressure flow studies in everyone suspected of having BOO, when an accurate diagnosis is critical before selecting potentially morbid procedures in selected patients and most experts agree it should be available.

References

1. de la Rosette JJ, et al. Relationship between lower urinary tract symptoms and bladder outlet obstruction. Results for the ICS-BPH study. Neurourol Urodyn. 1998;17(2):99–108.
2. Nitti VW. Pressure flow urodynamic studies: the gold standard for diagnosing bladder outlet obstruction. Rev Urol. 2005;7 Suppl 6:S14–21.
3. Abrams P, Cardozo L, Dall M, et al. The standardization of terminology of lower urinary tract function: report from the Standardisation Sub-Committee of the International Continence Society. Neurourol Urodyn. 2002;21:167–78.
4. Winters JC, Domchowski RR, Goldstein HB, Herndon CDA, Kobashi KC, Kraus SR, Lemack GE, Nitti VW, Rovner ES, Wein AJ. Urodynamic guidelines in adults: AUA/SUFU guideline. J Urol. 2012;188:2464–72.
5. Belal M, Abrams P. Noninvasive methods of diagnosing bladder outlet obstruction in men. Part 1: nonurodynamic approach. J Urol. 2006;176:22–8.
6. Brucker BM, Fong EDM, Shah SR, Kelly C, Rosenblum N, Nitti VW. Urodynamic differences between dysfunctional voiding and primary bladder neck obstruction in women. Urology. 2012;1(80):55–60.
7. Arnolds M, Oelke M. Positioning invasive versus noninvasive urodynamics in the assessment of bladder outlet obstruction. Curr Opin Urol. 2009;19:55–62.
8. Griffiths D, et al. Standardization of terminology of lower urinary tract function: pressure-flow studies of voiding, urethral resistance, and urethral obstruction. International Continence Society Subcommittee on Standardization of Terminology of Pressure-Flow Studies. Neurourol Urodyn. 1997;16(1):1–18.

9. Sonke GS, et al. Variability of pressure-flow studies in men with lower urinary tract symptoms. Neurourol Urodyn. 2000;19(6):637–51 (discussion 651–656).
10. Akikwala TV, Fleischman N, Nitti VW. Comparison of diagnostic criteria for female bladder outlet obstruction. J Urol. 2006;176:2093–7.
11. Chassagne S, Bernier PA, Haab F, Roehrborn CG, Reisch JS, Zimmern PE. Proposed cutoff values to define bladder outlet obstruction in women. Urology. 1998;51(3):408–11.
12. Nitti V, Tu L, Gitlin J. Diagnosing bladder outlet obstruction in women. J Urol. 1999;161(5): 1535–40.
13. Blaivas JG, Groutz A. Bladder outlet obstruction nomogram for women with lower urinary tract symptomatology. Neurourol Urodyn. 2000;19(5):553–64.
14. Defreitas GA, Zimmern PE, Lemack GE, Shariat SF. Refining diagnosis of anatomic female bladder outlet obstruction: comparison of pressure-flow study parameters in clinically obstructed women with those of normal controls. Urology. 2004;64(4):675–9.
15. Haylen BT, de Ridder D, Freeman RM, et al. An International Urogynaecological Association (IUGA)/International Continence Society (ICS) joint report on the terminology for female pelvic floor dysfunction. Int Urogynecol J. 2010;21:5–26.
16. National Clinical Guidelines Center at the Royal College of Physicians; a report commissioned by the NICE 201. Lower urinary tract symptoms in men. Clinical Guideline 97.
17. Klingler HC, Madersbacher S, Djavan B, et al. Morbidity of the evaluation of the lower urinary tract with transurethral multichannel pressure flow studies. J Urol. 1998;159:191–4.
18. Madersbacher S, Alivizatos G, Nordling J, et al. EAU 2004 guidelines on assessment, therapy and follow-up of men with lower urinary tract symptoms suggestive of benign prostatic obstruction (BPH guidelines). Eur Urol. 2004;46:547–54.
19. Schafer W, Abrams P, Liao L, et al. Good urodynamic practices: uroflowmetry, filling cystometry and pressure flow studies. Neurourol Urodyn. 2002;21:261–74.
20. Stocchi F, Carbone A, Inghilleri M, Monge A, Ruggieri S, Berardelli A, Manfredi M. Urodynamic and neurophysiological evaluation in Parkinson's disease and multiple system atrophy. J Neurol Neurosurg Psychiatry. 1997;62(5):507–11.

Part III
Final Examination: Unknowns

Chapter 20
Test Tracings: Final Exam

Eric S. Rovner and Michelle E. Koski

Test Question 1

Clinical history: A 50-year-old female presents complaining of urinary frequency, urgency, and nocturia. Physical exam shows normal genitalia without evidence of pelvic organ prolapse or urethral hypermobility. During urodynamic testing the patient reports early first sensation at a volume of 10 cc and reaches maximum cystometric capacity at 130 cc (filling volume tracing, Vinf, not shown.) (Fig. 20.1).

This study demonstrates:

1. Detrusor overactivity
2. Stress urinary incontinence
3. Impaired compliance
4. Detrusor sphincter dyssynergia (DSD)
5. Increased bladder sensation

Answer 5. Increased bladder sensation is demonstrated with early first sensation, early first desire to void, early strong desire to void and diminished maximum cystometric capacity. Detrusor overactivity is not seen on this tracing nor is stress urinary incontinence, impaired compliance, or an obstructed voiding pattern to suggest DSD.

E.S. Rovner, MD (✉)
Department of Urology, Medical University of South Carolina,
96 Jonathan Lucas St., CSB 644, Charleston, SC 29425, USA
e-mail: rovnere@musc.edu

M.E. Koski, MD (✉)
Department of Urology, Medical University of South Carolina,
96 Jonathan Lucas St., CSB 644, Charleston, SC 29425, USA

Department of Urology, Kaiser Permanente Southern California,
400 Craven Road, San Marcos, CA 92078, USA
e-mail: mkoski82@hotmail.com

© Springer Science+Business Media New York 2015
E.S. Rovner, M.E. Koski (eds.), *Rapid and Practical Interpretation
of Urodynamics*, DOI 10.1007/978-1-4939-1764-8_20

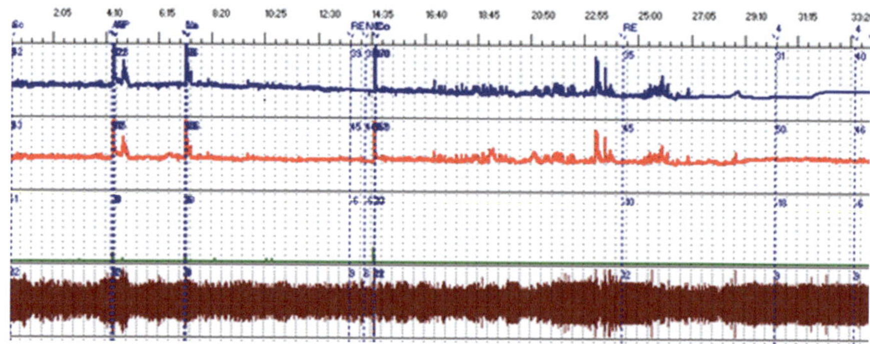

Fig. 20.1

Test Question 2

Clinical history: A 60 year old female presents with complaints of urgency, frequency, nocturia, and urgency-related incontinence. Physical exam is notable for a Grade IV cystocele, Grade III uterine prolapse, and Grade II rectocele. No stress incontinence is elicited with reduction of the prolapse. During urodynamic testing the patient reported urgency and a strong desire to void at 185 cc which she attempted to suppress (Fig. 20.2).

This study demonstrates:

1. Detrusor overactivity with leakage
2. Stress urinary incontinence
3. Impaired compliance
4. Striated sphincter dyssynergia
5. Detrusor overactivity without leakage

Answer 5. Detrusor overactivity without leakage is demonstrated with the rise in detrusor pressure and vesical pressure during the filling phase. No corresponding leakage is recorded by the uroflometer.

Test Question 3

The videofluoroscopic image (Fig. 20.3) is obtained in the patient described in Test Question 2.

This demonstrates:

1. Bladder diverticulum
2. Significant cystocele
3. Urethral hypermobility
4. Neurogenic bladder
5. Mild cystocele

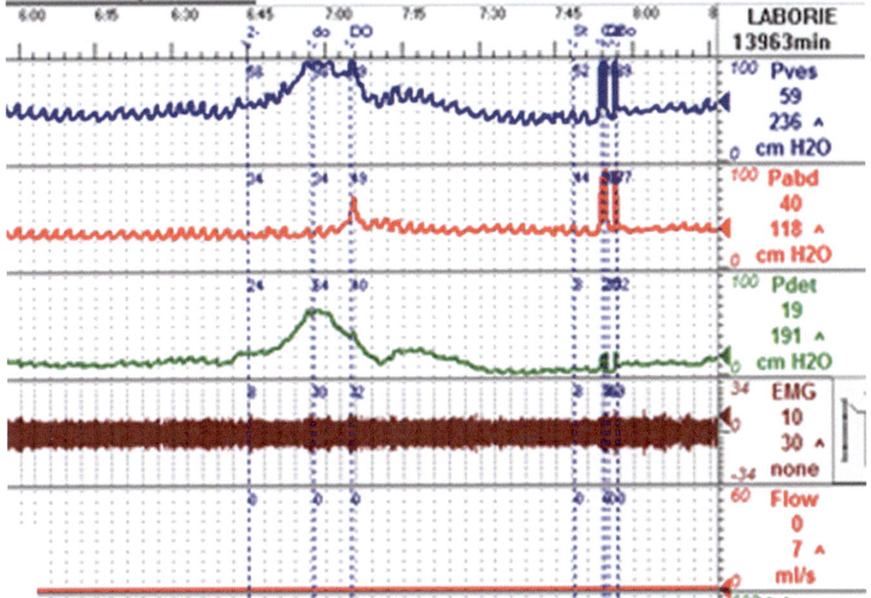

Fig. 20.2

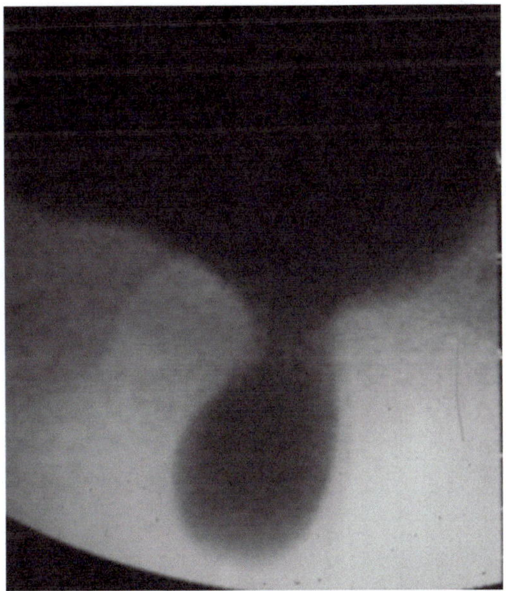

Fig. 20.3

Answer 2. Significant cystocele. The base of the bladder is descended well below the pubic symphysis.

Test Question 4

Clinical history: A 55-year-old female with multiple sclerosis presents with complaints of urgency, frequency, nocturia, and urgency-related incontinence. Physical exam reveals normal genitalia without evidence of prolapse. No stress incontinence is elicited with cough stress test. During urodynamic testing the patient reported urgency and a strong desire to void at 79 cc which she attempted to suppress (Fig. 20.4).

This study demonstrates:

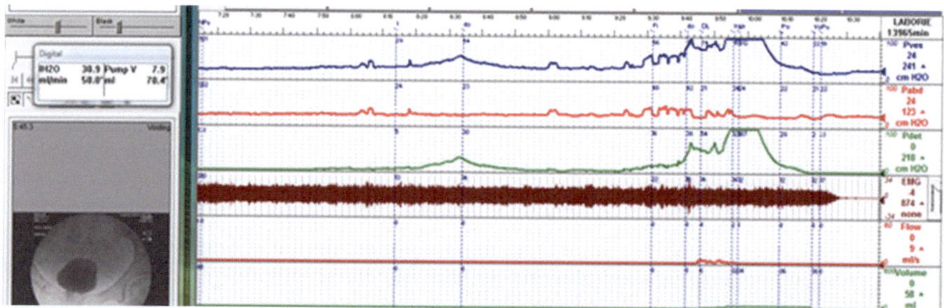

Fig. 20.4

1. Detrusor overactivity with leakage
2. Stress urinary incontinence
3. Impaired compliance
4. Detrusor overactivity without leakage
5. Both 1 and 4

Answer 5. Detrusor overactivity without leakage is noted first then detrusor overactivity with leakage is demonstrated with the rise in detrusor pressure and vesical pressure during the filling phase. Corresponding leakage is recorded by the uroflometer.

Test Question 5

Clinical history: A 65-year-old white male with a history of Parkinson's disease presents with a chief complaint of new onset urinary urgency. Urodynamics are shown in Fig. 20.5. He presents with a voiding diary showing volumes of 400–500 mL. Which of the following would be the best next step?

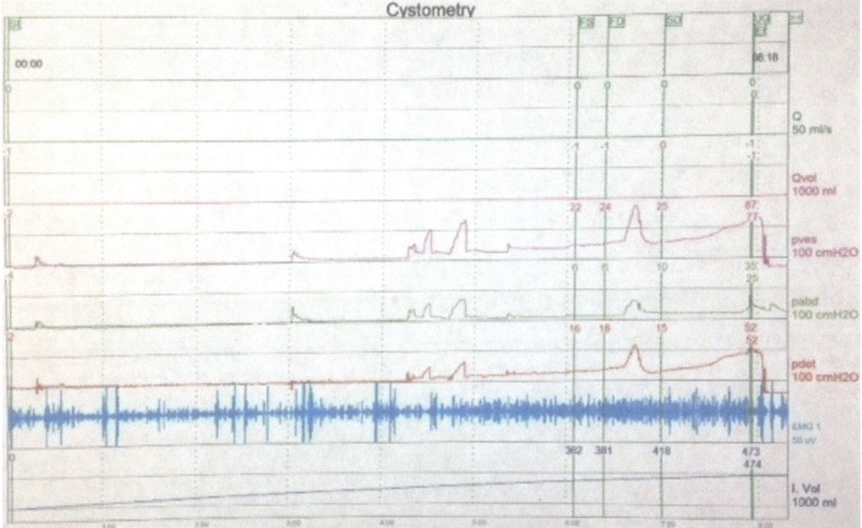

Fig. 20.5

1. Timed voiding and antimuscarinics
2. Intravesical botulinum toxin injection
3. Alpha-blocker therapy
4. Observation

Answer 1. Timed voiding and antimuscarinics. This patient demonstrates poor bladder compliance on his urodynamic tracing. His detrusor leak point pressure is >40 mm H_2O at bladder volumes >380 cc. Therefore, an appropriate next step would be timed voiding. His voided volumes theoretically should be 200–300 cc in order to maintain a normal detrusor pressure. Observation is not an appropriate next step due to the risk of upper tract damage. Alpha-blocker therapy will not improve his abnormal compliance. This patient may ultimately progress and require botulinum toxin injections, but on initial presentation, the least invasive approach should be tried first.

Test Question 6

Clinical History: A 30-year-old male with a history of T11 spinal cord injury is managed with CIC four times daily and maximum anticholinergic therapy. His catheterization diary shows volumes of 250–300 mL. His urodynamic tracing is seen in Fig. 20.6. He still complains of urinary leakage between catheterizations. Which of the following statements is *false*?

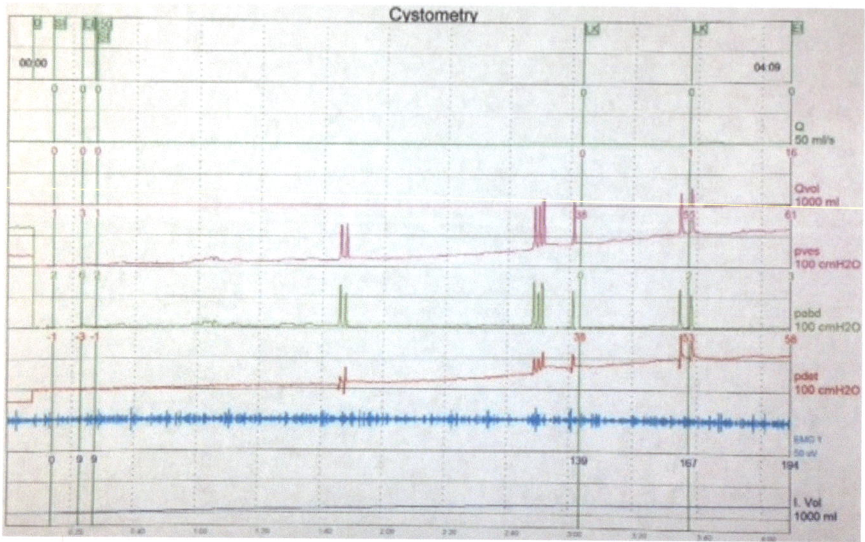

Fig. 20.6

1. The patient is at risk of upper tract damage due to an elevated abdominal leak point pressures during filling.
2. Botulinum toxin injections would be an appropriate next step in therapy.
3. Upper tract imaging should be performed on this patient.
4. This tracing demonstrates a compliance abnormality.

Answer 1. The patient is at risk of upper tract damage due to an elevated abdominal leak point pressures during filling. This patient's tracing shows abnormal bladder compliance and an elevated *detrusor* leak point pressure during filling. Abdominal leak point pressures are not generally related to the risk of upper urinary tract deterioration but detrusor leak point pressures are related to such a risk. Elevations in detrusor pressure, especially a tonic rise as demonstrated in this tracing, are worrisome for upper tract damage. This patient's clinical presentation and urodynamic tracing should warrant an upper tract evaluation. A renal ultrasound at a minimum should be performed. This patient would be an excellent candidate to study using videourodynamics to assess for a "pop-off" mechanism. Botulinum toxin injection would be a reasonable next step. However, if his detrusor pressure does not subsequently improve, he may ultimately require an augmentation cystoplasty.

Test Question 7

Clinical History: A 68-year-old male with benign prostatic hypertrophy undergoes urodynamics (Fig. 20.7).

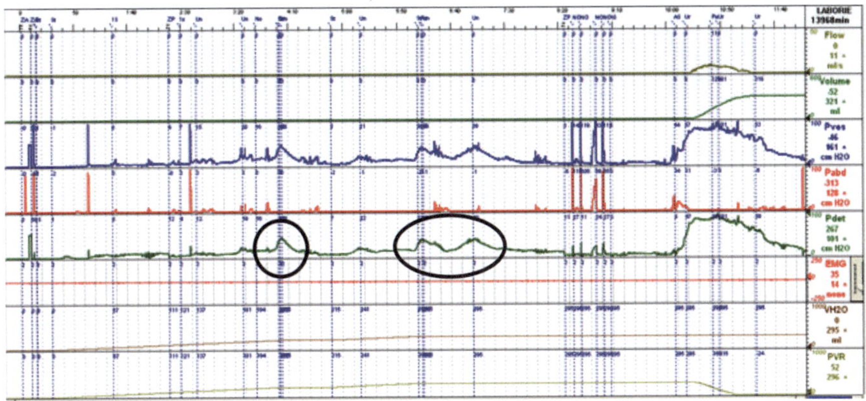

Fig. 20.7

The circles in this study represent:

1. Detrusor overactivity
2. Detrusor underactivity
3. Provocative maneuver (coughing)
4. Artifact
5. Impaired compliance

Answer: 1. Involuntary detrusor contractions produce a rise in pressure in the P_{ves} and P_{det} leads and not in the P_{abd} lead. The circles in this study represent detrusor overactivity. This is not detrusor underactivity as this is related to voiding pressures. A provocative maneuver such as coughing would generally appear as a sharp increase in the P_{ves} and P_{abd} leads due to the sudden increase in pressure generated with the cough. This does not represent an artifact; an increase in pressure in both the P_{ves} and the P_{det} lead in the face of a quiescent P_{abd} represents a bona fide detrusor contraction. Impaired compliance would appear as a slow increase in the P_{det} and P_{ves} signals as the volume in the bladder increases.

Test Question 8

Clinical History: A 57-year-old female with complaints of urinary incontinence undergoes urodynamics (Fig. 20.8).

The circles in this study represent detrusor overactivity: TRUE OR FALSE?

Answer: False. The areas indicated by the circles do not represent detrusor overactivity. They highlight the provocative maneuver of coughing as demonstrated by the sharp increase in pressure in the P_{ves} and P_{abd} leads. The spike-like increase in the P_{det} lead is not consistent with the characteristic wave form of a detrusor contraction which typically has a smoother rise and fall akin to that of a bell shaped curve.

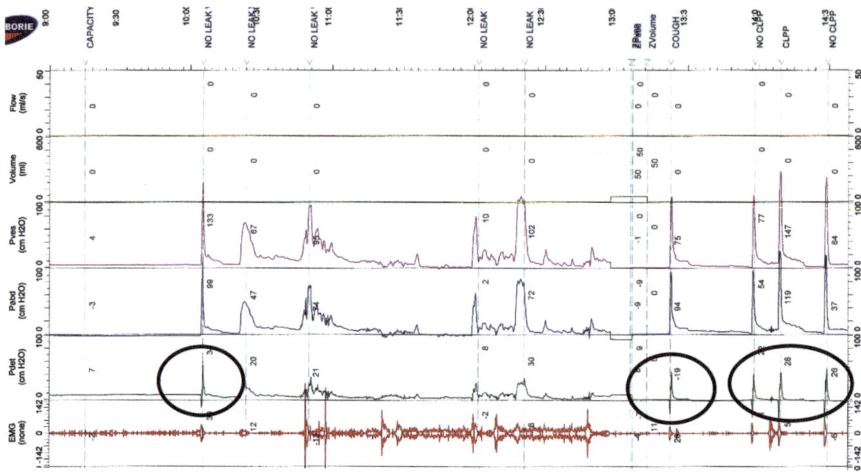

Fig. 20.8

These spikes in the P_{det} actually represent an artifact of urodynamic studies resulting from catheter transducer mismatch between the P_{ves} and P_{det} transducers. This is an important form of artifact in urodynamic studies.

Test Question 9

Clinical History: A 57-year-old female with urinary incontinence. The patient reports leakage with physical activity, such as playing soccer, working out at the gym, and lifting weights, and also reports leakage preceded by the urge to urinate. This sometimes occurs at night while she is sleeping. She wears two pads per day. The patient was prescribed an antimuscarinic medication at her last office visit, which she reports is helping with her urgency, but not with her urinary incontinence (Fig. 20.9a, b).

1. Based on the urodynamics study, what is the primary diagnosis?

   a. Stress urinary incontinence only
   b. Urgency urinary incontinence only
   c. Mixed urinary incontinence
   d. Neither stress nor urge urinary incontinence

2. At approximately 67 mL H_2O, the urethral tracing indicates

   a. A rise in maximum urethral pressure (MUP)
   b. A rise in maximum urethral closure pressure (MUCP)
   c. An artifact due to repositioning of the catheter

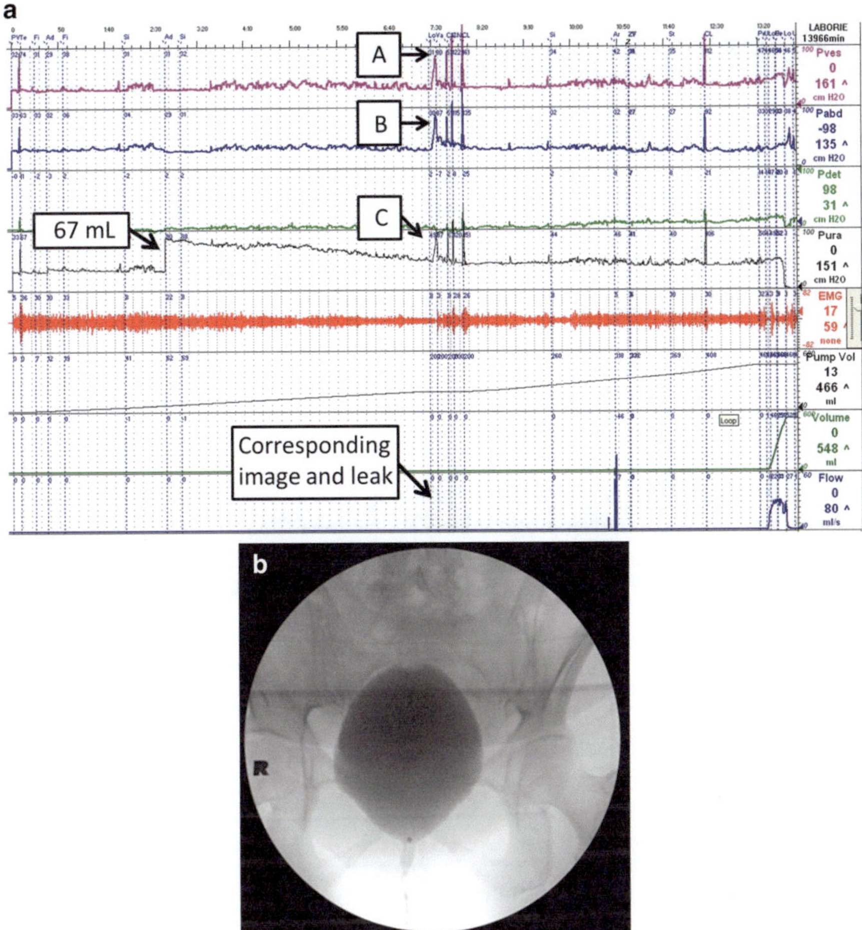

Fig. 20.9

3. Which arrow points to the ALPP?

    a. A
    b. B
    c. C
    d. A and B

Answers (1A, 2C, 3B)

1. The correct answer is A, stress urinary incontinence only. The study indicates that the patient leaks with stress maneuvers. Leakage is not associated with an involuntary detrusor contraction, which means that there is no urgency incontinence and furthermore, no mixed urinary incontinence.

2. The correct answer is C, an artifact due to repositioning of the catheter, represented by a sudden vertical change in the Pura catheter tracing. Urethral pressure measurements, on the other hand, occur as the urethral catheter is removed from the bladder. Typically, these pressures are exerted over time, and not just at one moment in time, as exhibited on this tracing.
3. The correct answer is D, indicating that ALPP is measured by the pressure measurement on P_{ves} or P_{abd}. As discussed in Chap. 16, however, this is controversial and in reality either measurement, P_{ves}, or P_{abd}, is acceptable and could be used for ALPPs. The most important point is that ALPPs are measured with the same type of catheter each time in a standardized fashion.

Test Question 10

Clinical History: A 61-year-old female presents with a complaint of urinary incontinence that has been getting progressively worse over the last 4 years. She reports symptoms of both stress and urge incontinence and has tried an antimuscarinic without improvement of her symptoms. Please note, there is no voiding phase in this study (Fig. 20.10a, b).

1. Fluoroscopy shows

    a. A smooth-walled bladder
    b. An open bladder neck
    c. Vesicoureteral reflux
    d. a and b
    e. All of the above

2. Leakage of urine was demonstrated at a volume of

    a. 53 mL H_2O
    b. 179 mL H_2O
    c. 220 mL H_2O
    d. B and C
    e. All of the above

3. The patient has videourodynamic signs of

    a. Stress urinary incontinence
    b. Urge urinary incontinence
    c. Open bladder neck
    d. A and C
    e. All of the above

    Answers (1D, 2D, 3E)

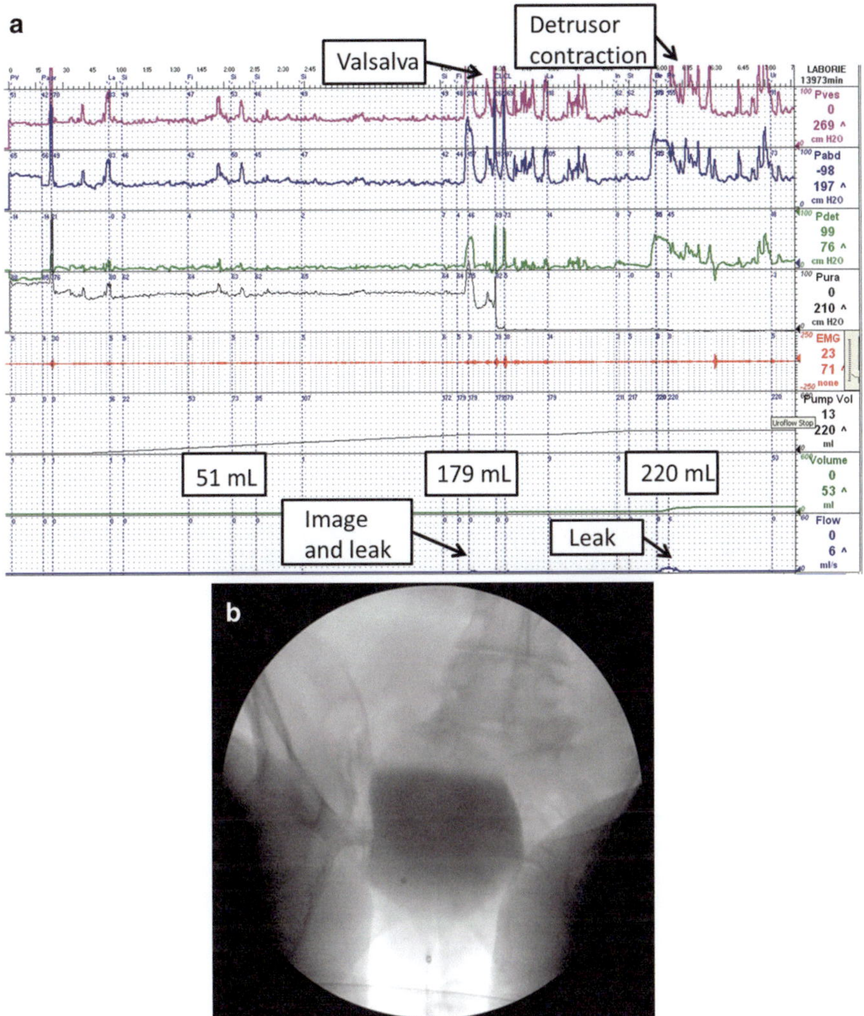

Fig. 20.10

1. The correct answer is D, both a smooth-walled bladder and an open bladder
   neck, as represented by the "beaked" appearance of the bladder neck. No vesicoureteral reflux is present.
2. The correct answer is D, leakage occurred at both 179 mL H_2O and at 220 mL
   H_2O. There is no leakage of urine at 53 mL H_2O.
3. The correct answer is E, all of the above. Stress urinary incontinence is shown at
   179 mL H_2O, urgency urinary incontinence at 220 mL H_2O, and the fluoroscopic
   image shows an open bladder neck during a leak, as indicated by the "beaked"
   appearance,

Test Question 11

Clinical history: A 53-year-old female complains of frequency, a weak stream, and sensation of incomplete emptying. Patient denies prior surgery except for hysterectomy. Patient denies history of UTI or other known neurological disease (Fig. 20.11).

This study demonstrates:

1. Detrusor overactivity
2. Stress urinary incontinence
3. Valsalva voiding
4. Impaired compliance
5. Striated sphincter dyssynergia

The correct answer is 3. The study demonstrates Valsalva voiding with a characteristic sawtooth pattern producing a flow that is prolonged and intermittent. SUI was assessed and not demonstrated. Compliance is normal. The rises in detrusor pressure are a result of slightly unequal transmission in vesical and abdominal pressures (artifact).

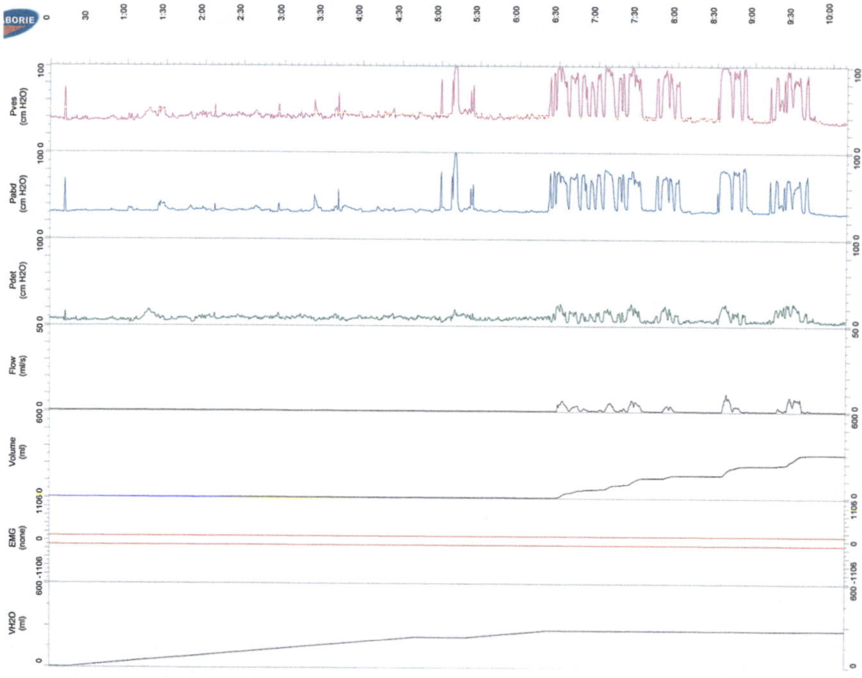

Fig. 20.11

Test Question 12

Clinical history: A 73-year-old female complains of frequency, incontinence, and sensation of incomplete emptying. She has no prior history of GU surgery. Her past medical history is significant for diabetes and hypertension. She wears three incontinence pads per day. Patient was asked to cough and strain several times during filling to assess for SUI (Black arrow denotes permission to void) (Fig. 20.12).

This study demonstrates:

1. Detrusor aftercontraction
2. Instrinsic sphincter deficiency
3. Detrusor overactivity with impaired contractility
4. Impaired compliance
5. Stress urinary incontinence

The correct answer is 3. The study demonstrates that the patient has urgency incontinence. SUI was not seen with cough or valsalva during filling. After permission to void, she voids primarily by straining and does not generate very high detrusor pressures producing an intermittent stream. This picture is suggestive of detrusor overactivity with impaired contractility.

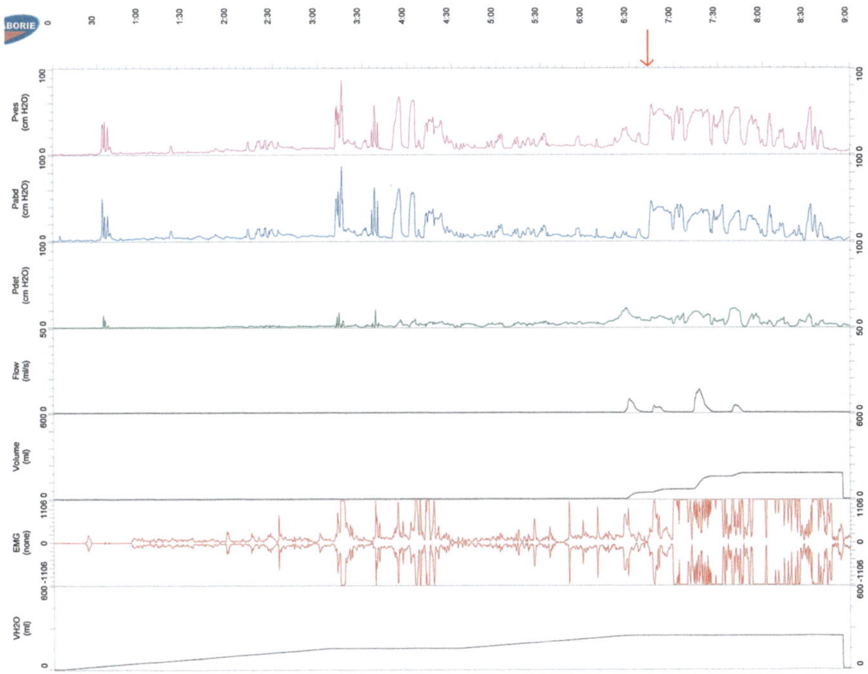

Fig. 20.12

Test Question 13

Clinical History: A 37-year-old female with past medical history of multiple sclerosis (MS) with complaint of urinary frequency and urge incontinence undergoes urodynamics. Based on the tracing (Fig. 20.13), the diagnosis is:

1. DSD
2. Bladder outlet obstruction
3. Intrinsic sphincteric deficiency
4. Normal voiding pattern

The answer is 1 DSD. Normal voiding is characterized by sphincter relaxation prior to detrusor contraction. DSD is diagnosed via urodynamics by involuntary increased EMG activity during a bladder contraction due to a neurologic condition. EMG activity during detrusor contraction must be in the absence of Valsalva and Crede maneuvers. There is no rise of P_{abd} consistent with increased intra-abdominal pressure and the patient in this case carries a diagnosis of MS. A similar pattern of EMG activity can be seen in patients attempting to suppress urge associated with involuntary detrusor contraction. Voluntarily contracting pelvic floor helps to abort the detrusor contraction and remain continent. In patients with DSD, the EMG activity is due to involuntary contraction of pelvic floor and external sphincter.

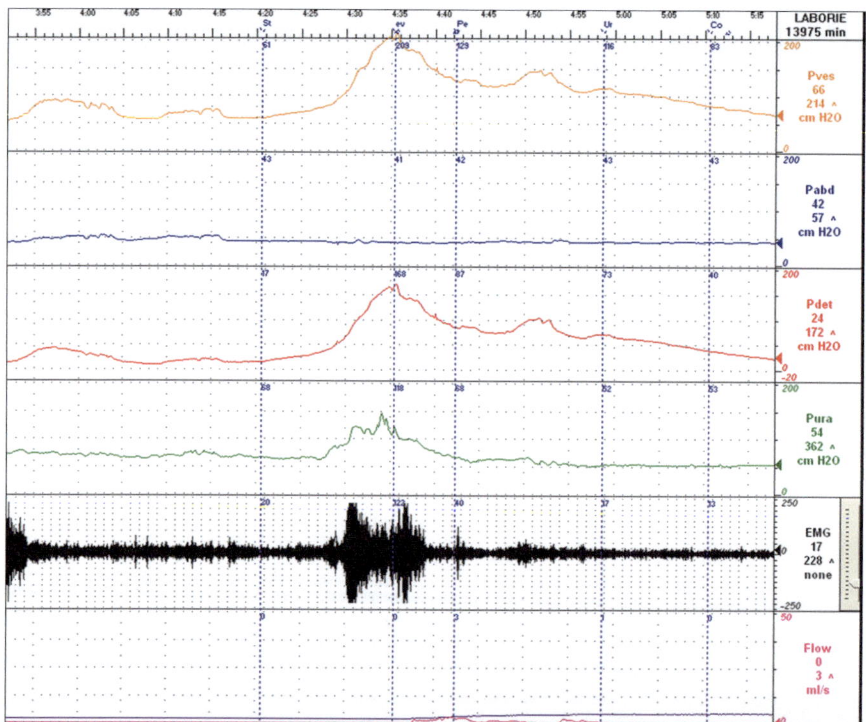

Fig. 20.13

Test Question 14

Clinical History: A 25-year-old female presents with a complaint of urge urinary incontinence. Patient has a long standing history of encoperesis and constipation. Physical exam reveals a tense pelvic floor with a large amount of stool in rectum. Patient has been evaluated by neurology with a negative work-up including normal MRI of spine. Urodynamic evaluation is represented in Fig. 20.14.

This study demonstrates:

1. DSD
2. Primary Bladder Neck Obstruction
3. Dysfunctional Voiding (Non-neurogenic neurogenic bladder)
4. Valsalva voiding

The answer is (3) Dysfunctional voiding. EMG activity during a detrusor contraction can be voluntary or involuntary contraction such as that seen in patients with neurologic disorders. The patient in this study had an involuntary detrusor contraction noted as a rise in P_{det} prior to permission to void. The patient voluntarily

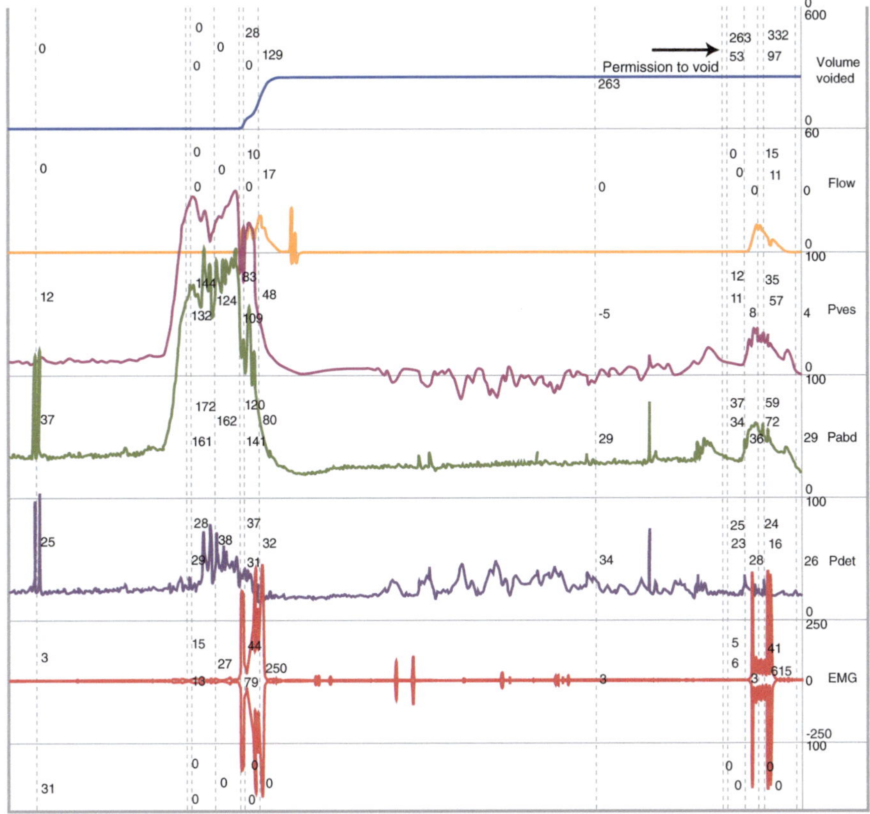

Fig. 20.14

contracted their sphincter complex to prevent leakage of urine seen as a rise in EMG activity. Once permission to void is given, the patient generates a detrusor contraction and flow is generated at which time increased EMG activity is noted, consistent with a diagnosis of dysfunctional voiding. The history of constipation and urinary incontinence also leads one to a diagnosis of global pelvic floor dysfunction. The patient does not have a neurologic diagnosis which would be necessary for diagnosis of DSD. Wet EMG leads can lead to an artifactual reading after initiation of flow, but the EMG soon dampens in this tracing, making artifact unlikely.

Test Question 15

Clinical history: A 28-year-old woman presents with stress urinary incontinence. She has no other storage symptoms, no pelvic organ prolapse on pelvic exam, and a positive cough stress test. Her uroflow tracing is below. The post-void residual was 5 mL (Fig. 20.15).

Which of the following is true about the uroflow pattern?

1. The flow curve is intermittent
2. Obstruction is ruled out by this uroflow curve
3. The patient is straining at the end of the uroflow
4. The voided volume is inadequate for interpretation
5. The flow curve is continuous

Answer: 5

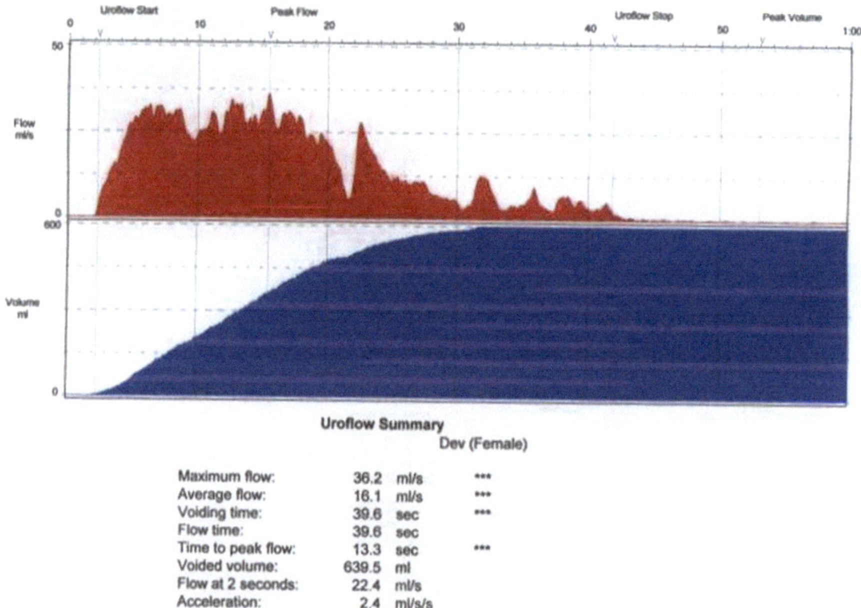

Fig. 20.15

The correct answer is 5. The study demonstrates a continuous flow curve, rather than an intermittent one. Abdominal straining and obstructed urination cannot be diagnosed solely from a non-invasive uroflow. A pressure-flow study that evaluates simultaneous detrusor and abdominal pressures during urination is required to diagnose both of these. In adults, flow events of less than 100–150 mL should be interpreted with caution.

Test Question 16

Clinical history: A 53-year-old male with Parkinson's disease presents with storage and voiding lower urinary tract symptoms (LUTS). He has failed conservative therapy with behavioral modification and is considering medical therapy with antimuscarinic drugs and alpha-adrenergic blockers. He undergoes urodynamics and his tracing is seen in Fig. 20.16.

This study demonstrates:

1. Detrusor overactivity
2. Low pressure, low flow voiding
3. Low compliance
4. Options 1 and 2 are correct
5. Obstruction per the Abrams–Griffith number

Answer: 4

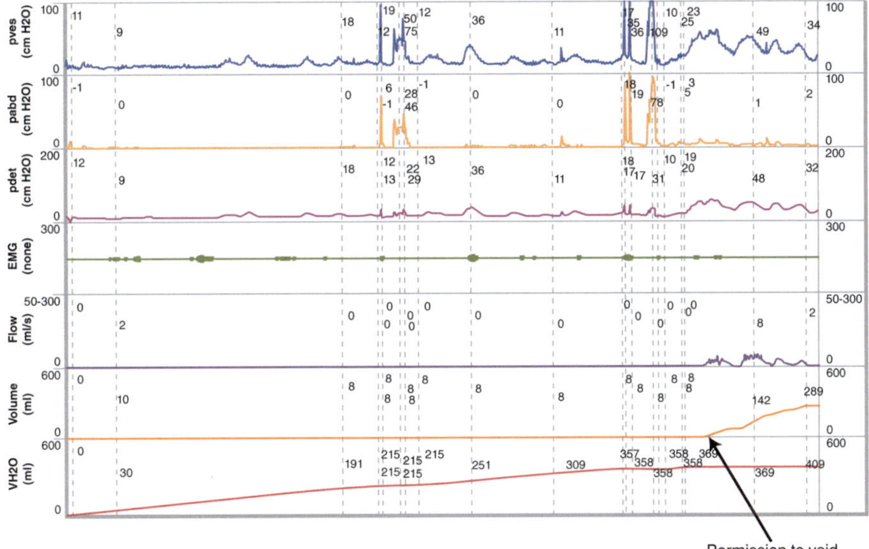

Fig. 20.16

The correct answer is 4. The study demonstrates frequent involuntary detrusor contractions and a low normal pressure ($P_{det}Q_{max} = 48$ cm H_2O), low flow ($Q_{max} = 8$ mL/s), volitional voiding pattern. Normal adult males typically void with detrusor pressures between 40 and 60 cm H_2O. The AG number = $P_{det}Q_{max} - 2Q_{max}$, with AG > 40 indicating a high chance of obstruction, AG < 15 unlikely obstruction, and AG = 15–40 indicating an equivocal result (this patient had an AG number = 32). Normal compliance (large change in volume/small change in pressure) is present, making option 3 incorrect.

Appendix

Differential Diagnosis and Pattern Recognition: Causes of Commonly Encountered Patterns on PFUD Tracings

Multichannel pressure flow urodynamic tracings may have an infinite number of different patterns encountered between the various recording channels. What follows is a list of common signal patterns seen on PFUD tracings and their possible cause: some of which are clinically relevant/important and some of which are related to the circumstances of the study or artifactual. This is not meant to be a complete exhaustive list nor a diagnostic list, but rather a practical list of some of the most commonly seen signal patterns on the tracing and their potential explanations.

1. Changes in Pves (P1):

   Sudden rise in Pves with concomitant rise in Pabd (Fig. A.1[1]):

   - cough
   - valsalva
   - extrinsic compression on abdomen
   - patient movement during study
   - artifact (rare)

   Sudden transient rise in Pves without concomitant rise in Pabd during cough/valsalva (Fig. A.2):

   - Artifact only:

     non-functioning or absent Pabd transducer
     acute transient obstruction of Pves transducer

---

[1] Figures courtesy of Brett Lebed, M.D.

© Springer Science+Business Media New York 2015
E.S. Rovner, M.E. Koski (eds.), *Rapid and Practical Interpretation of Urodynamics*, DOI 10.1007/978-1-4939-1764-8

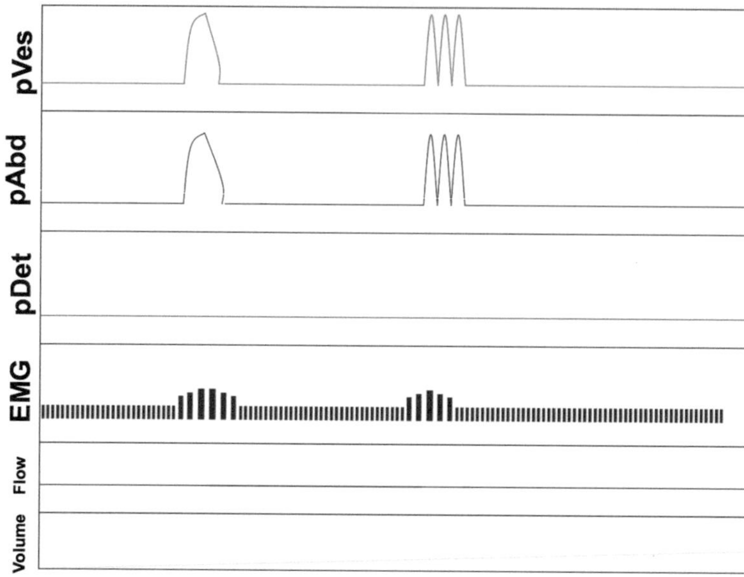

Fig. A.1 Sudden rise in Pves with concomitant rise in Pabd

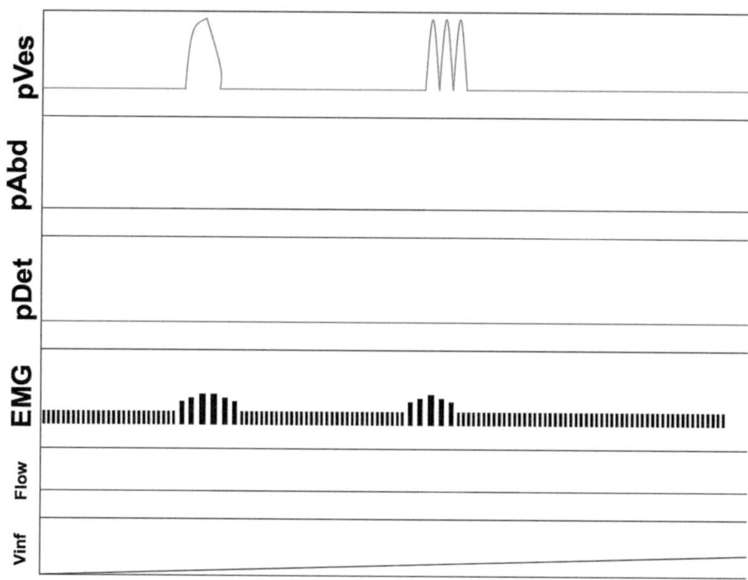

Fig. A.2 Sudden transient rise in Pves without concomitant rise in Pabd during cough/valsalva

Sudden drop in Pves with sudden rise in Pdet (Fig. A.3):

– Artifact only:

   Pves catheter is dislodged or migrated or voided out
   Movement, blockage, or disconnection of Pves catheter

Sudden sustained rise in Pves without concomitant rise in Pabd (Fig. A.4):

– Sustained tetanic detrusor contraction (rare)
– Artifact

   migration of Pves into urethra/bladder neck

Gradual and sustained rise in Pves without rise in Pabd (Fig. A.5):

– Decreased compliance

   Neurogenic bladder
   Infection
   Long-term indwelling catheter with recent removal

– Artifact secondary to supra-physiologic filling

Gradual decrease in Pves with gradual decrease in Pdet (Fig. A.6)

– Artifact only:

   Migration of Pves caudad/inferiorly
   loss of signal from Pves

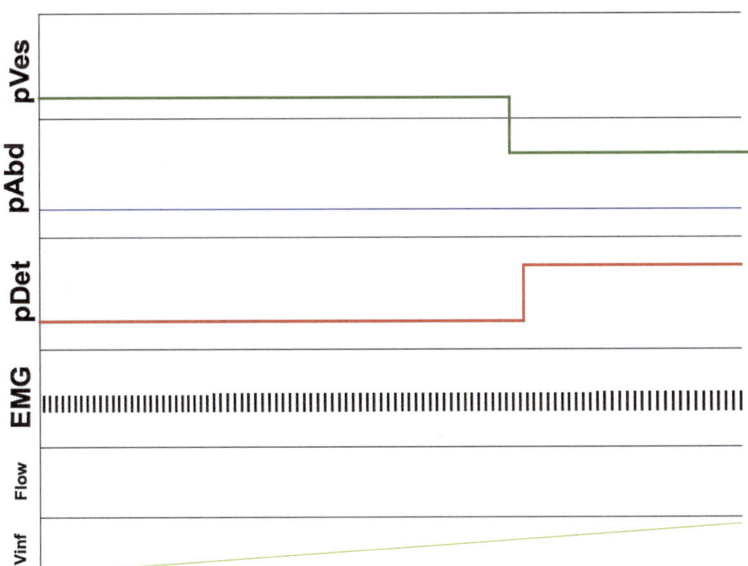

Fig. A.3 Sudden drop in Pves with sudden rise in Pdet

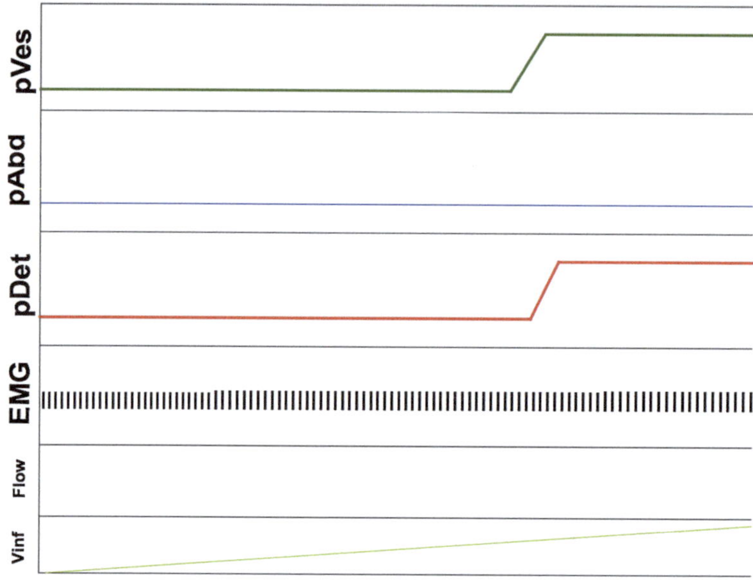

Fig. A.4 Sudden sustained rise in Pves without concomitant rise in Pabd

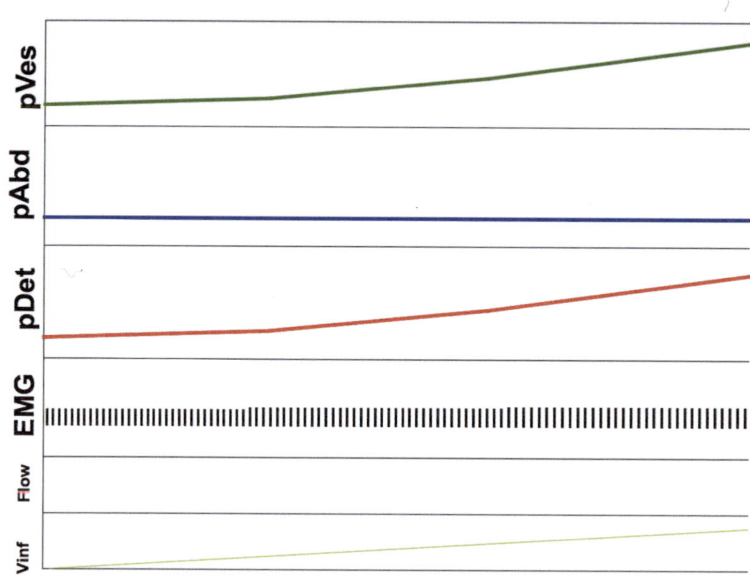

Fig. A.5 Gradual and sustained rise in Pves without rise in Pabd

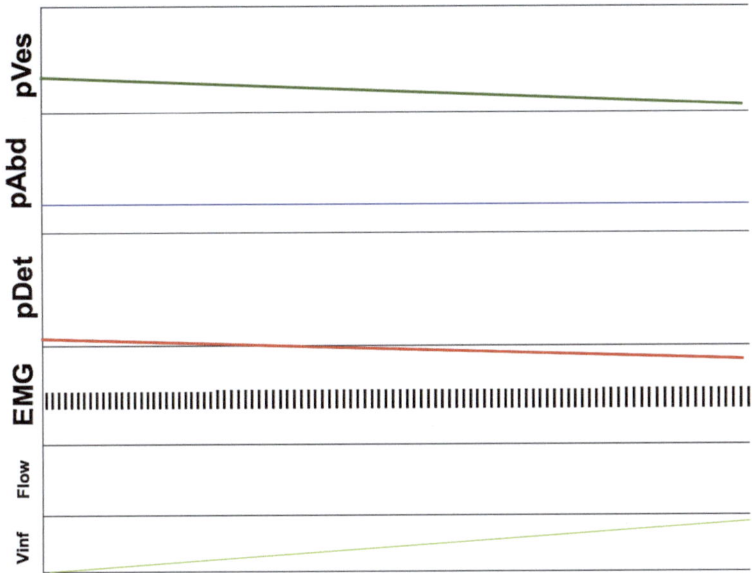

Fig. A.6 Gradual decrease in Pves with gradual decrease in Pdet

Phasic rise in Pves and Pdet without change in Pabd (Fig. A.7)

– Detrusor overactivity

2. Changes in Pdet (detrusor pressure)

Decrease in Pdet without change in Pves (Fig. A.8):

– Artifact only

   migration of Pabd cephalad

Increase in Pdet without increase in Pves (Fig. A.9):

– Artifact only

   migration of Pabd caudad (inferiorly)
   gradual loss of signal from Pves or Pves migration caudad/inferiorly (see Fig. A.6)

Transient/sudden decrease in Pdet without rise in Pves (Fig. A.10)

– Artifact only

   rectal contraction
   Pabd signal transduction problems
   non-functioning Pves catheter during valsalva/cough

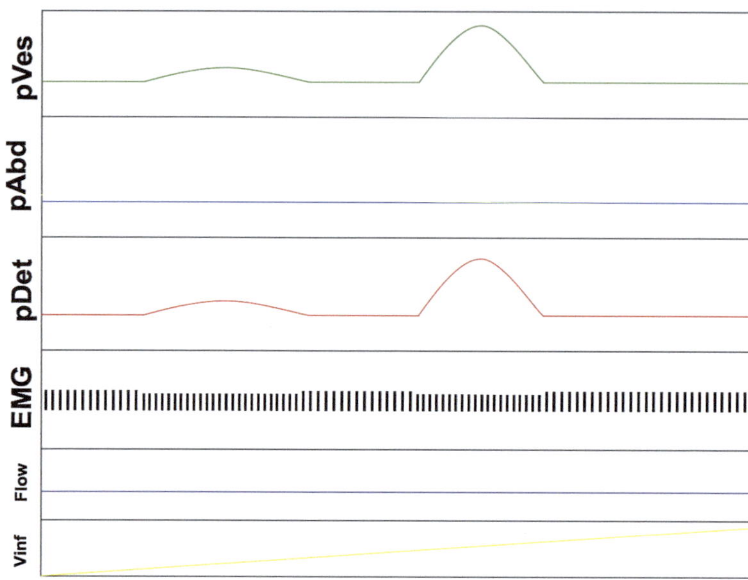

Fig. A.7 Phasic rise in Pves and Pdet without change in Pabd

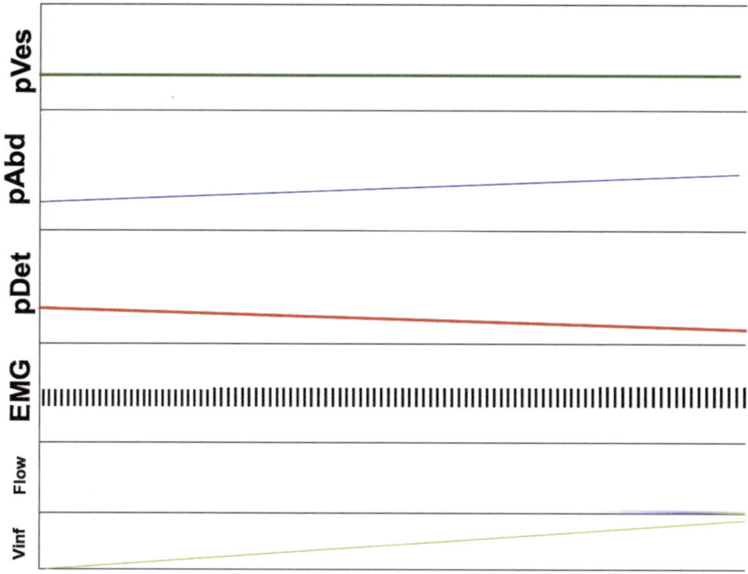

Fig. A.8 Decrease in Pdet without change in Pves

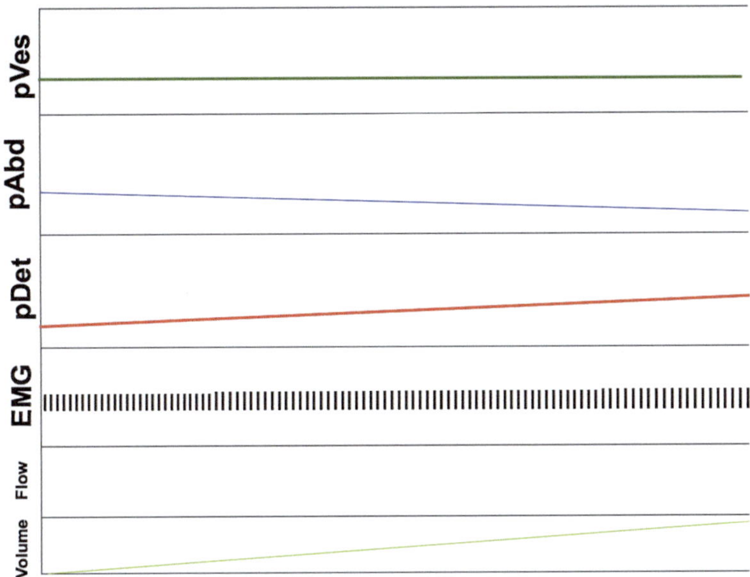

Fig. A.9 Increase in Pdet without increase in Pves

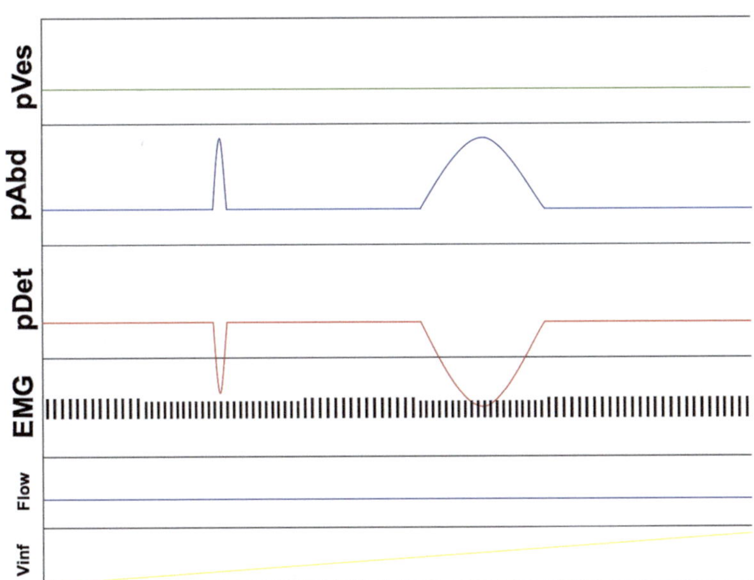

Fig. A.10 Transient/sudden decrease in Pdet without rise in Pves

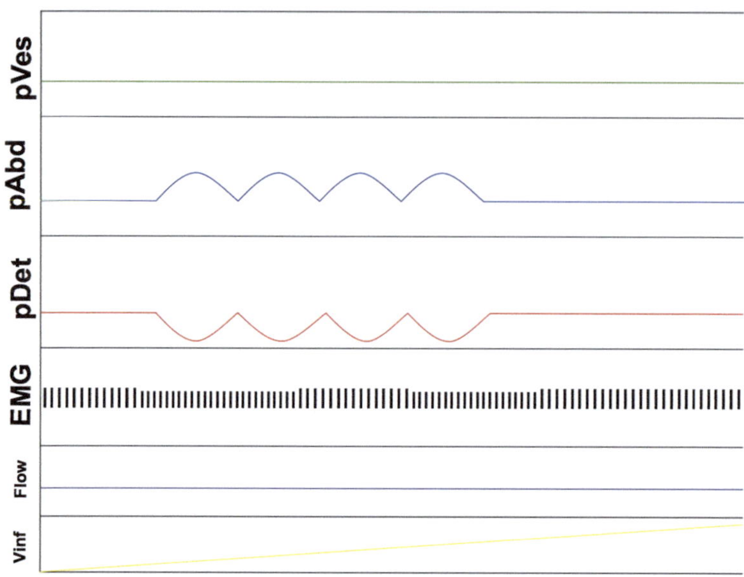

Fig. A.11 Phasic "increases" in Pdet without a rise in Pves

Phasic "increases" in Pdet without a rise in Pves (Fig. A.11)

– Artifact only

　multiple consecutive rectal contractions

Index

© Springer Science+Business Media New York 2015

343

E.S. Rovner, M.E. Koski (eds.), *Rapid and Practical Interpretation
of Urodynamics*, DOI 10.1007/978-1-4939-1764-8

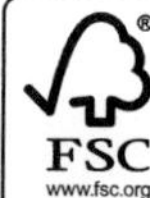

MIX
Papier aus verantwortungsvollen Quellen
Paper from responsible sources
FSC® C105338

If you have any concerns about our products,
you can contact us on
ProductSafety@springernature.com

In case Publisher is established outside the EU,
the EU authorized representative is:
Springer Nature Customer Service Center GmbH
Europaplatz 3, 69115 Heidelberg, Germany

Printed by Libri Plureos GmbH
in Hamburg, Germany